CRC SERIES IN AGING

Editors-in-Chief

Richard C. Adelman, Ph.D.
Director
Aging Research Program
Temple University School of Medicine
Philadelphia, Pennsylvania

George S. Roth, Ph.D.
Research Biologist
Gerontology Research Center
National Institute on Aging
Baltimore City Hospitals
Baltimore, Maryland

HANDBOOK OF BIOCHEMISTRY IN AGING
Editor
James Florini
Department of Biology
Syracuse University
Syracuse, New York

HANDBOOK OF PHYSIOLOGY IN AGING
Editor
Edward J. Masoro
Department of Physiology
University of Texas
Health Science Center
Houston, Texas

HANDBOOK OF IMMUNOLOGY IN AGING
Editors
Marguerite M.B. Kay and
Takashi Makinodan
Geriatric Research Education and
Clinical Center
Wadsworth Veterans Administration
Hospital
Los Angeles, California

IMMUNOLOGICAL TECHNIQUES APPLIED TO AGING RESEARCH
Editors
William H. Adler and Albert A. Nordin
Gerontology Research Center
National Institute On Aging
Baltimore City Hospitals
Baltimore, Maryland

SENESCENCE IN PLANTS
Editor
Kenneth U. Thimann, Ph.D.
The Thimann Laboratories
University of California
Santa Cruz, California

CURRENT TRENDS IN MORPHOLOGICAL TECHNIQUES
Editor
John E. Johnson, Jr.
Gerontology Research Center
National Institute on Aging
Baltimore City Hospitals
Baltimore, Maryland

Additional topics to be covered in this series include Cell Biology of Aging, Microbiology of Aging, Pharmacology of Aging, Evolution and Genetics Animals Models for Aging Research, Hormonal Regulatory Mechanisms, Detection of Altered Proteins, Insect Models, Lower Invertebrate Models, Testing the Theories of Aging, and Nutritional Approaches to Aging Research

Immunological Techniques Applied to Aging Research

Editors

William H. Adler, M.D.
Section Chief
Clinical Immunology Section
Gerontology Research Center
National Institute on Aging
Baltimore City Hospital
Baltimore, Maryland

Albert A. Nordin, Ph.D.
Senior Scientist
Clinical Immunology Section
Gerontology Research Center
National Institute on Aging
Baltimore City Hospitals
Baltimore, Maryland

CRC Series in Aging
Editors-in-Chief

Richard C. Adelman, Ph.D
Director
Aging Research Program
Temple University School of Medicine
Philadelphia, Pennsylvania

George S. Roth, Ph.D.
Research Biochemist
Gerontology Research Center
National Institute on Aging
Baltimore City Hospitals
Baltimore, Maryland

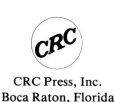

CRC Press, Inc.
Boca Raton, Florida

Library of Congress Cataloging in Publication Data

Main entry under title:

Immunological techniques applied to aging research

   (Methods in aging research ; v. 5)
   Bibliography: p.
   Includes index.
   1. Aging. 2. Immunity. I. Adler, William H.
II. Nordin, Albert A. III. Series. {DNLM:
1. Aging. 2. Allergy and immunology. WT20 M592
v. 5}
QP86.15   599.03'72   80-16442
ISBN 0-8493-5809-4

Direct all inquiries to CRC Press, Inc., 2000 N.W. 24th Street, Boca Raton, Florida 33431.

© 1981 by CRC Press, Inc.

International Standard Book Number 0-8493-5809-4

Library of Congress Card Number 80-16442
Printed in the United States

PREFACE

The application of immunologic techniques to the study of aging processes is a recent development. The suggestion that immunologic function declines with age has prompted research into the mechanism of the decline. The goal that has been stated is that by understanding the decline in function certain remedies may be applicable for the augmentation or restoration of immune activity in the elderly with the resulting benefit of changes in the prevalence of certain age-associated disease patterns.

On a basic level, immune function of the host has been studied to help elucidate the process of aging itself. The immune system allows the study of organ, tissue, and cellular function along with protein structure and cellular interactions. Therefore, in the field of aging research, immunology has attracted a great interest.

This book is a collection of descriptions of immunological techniques used to investigate lymphocyte function, and basic considerations of problems of immunology/aging research. The contributions are varied but in no way all-inclusive. Due to space considerations there are important areas which have been left out. However, most of the commonly used immunologic techniques have been covered and if the author(s) had a background in aging research the special problems associated with the applications of these techniques in aging research have been explored. It is hoped that this volume will provide a more trouble-free and easy introduction into aging research for individuals attracted into the field by the stimulating unique problems and the availability of scientific knowledge on immune function.

The enthusiastic particpation of the contributors to this volume has been of great help and has allowed the editors to proceed with organization with a minimum of problems. We acknowledge their effort and assume any responsibility for any criticisms of bias in our assignments of priority.

William H. Adler
and
Albert A. Nordin

EDITORS-IN-CHIEF

Dr. Richard C. Adelman is currently Executive Director of the Temple University Institute on Aging, Philadelphia, Penn., as well as Professor of Biochemistry in the Fels Research Institute of the Temple University College of Medicine. An active gerontologist for more than 10 years, he has achieved international prominence as a researcher, educator, and administrator. These accomplishments span a broad spectrum of activities ranging from the traditional disciplinary interests of the research biologist to the advocacy, implementation, and administration of multidisciplinary issues of public policy of concern to elderly people.

Dr. Adelman pursued his pre- and postdoctoral research training under the guidance of two prominent biochemists, each of whom is a member of the National Academy of Sciences: Dr. Sidney Weinhouse as Director of the Fels Research Institute, Temple University, and Dr. Bernard L. Horecker as Chairman of the Department of Molecular Biology, Albert Einstein College of Medicine, Bronx, N.Y. His accomplishments as a researcher can be expressed in at least the following ways. He is the author and/or editor of more than 70 publications, including original research papers in referred journals, review chapters, and books. His research efforts have been supported by grants from the National Institutes of Health for the past 10 consecutive years, at a current annual level of approximately $300,000. He continues to serve as an invited speaker at seminar programs, symposiums, and workshops all over the world. He is the recipient of the IntraScience Research Foundation Medalist Award, an annual research prize awarded by peer evaluation for major advances in newly emerging areas of the life sciences. He is the recipient of an Established Investigatorship of the American Heart Association.

As an educator, Dr. Adelman is also involved in a broad variety of activities. His role in research training consists of responsibility for pre- and postdoctoral students who are assigned specific projects in his laboratory. He teaches an Advanced Graduate Course on the Biology of Aging, lectures on biomedical aspects of aging to medical students, and is responsible for the biological component of the basic course in aging sponsored by the School of Social Administration. Training activities outside the University include membership in the Faculty of the National Institute on Aging summer course on the Biology of Aging; programs on the biology of aging for AAA's throughout Pennsylvania and Ohio; and the implementation and teaching of Biology of Aging for the Nonbiologist locally, for the Gerontology Society and other national organizations, as well as for the International Association of Gerontology.

Dr. Adelman has achieved leadership positions across equally broad areas. Responsibilities of this position include the intergration of multidisciplinary programs in research, consultation and education, and health service, as well as advocacy for the University on all matters dealing with aging. He coordinates a city-wide consortium of researchers from Temple University, the Wistar Institute, the Medical College of Pennsylvania, Drexel University, and the Philadelphia Geriatric Center, conducting collaborative research projects, training programs, and symposiums. He was a past President of the Philadelphia Biochemists Club. He serves on the editorial boards of the *Journal of Gerontology, Mechanisms of Ageing and Development, Experimental Aging Research,* and *Gerontological Abstracts.* He was a member of the Biomedical Research Panel of the National Advisory Council of the National Institute on Aging. He chairs a subcommittee of the National Academy of Sciences Committee on Animal Models for Aging Research. As an active Fellow of the Geronological Society, he is a past Chairman of the Biological Sciences section; a past Chairman of the Society Public Policy Committee for which he prepared Congressional testimony and represented the Society on the Leadership Council of the Coalition of National Aging Organizations; and is Secretary-Treasurer of the North American Executive Committee of the International Association of Gerontology. Finally, as the highest testimony of his leadership capabilities, he continues to serve on National Advisory Committees which impact on diverse key issues dealing with the elderly. These include a 4-year appointment as member of the NIH Study Section on Pathobiological Chemistry; the Executive Committee of the Health Resources Administration Project on publication of the recent edition of *Working with Older People — A Guide to Practice;* a recent appointment as reviewer of AOA applications for Career Preparation Programs in Gerontology; and a 4-year appointment on the Veterans Administration Long-Term Care Advisory Council responsible for evaluating their program on Geriatric Research, Education, and Clinical Centers (GRECC).

George S. Roth, Ph.D., is a research chemist at the Gerontology Research Center of the National Institute on Aging, Baltimore, Md.

Dr. Roth received his B.S. in Biology from Villanova University in 1968 and his Ph.D. in Microbiology from Temple University School of Medicine in 1971. He received post-doctoral training in Biochemistry at the Fels Research Institute in Philadelphia, Pa. Since coming to NIA in 1972, Dr. Roth has also been affiliated with the Graduate Schools of Georgetown University and George Washington University.

He is an officer of the Gerontological Society of America, a co-editor of the CRC series, "Methods of Aging Research", an associate editor of "Neurobiology of Aging", and a referee for numerous other journals. Dr. Roth has published extensively in the area of hormone action and aging and has lectured throughout the world on this subject.

THE EDITORS

William H. Adler, M.D. is Section Chief of the Clinical Immunology Section, Clinical Physiology Branch at the National Institute on Aging, National Institutes of Health, Department of Health, Education and Welfare.

Dr. Adler received his A.B. degree from Harvard University in 1961 and his M.D. from the State University of New York at Buffalo in 1965. His professional experience includes serving as an intern and resident in pediatrics at the University of Florida from 1966 to 1968, Fellow in Immunology from 1965 to 1966 and 1968 to 1969 in the Department of Pediatrics and Pathology at the University of Florida. He was an Assistant Professor of Pediatrics and Pathology at the University of Florida from 1969 to 1970. From 1970 to 1972 he served in the U.S. Army Medical Corp at the Army Medical Research Institute for Infectious Disease at Fort Detrick, Maryland. From 1972 to 1973 Dr. Adler was a Fellow of the New York Cancer Research Institute at the Clinical Research Center, Harrow, England. Dr. Adler joined the NIH in 1973.

Dr. Adler is a member of the American Association of Immunologists and the Society for Pediatric Research.

His current research concerns the developmental changes in immune function throughout the life span in humans and experimental animals.

Albert A. Nordin, Ph.D. is a Senior Scientist in the Clinical Immunology Section, Clinial Physiology Branch at the National Institute on Aging, National Institutes of Health, Department of Health, Education and Welfare.

Dr. Nordin received his B.S. degree from the University of Pittsburgh in 1956 and his Ph.D. from the University of Pittsburgh School of Medicine in 1962. His professional experience includes an Assistant Professorship in the Department of Microbiology at the University of Pittsburgh School of Medicine, from 1963 to 1966, and he was an Associate Professor in the Department of Microbiology at the University of Notre Dame from 1966 to 1972. He was an invited Visiting Scientist of the Swiss Institute for Experimental Cancer Research, Lausanne, Switzerland from 1969 to 1970, a guest Professor of the Basel Institute of Immunology, Basel, Switzerland in 1975 and 1980 to 1981. Dr. Nordin joined the NIH in 1972.

Dr. Nordin is a member of the American Association of Immunologists.

His current research concerns the cellular interactions of the immune response and the effect of age on the immune mechanism.

CONTRIBUTORS

William H. Adler, M.D.
Head, Immunology Section
Gerontology Research Center
NIA, NIH
Baltimore City Hospitals
Baltimore, Maryland

Mary Anne Brock, Ph.D.
Research Biologist
Gerontology Research Center
NIA, NIH
Baltimore City Hospitals
Baltimore, Maryland

K. T. Brunner, D.V.M.
Head, Department of Immunology
Swiss Institute for Experimental
Cancer Research
Epalinges, Switzerland

M. A. Buchholz
Geronotology Research Center
NIA, NIH
Baltimore City Hospitals
Baltimore, Maryland

Francis J. Chrest, B.S.
Biologist
Gerontology Research Center
NIA, NIH
Baltimore City Hospitals
Baltimore, Maryland

Ronald W. Gillette, Ph.D.
Director Special Projects Laboratory
Meloy Laboratories, Inc.
Springfield, Virginia

J. J. Haaijamn, Ph.D.
Institute for Experimental Gerontology
TNO
Rijswijk, The Netherlands

David E. Harrison, Ph.D.
The Jackson Laboratory
Bar Harbor, Maine

John M. Hefton, Ph.D.
Assistant Professor of Anatomy
The New York Hospital
Cornell Medical Center
New York, New York

Jochen W. Heine, Ph.D.
Senior Cancer Research Scientist
Abbott Laboratories
North Chicago, Illinois

W. Hijmans, M.D.
Professor of Medicine
Study Group for Medical Gerontology
Department of Pathology
Leiden University Medical Center
Leiden, The Netherlands

C. F. Hollander, M.D., Ph.D.
Director, Institure for Experimental
  Gerontology TNO
Rijswijk, The Netherlands

Paul W. Kincade, Ph.D.
Associate Member, Sloan-Kettering
  Institute for Cancer Research
Rye, New York

Ada M. Kruisbeek, Ph.D.
Institute for Experimental Gerontology
  TNO
Rijswijk, The Netherlands

H. R. MacDonald, Ph.D.
Unit of Human Cancer Immunology
Ludwig Institute for Cancer Research
Epalinges, Switzerland

James E. Nagel, M.D.
Immunology Section
Gerontology Research Center
NIA, NIH
Baltimore City Hospitals
Baltimore, Maryland

Albert A. Nordin, Ph.D.
Research Immunologist
Gerontology Research Center
NIA, NIH
Baltimore City Hospitals
Baltimore, Maryland

Jiri Radl, M.D., Ph.D.
Institute for Experimental Gerontology
 TNO
Rijswijk, The Netherlands

Henrica R.E. Schuit
Study Group for Medical Gerontology
Department of Pathology
Leiden University Medical Center
Leiden, The Netherlands

H. A. Solleveld, D.V.M.
Institute for Experimental Gerontology
 TNO
Rijswijk, The Netherlands

C. Taswell
Unit of Human Cancer Immunology
Ludwig Institute for Cancer Research
Epalinges, Switzerland

M. J. van Zwieten, D.V.M.
Institute for Experimental Gerontology
 TNO
Rijswijk, The Netherlands

Marc E. Weksler, M.D.
Director Division of Geriatrics and
 Gerontology
Department of Medicine
Cornell University Medical College
New York, New York

C. Zurcher, M.D., Ph.D.
Institute for Experimental Gerontology
 TNO
Rijswijk, The Netherlands

TABLE OF CONTENTS

Chapter 1

PATHOLOGY

M. J. van Zwieten, C. Zurcher, H. A. Solleveld, and C. F. Hollander

TABLE OF CONTENTS

I. INTRODUCTION

A great deal of effort emanating from a number of scientific disciplines, including immunology, has been expended in recent years towards an understanding of the basic mechanisms underlying the aging process. It has been stated that a primary goal of understanding these fundamental mechanisms should ultimately be to increase the quality, and not necessarily the quantity, of man's final years.[1] To test many of the hypotheses put forward concerning the aging process, investigations must be carried out in animals. Most aging research on animals is currently being performed in rodents primarily for the reasons that (1) they are mammals and therefore more comparable to man than are non-mammalian systems, (2) they have relatively short life spans, (3) well-established inbred strains are available, (4) they can be housed and manipulated relatively easily under carefully controlled conditions, and (5) their cost is relatively low as compared to that of the larger domestic animals and primates. It has been repeatedly emphasized[2-6] that for the proper use of rodents in aging studies, a thorough knowledge of the spontaneous age-associated lesions in the specific strains or stocks used is required. The reasons for this will become evident from the following sections.

Many excellent comprehensive studies on the pathological changes during aging of a number of different rodent species and strains have been published.[6-24] It is not the intent of this chapter to review exhaustively the findings of these investigations; the interested reader is referred to the appropriate studies for details. Rather, the purpose of this chapter, after briefly discussing the definition of an aged animal, is to give an introduction to some of the age-related pathological changes an investigator may encounter when using rodents for aging research, and in particular, those changes which may affect the tissues of the immune system. Data will also be included, where available, on the specific effects of infectious and parasitic diseases on immune functions and immunological assays. Finally, consideration will be given to various aspects of the health status of rodents in aging research, followed by a brief presentation of a health-monitoring program designed to provide the investigator with information on the quality of the experimental animals in his colony.

II. DEFINING THE AGED ANIMAL

As a prerequisite for the study of age-related changes in the functioning of the immune system in laboratory animals, one must first define what is meant by an aged animal. When the mortality of inbred mice or rats which are kept under controlled environmental conditions (such as barrier system, housing, nutrition, etc.) is estimated with the passage of time, the percentage surviving from a cohort (here defined as a group of animals of the same strain and sex, introduced into the colony at the same time) can be plotted against time and a survival curve constructed. In order to exclude the variable and sometimes appreciable preweaning mortality, it is advisable to use only postweaning mortality data (>3 weeks after birth) for calculation of the survival curve.

If all environmental and genetic factors within a strain or substrain were identical for each individual mouse or rat, all animals would be expected to age in the same way and to die at the same time. The survival curve would then show a rectangular form (Figure 1). If one allows for some variability in the response of each individual to its environment the curve will acquire a more sigmoidal form.[25] The maximum age attained indicates the lifespan of the males or females of the specific strain under those specific laboratory conditions. This more or less rectangular type of survival curve is found when all deaths in a population are due to aging. However, a curve with a

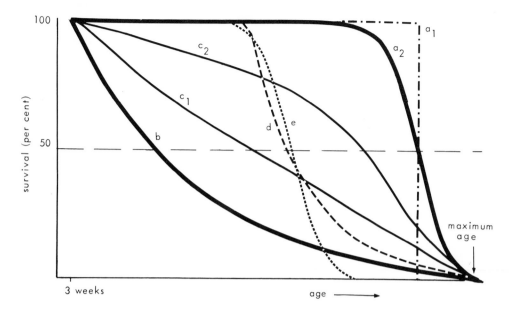

FIGURE 1. Hypothetical survival curves for a population: when all genetic and environmental factors are identical and death occurs in all individuals at the same time (a_1); when mortality is due to aging alone, allowing for some interindividual variability (a_2); when mortality is mainly due to random causes (b); when mortality is substantially influenced by both aging and random causes (c_1 and c_2); when mortality is influenced by the introduction of a life-shortening disease process, causing either a random loss pattern of decline (d) or a sigmoidal pattern of decline (e).

similar shape, but exhibiting a much earlier decline and leading to a decreased maximum life span, may be observed when, for instance, a rapidly fatal infectious disease affects a cohort which previously had been free of disease.

If, on the other hand, one assumes that all deaths occurring in a population are totally independent of the age of the animal, then each group of animals alive at the beginning of a certain interval will have a certain chance of dying during that interval and this chance will be the same for each succeeding time interval. The survival curve will then show an exponential decline. Most survival patterns will reflect a combination of these factors although to different degrees. The resultant curves will therefore fit in between the two extremes formed by the "rectangular" curve due to aging alone, and the exponential one due to random loss alone. The most important points which may give an approximation of the shape of the survival curve are the 90%, 50%, 10% and maximum survival ages.

The shape of the survival curve indicates whether random loss is an important factor in the mortality observed in a certain population. In case of a more or less rectangular decline, it is still quite possible that this form is caused by death from intercurrent diseases[3] such as infections, or, in general, by any single specific cause of death manifesting itself after a disease-free period, (e.g., malignant lymphoma in AKR mice or chronic respiratory disease in rats). This would prevent the development of multiple pathological changes (so-called "multiple pathology"), characteristic for the aging process, from becoming apparent. Therefore, a complete necropsy and histological examination must be performed on those animals dying spontaneously or killed when moribund to exclude death due to causes other than aging alone.

Assuming that one is dealing with an aging population characterized by a more or less rectangular survival curve and dying with multiple pathological changes, then an aged animal may be defined in several ways. One can select as a definition the age at which the curve starts its phase of rapid decline, the mean age (i.e., the summation of the age at death of each animal when the last animal of the cohort has died, divided by the initial number of animals present in the cohort), the 90%, 50% (or median age), or 10% survival ages, or the age at which the probability of dying starts increasing exponentially. Of these possibilities, the 50% survival age is not easily influenced by fluctuations in random loss, contrary to the situation at the 90% survival age or the mean age. Those criteria which are based on the form of the downward bend of the survival curve are relatively inaccurate and therefore less suitable for the purposes of a definition. At the 10% survival age one is certain to be dealing with aged animals, but, for economical reasons, adhering to such a strict criterion would be impractical.[4] A workable definition of an aged animal therefore might be formulated follows. An animal past the 50% survival age derived from a population which has a more or less rectangular survival curve, and in which the pathological changes are characterized by multiple lesions with no single cause of death dominating the spectrum of pathological findings. One must realize that when studying one particular age group past the 50% survival age one is dealing with a homogeneous population in terms of chronological age, but an heterogenous population with respect to biological age (or life expectancy), since the population consists both of animals that are about to die and animals that will die only after several months. Comparison of the pathology data derived from killed versus spontaneously dying animals of the same chronological age has revealed considerable differences between the two groups.[7] This may be explained by the fact that the aging process proceeds with different velocities in different animals of one inbred strain and that the severity and number of lesions ultimately causing death of the animal will therefore vary considerably between animals of the same chronological age. This heterogeneity with respect to the biological age may also be reflected in various immunological parameters.

III. DEFINING THE AGE-ASSOCIATED PATHOLOGY OF THE EXPERIMENTAL ANIMAL

Classically, the diseases in man most commonly regarded as being characteristically associated with aging are vascular diseases (particularly arteriosclerosis), neoplasia, autoimmune diseases, diseases characterized by degeneration and atrophy (such as of the central nervous, immune, and skeletal systems), and infectious diseases.[26] Various different species and strains of laboratory rodents serve as excellent models for the study of certain aspects of these diseases of aging. A detailed discussion of the animal models of age-associated diseases which have been published is not within the scope of this chapter. Selected references to this subject have been listed above. For the purposes of this chapter we will define "age-associated pathology" of experimental animals as those pathological changes found at necropsy in animals allowed to live out their natural life spans. Not included in this definition are those lesions resulting from intercurrent infectious diseases which are generally not a direct result of the aging process.

The investigator using aging rodents for in vitro or in vivo immunological studies should be aware of the "background noise" of pathological changes to be expected in the laboratory animals at his disposal. This information also may provide the means whereby he can select the appropriate species, strain, or sex that is best suited for his studies. Conversely, certain strains of rats or mice may be eliminated from a particular study due to a significant incidence of an undesirable lesion.

The investigator should also be aware of the effects of possible intercurrent infections in his laboratory animals on the tissues he may be using, as well as on the functional parameters he may be testing. Finally, researchers using rodent tissues (e.g., lymphoreticular organs) primarily for in vitro studies should be encouraged whenever possible to submit for histopathological examination any tissues which, in his opinion, are grossly abnormal or which yield experimental results which deviate markedly from those which could be anticipated. It is important to realize that gross alterations alone are often not sufficient for a diagnosis. Careful observations and an index of suspicion in this regard may obviate many needless hours of unrewarding research. Likewise, appropriate morphological studies may yield valuable additional information which may complement the functional studies.

In most research situations, close collaboration with veterinary or medical pathologists experienced in interpreting histological changes in laboratory animals is desirable and usually readily attainable, and will generally result in the generation of specific information regarding experimentally induced lesions or animal disease problems. However, the primarily "basic immunology" - oriented investigator who wishes to keep tabs on his experimental animals and/or animal tissues can do so by adhering to a few standard histopathological practices. It may be beneficial in this regard to briefly outline some general procedures followed in our laboratory which are intended to increase the quality and yield of the histological material.

Ideally, in aging studies where histopathological changes are being evaluated, laboratory rodents should be necropsied immediately after death. However, this is not always practicable especially since most deaths seem to occur at inopportune times (i.e., during the night and weekends) and since the autolysis rate for rodents is relatively high, this approach often results in the loss of much valuable animal material for further histopathological study. A more practical approach is that laboratory rodents on lifetime studies are examined frequently (at least once a day and usually more often) to identify those animals which are sick or moribund. Those are then removed to a "sick ward" for closer and more frequent observation and are sacrificed as shortly as possible (in the judgment of the experienced animal caretaker) before the animal's natural death. Even when using this approach, significant losses due to autolysis may be encountered.

Moribund animals are killed with ether and a complete necropsy is performed. Each animal is accessioned separately. Careful attention is paid to any gross alterations, and these are descriptively recorded on the necropsy card which is retained in a permanent file. A large number of tissues from all organ systems are routinely sampled, including a variety of lymph nodes (superficial and deep cervical, axillary/brachial, anterior mediastinal, mesenteric, lumbar and inguinal). All tissues are fixed in 10% neutral buffered formalin, trimmed, embedded in paraffin, and sectioned following standard procedures. During the necropsy, impression smears are sometimes made of lymphoreticular tissues especially when hematopoietic neoplasia is suspected. These smears are stained with May-Grünwald-Giemsa and form a valuable adjunct to the routine diagnostic material. Likewise, tissue samples may be frozen in liquid nitrogen at this time for later immunofluorescence, histochemical, or transplantation studies. Also, certain tissues, especially those with neoplastic lesions, are fixed in 2% glutaraldehyde and stored for subsequent electron microscopic examination.

Depending upon the specific needs of the investigator, of course, complete necropsies are not always performed. The procedure described above is valid for many studies including life span studies where information on the age-associated lesions within a particular strain or stock is required. Quite frequently, investigators using tissues from aging rodents for in vitro studies submit samples of their test material for histopathological examination to provide a morphological parameter to their studies. Also, samples are submitted to check on the success or completeness of an experimental procedure, such as thymic implantation or thymectomy.

In general, however, a complete necropsy is necessary when aged animals are involved and multiple pathological changes can be expected. As will be discussed later, many age-related lesions can influence tests of immunological functions. In animals used for short-term studies, a complete necropsy is preferred in at least a representative sampling of the test animals to exclude interference by infectious diseases or environmental disturbances.

IV. CONDITIONS WHICH MAY INFLUENCE IMMUNOLOGICAL STUDIES

A. Age-Related Diseases

As has been stated above, a prerequisite for any experimental study on aging is the availability of survival data and baseline pathological data of the particular species and strain of laboratory animal used. Unfortunately, immunological studies are all too frequently carried out without an appreciation of the possible influences that various age-related lesions in the experimental animal may have on immunological functions. The following section is not meant to give a detailed account of lesions which may generally be found in aged animals but to stress only those points which may be important for those studying immune functions in aged animals.

That age-associated pathology of the lymphoid tissues is often associated with disturbances in immune function is clearly recognized.[27,28] Aging affects all organ systems, however, although the pattern and severity of lesions may differ between species, strains, and substrains. Some of these age-related diseases may secondarily affect the lymphoid tissues and thereby also immune functions; others leave those tissues apparently undisturbed (at least histologically), but in this last instance functional studies are clearly needed for definitive proof.

As the interaction between immune system and age-related diseases is manifold, each investigator must know which lesions may occur in his specific animal model and to what extent they may influence his interpretation of the results.

In the following pages we will give examples of the different ways by which age-related diseases may interfere with the integrity of the immune system. To this end we used data obtained on three mouse strains often used for immunological studies. The three strains differ from each other in several immune parameters[29] but also in other important respects. Very brief mention will also be made of several conditions which affect tissues of the immune system of rats.

1. Mice

The three mouse strains studied were the C57BL/KaLwRij, the NZB/Lac, and the CBA/BrARij. These strains, which will be referred to hereinafter as C57BL, NZB and CBA, were inbred at the REP*-Institutes TNO by brother - sister mating in a closed colony system. They were bred and reared under conventional conditions, and cohort groups born during the same week were transferred to the animal quarters of the Institute for Experimental Gerontology TNO for longevity studies when 4 to 12 weeks of age. All mice were housed under well-controlled conventional conditions[30] in polycarbonate (Makrolon®) cages with a bedding of sterilized wood shavings and they were fed a commercial pelleted diet (AM II®, Hope Farms, Woerden, The Netherlands). Food and tap water were provided *ad libitum.* The mice were kept approximately 15 to a cage. The animals were allowed to live their natural life spans, and when killed

---

*   REP stands for Radiobiological Institute, Institute for Experimental Gerontology, and Primate Center TNO.

Table 1
SURVIVAL DATA OF CBA, C57BL AND NZB MICE

Strain	Sex	Number of cohorts[a]	Percent survival age (months)			Maximum survival (months)
			90	50	10	
CBA	Male	5	15 ± 3[b]	29 ± 2	33 ± 2	34 ± 2
			(11 — 17)	(28 — 30)	(30 — 35)	(31 — 36)
	Female	5	18 ± 3	29 ± 3	33 ± 1	36 ± 3
			(13 — 22)	(25 — 31)	(32 — 35)	(34 — 40)
C57BL	Male	7	16 ± 5	24 ± 2	29 ± 1	31 ± 2
			(8 — 21)	(21 — 27)	(28 — 30)	(29 — 33)
	Female	6	16 ± 3	22 ± 1	27 ± 1	29 ± 2
			(13 — 20)	(21 — 23)	(26 — 28)	(26 — 30)
NZB	Male	5	13 ± 1	19 ± 1	23 ± 1	25 ± 2
			(12 — 14)	(18 — 20)	(21 — 24)	(23 — 28)
	Female	5	9 ± 3	13 ± 2	17 ± 1	20 ± 2
			(5 — 12)	(11 — 16)	(15 — 18)	(16 — 21)

[a]   Each cohort consisted of approximately 30 mice.
[b]   Mean ± standard deviation; range of the values between parentheses.

After Blankwater, M. J., *Ageing and the Humoral Immune Response in Mice,* Institute for Experimental Gerontology TNO, Rijswijk, The Netherlands, 1978. With permission.

moribund, or found dead, a complete necropsy was done as described in Section III. Autolyzed or partially cannibalized mice were discarded.

The survival data of male and female mice of the three strains are given in Table 1, and includes the 90%, 50%, 10%, and maximum survival ages as observed under our husbandry conditions. Survival curves of representative cohorts of 30 mice of each sex and strain are shown (Figure 2). Additional data on the survival patterns of these mice with a comparison to the longevity of similar mouse strains from other laboratories have been published.[29]

a. Neoplastic Lesions

The neoplastic lesions found in mice of these three strains are listed in Table 2. The mean ages and number of mice examined of each strain and sex are also included.

The most common neoplasms in C57BL mice involved the lymphoreticular system. Approximately 50% of all C57BL mice in this study died with a lymphoreticular tumor. Tumors compatible with reticulum cell sarcoma type B as described by Dunn[31] occurred most frequently, being observed in 28% and 23% of male and female C57BL mice, respectively. The site most frequently involved by this tumor was the mesenteric lymph node, but spleen, other lymph nodes, liver, and lung were also commonly involved. The affected tissues were enlarged, firm, and pale, and the lymph nodes and spleen often had a slightly nodular appearance. Histologically, this neoplasm was characterized by a nodular or diffuse proliferation of a mixture of cells including lymphoblasts, lymphocytes, plasma cells, histiocytes, and to a lesser extent, polymorphonuclear leukocytes (Figure 3). Giant cells were usually present, although generally not numerous. In some cases a mixed pattern of malignant lymphoma and reticulum cell sarcoma type B was found. In other cases, the tumor was difficult to distinguish from a malignant plasma cell tumor. Preliminary electron microscopic studies of this tumor indicate that the neoplastic cells are of lymphoid origin.[31a] This tumor, as well as other tumors originating in the lymphoreticular tissues, may cause a severe reduction of the

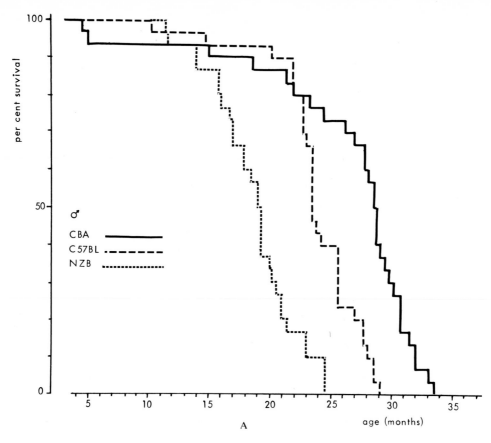

FIGURE 2.   Survival curves of representative cohorts of male (A) and female (B) CBA, C57BL, and NZB mice.

amount of normal lymphoid tissue (Figure 4), and may presumably thereby influence the immunological capacities of such tissues.

Reticulum cell sarcoma type A[31] was found in 18% and 4% of females and males, respectively, and involved primarily the liver and less frequently spleen, lymph nodes, lungs, and genital organs. The characteristic localization of tumor cells in hepatic sinusoids (Figure 5), splenic red pulp (Figure 6), and lymph node sinuses, the frequently observed erythrophagocytosis by tumor cells, and the occasionally biphasic (polygonal and fusiform) but generally monomorphic appearance of these cells are suggestive for a monocytic-histiocytic origin of this tumor. The question of cellular origin has recently come under close scrutiny, however, and it is possible that a number of these tumors, especially those originating in the genital tract, are of Schwann cell origin.[32] Reticulum cell sarcoma type A may affect the lymphoid tissues either by direct involvement or indirectly since the associated excessive erythropoiesis causes severe atrophy of the splenic white pulp (Figure 6).

In 16% and 11% of female and male C57BL mice, respectively, other forms of lymphoreticular tumors were found, including malignant lymphoblastic lymphomas, plasmacytomas, and unclassifiable lymphoid tumors (poorly differentiated lymphoid tumors and tumors with mixed patterns).

In this context, mention should be made of an entity resembling idiopathic paraproteinemia of man, which was recently described in C57BL mice, and which may represent a benign lymphoproliferative disorder. This condition is discussed more fully elsewhere in this volume (Chapter 8, J. Radl).

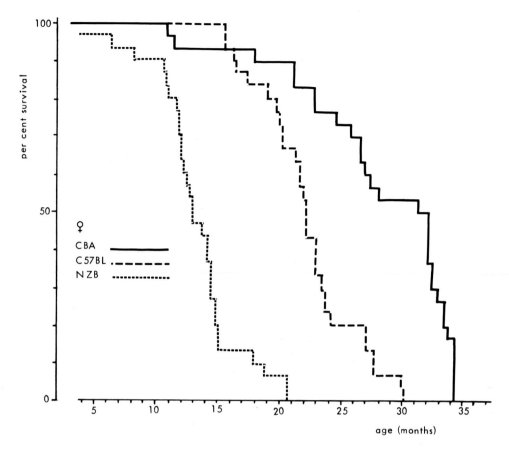

FIGURE 2B

Other tumors found in this strain included testicular interstitial cell tumors in 13% of the males, thyroid follicular adenomas in 9% of the males and 2% of the females, and hepatocellular neoplasms (type A and B nodules)[33] in 6% of the males. Pulmonary alveologenic carcinomas were relatively uncommon, occurring in only 3% of the males. Seven per cent of the females had sarcomas of various types. It is unknown whether these tumors influence immune function, but generally no important changes of the lymphoid tissues were observed.

In NZB mice, the most frequently occurring neoplasms were also of the lymphoreticular and hemopoietic tissues. Reticulum cell sarcomas, both types A and B, were similar histologically to those found in the C57BL mice, and together they were observed in 18% of males and 9% of female NZB mice. Twelve per cent of the males and 12% of the females had other types of lymphoreticular and hemopoietic neoplasms, including lymphoblastic lymphoma, (four cases), unclassifiable lymphomas (five cases), myeloid leukemia (two cases) and mast cell tumor (one case). Other neoplasms were relatively rare in this series of mice, although sarcomas of several types were diagnosed in 12% of the males (Table 2). With regard to immune function the same considerations as mentioned for C57BL mice can apply here.

The most common tumors found in CBA mice were tubular adenomas and granulosa-theca cell tumors of the ovary, which occurred in 79% of the females. Hepatocellular neoplasms were also common and occurred in about a third of the males and 19% of the females. Tumors of the lymphoreticular and hemopoietic systems were

Table 2
NEOPLASTIC LESIONS IN AGING CBA, C57BL, AND NZB MICE

Type of tumor	Prevalence in males (%)			Prevalence in females (%)		
	CBA	C57BL	NZB	CBA	C57BL	NZB
Lymphoreticular and hemopoietic tissue						
Reticulum cell sarcoma type A[a]	—[b]	4	10	5	18	7
Reticulum cell sarcoma type B	—	28	8	5	23	2
Other[c]	4	11	12	2	16	14
Hepatocellular neoplasm type A[d]	23	3	2	12	—	—
Hepatocellular neoplasm type B	11	3	—	7	—	—
Thyroid follicular adenoma	—	9	6	—	2	—
Sarcoma[e]	—	1	12	5	7	—
Ovarian tumors[f]	—	—	79	79	—	5
Testis: interstitial cell tumor	12	13	—	—	—	—
Lung: alveologenic carcinoma	11	3	—	7	—	2
Uterus: adenocarcinoma				7		
Other tumors[g]	11	7	6	24	2	16
Number examined	44	105	50	41	44	44
Mean age (range) in months	28(17—36)	23(6—34)	17(4—27)	28(12—32)	20(8—29)	14(5—24)

Note: Only those lesions which occurred with a prevalence of 5% or more in one of the three strains are included.

a   According to the classification of Dunn.[31]
b   Lesions not observed.
c   Lymphoblastic lymphoma, plasmacytoma, unclassifiable lymphomas, myeloid leukemias, and mast cell tumors.
d   According to the classification of Walker, Thorpe, and Stevenson.[33]
e   Fibrosarcoma, rhabdomyosarcoma, osteosarcoma, undifferentiated hemangiosarcoma, liposarcoma.
f   Tubular adenoma and granulosa-theca cell tumor.
g   Includes cases of benign and malignant neoplasms in a variety of tissues.

After Blankwater, M. J., *Ageing and the Humoral Immune Response in Mice,* Institute for Experimental Gerontology TNO, Rijswijk, The Netherlands, 1978. With permission.

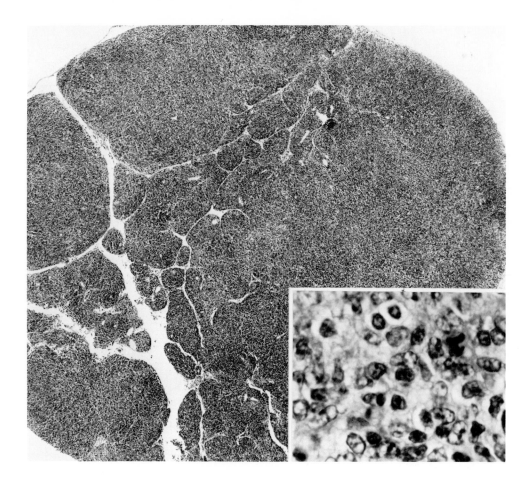

FIGURE 3. Typical pattern of reticulum cell sarcoma type B in mesenteric lymph node of a 16-month-old male C57BL mouse. The normal lymph node architecture has been replaced by a nodular proliferation of neoplastic cells. Hematoxylin-phloxine-saffron (HPS) × 32. Inset: Higher magnification showing mixture of mononuclear cells in the tumor, including cells resembling lymphoblasts, lymphocytes, and histiocytes. HPS × 800.

much less common than in the other two strains, being found in 12% of females and 4% of males. Alveologenic carcinomas occurred more frequently in this strain than in the other two strains, and were observed in 11% of males and 7% of females. Finally, testicular interstitial cell tumors were observed in 12% of the males. Thus, in this strain direct involvement of the lymphoid tissues by neoplasms was relatively rare and the effect of the other tumors on the immune system was not apparent from the histological appearance of the lymphoid tissues.

b. Nonneoplastic Lesions

The nonneoplastic lesion which dominated the age-related pathology of the C57BL strain was amyloidosis (see Table 3). In males, 83% had amyloid deposits in one or more organs, while 73% of the females were similarly affected. Amyloid deposition was frequently found in the lamina propria of the terminal ileum, followed in order of decreasing frequency by cecum, spleen, liver, kidney, lung, thyroid, and mesenteric lymph node. Grossly, affected spleen and liver appeared pale and had a somewhat opaque, glassy appearance. In the spleen, amyloid was first located around the periph-

Table 3
NONNEOPLASTIC LESIONS IN AGING CBA, C57BL, AND NZB MICE

Diagnosis	Prevalence in males (%)			Prevalence in females (%)		
	CBA	C57BL	NZB	CBA	C57BL	NZB
Amyloidosis	—[a]	83	12	5	73	—
Periarteritis nodosa	2	16	2	—	36	—
Fibrinoid vascular necrosis and hyalinization	—	—	12	—	2	27
Thrombosis (mainly atrial)	2	4	42	2	—	32
Ischemic liver necrosis						
Not due to torsion	—	1	26	—	4	33
Due to torsion	16	—	—	—	—	—
Focal myocardial necrosis and fibrosis	—	—	56	—	—	48
Gastrointestinal tract ulceration	—	—	10	—	2	18
Cystic endometrial hyperplasia				45	52	34
Endometrial polyp				10	2	2
Dystrophic calcinosis (cardiac and smooth muscle)	75	—	2	78	—	18
Multifocal liver necrosis	16	3	16	17	14	16
Serosal epithelial cysts	11	—	—	2	—	—
Thyroid cyst	36	10	19	51	4	17
Ovarian follicular cysts				50	34	2
Hydronephrosis	2	6	4	—	9	14
"Mesenteric disease"	7	10	—	—	18	—
Purulent inflammation[b]	5	6	22	—	9	20
Acidophilic macrophage pneumonia	5	30	—	2	16	—
Severe testicular atrophy	77	5	4			
Spermatocele	—	7	—			
Cystic sinuses of lymph nodes	—	—	8	—	—	9
Number examined	44	105	50	41	44	44
Mean age (range in months)	28(17—36)	23(6—34)	17(4—27)	28(12—32)	20(8—29)	14(5—24)

Note: Only those lesions which occurred with a prevalence of 5% or more in one of the three strains are included.

[a]   Lesions not observed.
[b]   Skin excluded.

After Blankwater, M. J., *Ageing and the Humoral Immune Response in Mice,* Institute for Experimental Gerontology TNO, Rijswijk, The Netherlands, 1978. With permission.

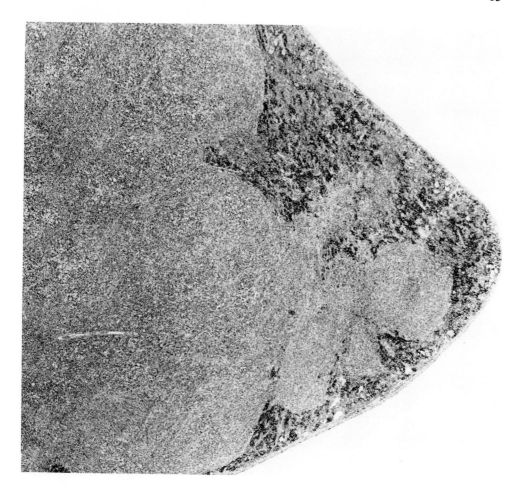

FIGURE 4. Photomicrograph of reticulum cell sarcoma type B originating in the white pulp of the spleen with characteristic nodular growth pattern. HPS × 32.

ery of the splenic follicles (Figure 7) from where it spread out in severe cases to involve nearly the entire spleen, resulting in nearly complete atrophy of the white pulp. In lymph nodes, amyloid was detected in and around macrophages located in the subcapsular sinus (Figure 8). In severely involved lymph nodes, amyloid deposits also affected the paracortical areas but never caused complete effacement of the original architecture.

Another nonneoplastic lesion which was especially common in female C57BL mice (36%) was periarteritis nodosa. Coronary, carotid, and mesenteric arteries were most often involved. Important sequelae were cardiac and cerebral infarction; the latter was often evident clinically as head tilt and circling to one side. The lesions were characterized by an intense infiltration of mixed inflammatory cells in the media and adventitia of arteries, and in the surrounding tissues (Figure 9). Although a direct effect of this disease on the lymphoid tissues was only rarely observed (e.g., splenic infarction), it may represent an abnormal response of the immune system to endogenous or exogenous antigens resulting in immune complex formation and deposition.[34,35]

A nonneoplastic lesion involving primarily the mesenteric lymph node deserves brief mention, since grossly it can sometimes be mistakenly identified as a primary or metastatic tumor. The lesion, well described by Dunn,[31] is termed "mesenteric disease",

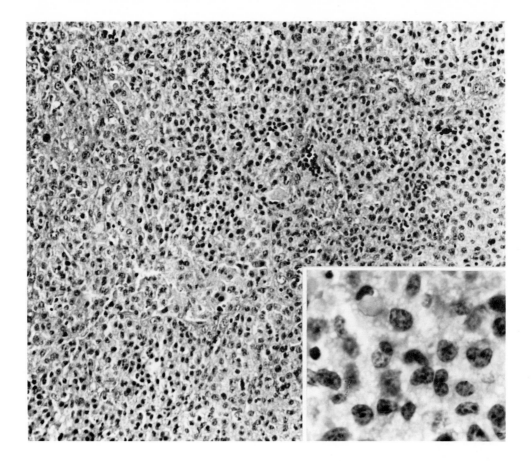

FIGURE 5.   Reticulum cell sarcoma type A growing diffusely in liver of a 24-month-old female C57BL mouse. Remnants of original hepatic architecture can be seen in the left side of the photomicrograph. HPS × 210. Inset: Higher magnification showing monomorphic appearance of tumor cells with foamy cytoplasm and oval or beanshaped nuclei. HPS × 800.

and grossly the lymph node was enlarged and focally or diffusely reddened. Histologically, the lesion was characterized by cystic dilation of sinusoidal-like spaces (Figure 10) which were lined by flattened endothelial-like cells. The cysts were filled either with relatively acellular proteinaceous fluid or with blood. It was usually not possible to determine whether the cysts originated from dilated sinuses or from blood vessels. This lesion, which may also affect mediastinal lymph nodes, was observed in 18% of females and 10% of males in our series of C57BL mice. The resultant atrophy of normal lymphoid structures in the affected lymph nodes may severely influence functional studies performed with cells derived from such lymph nodes.

A lung lesion characterized by a focal to widespread intra-alveolar accumulation of large acidophilic macrophages (Figure 11) was observed in 30% and 16% of male and female C57BL mice, respectively. The macrophages, which frequently contained several nuclei, contained needle-like to rhomboid crystals of varying sizes, which were either colorless or deeply acidophilic, and similar crystals were found free in alveoli and occasionally in bronchioles. In the more severe cases, neutrophils were a part of the intra-alveolar cellular infiltrate. The etiology of this lesion, which we have termed "acidophilic macrophage pneumonia", is unknown and the exact nature of the crystals has not been defined. The possibility that this represents a defective processing of an

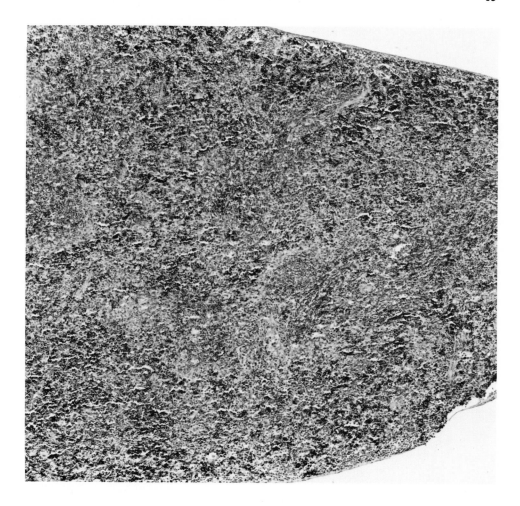

FIGURE 6.   Reticulum cell sarcoma type A (lightly stained cells) diffusely infiltrating the splenic red pulp, accompanied by prominent erythropoiesis (darkly stained cells). Note severely atrophic white pulp. HPS × 65.

endogenous substance(s) by macrophages has yet to be explored. Similar crystal-containing acidophilic macrophages have been observed in bone marrow, lymph nodes, and spleen of C57BL mice, although less frequently than in lung. Others have reported similar lung lesions in mice[36] as well as comparable crystal-containing macrophages in mouse bone marrow.[37]

The majority of the lesions observed in this series of NZB mice tended to be either of a degenerative or inflammatory nature. Nearly all mice examined had evidence of glomerulopathy (not shown in table) characterized by the frequent occurrence of hyaline thrombi in glomerular capillaries and by thickened, hyalinized glomerular basement membranes (GBM) with an increased amount of mesangial matrix. These changes varied from uniform diffuse thickening of the GBM to severe segmental hyalinization and sclerosis of glomerular tufts, often with prominent fibrinoid necrosis of a portion of a tuft (Figure 12). In some animals the renal lesions were limited to the changes just described, but in most mice they were accompanied by tubular changes which varied from mild focal dilatation to severe, widespread tubular dilatation accompanied by atrophy and collapse of tubules. Casts were prominent in these kidneys as were interstitial fibrosis and chronic inflammation resulting in "endstage" renal disease.

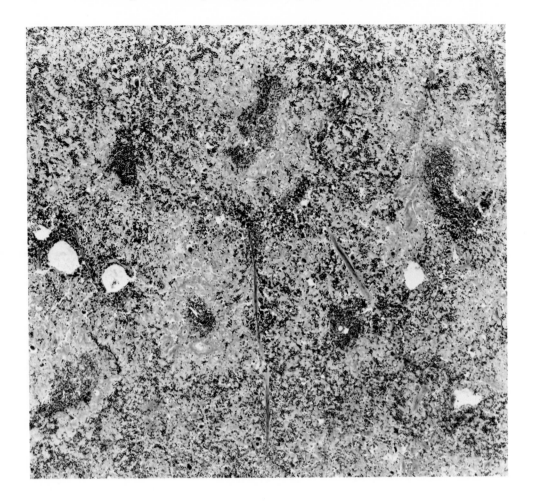

FIGURE 7.   Splenic amyloidosis in a 24-month-old male C57BL mouse. Note perifollicular location of amyloid, and accompanying atrophy of splenic follicles. HPS × 48.

Hyalinization and fibrinoid necrosis of small muscular arteries in various organs of the body was observed in 27% and 12% of females and males, respectively. Such arterial changes were found predominantly in spleen (Figure 13), lymph nodes, and gastrointestinal tract. Localized or widespread vascular thrombosis was seen in 32% and 42% of female and male NZB mice, respectively. Large atrial or auricular thrombi were present in many of these mice. Important sequelae of those vascular lesions were focal ischemic necrosis primarily of heart and liver. The effect of these severe vascular lesions on the immune system is difficult to estimate when no clearcut infarction of those tissues is observed.

In addition, mild to severe purulent inflammation of unknown etiology involving mainly organs of the genito-urinary tract, but other organs as well, was seen in 22% of the males and 20% of the females examined.

Extensive extramedullary hematopoiesis in various tissues was also a typical finding in NZB mice. This was the cause of the splenic enlargement often noted on gross examination (Figure 14). Marked hemosiderosis primarily of spleen and liver was also present in most of these mice. These latter changes are considered to be related to the Coombs' positive hemolytic anemia present in NZB mice.[38]

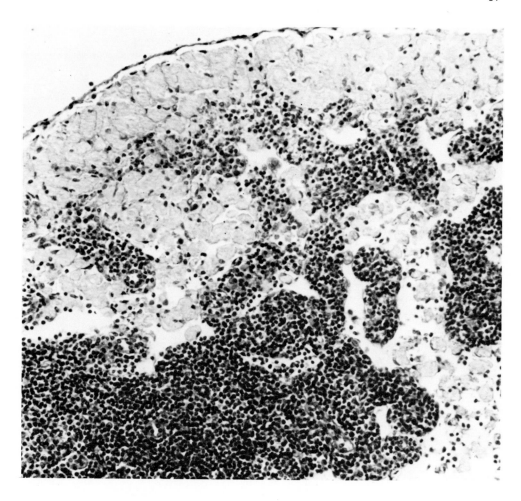

FIGURE 8.   Intracellular amyloid in macrophages located in subcapsular and cortical sinuses of mesenteric lymph node from a 16-month-old male C57BL mouse. HPS × 256.

Large, active lymphoid follicles with prominent germinal centers were common in lymph nodes and spleens of NZB mice, and numerous plasma cells were present in the splenic cords and medullary cords of lymph nodes, presumably reflecting the increased reactivity of the B cell system known for this strain.

The nonneoplastic lesions in the CBA mice of this series were dominated by dystrophic calcinosis[39] of cardiac muscle, gastrointestinal smooth muscle, and in renal tubules (75% of males and 78% of females), and testicular atrophy in 77% of males. In addition, the formation of cysts in a number of organs and tissues, including thyroid, ovary, thymus (Figure 15), and visceral peritoneum, was commonly seen. No association between these lesions and the histological appearance of the lymphoid tissues was observed.

Other common histological changes not listed in the table which were observed in all three strains of mice, although varying in extent and severity among the strains and among individual mice of a single strain, included the following: glomerulonephritis (mentioned above for NZB mice), fibromyxomatous change of cardiac valves, focal adrenocortical atrophy with fibrosis, ceroid deposition, especially in ovaries and adrenal glands, and sparse to moderate infiltration by lymphocytes and plasma cells of a

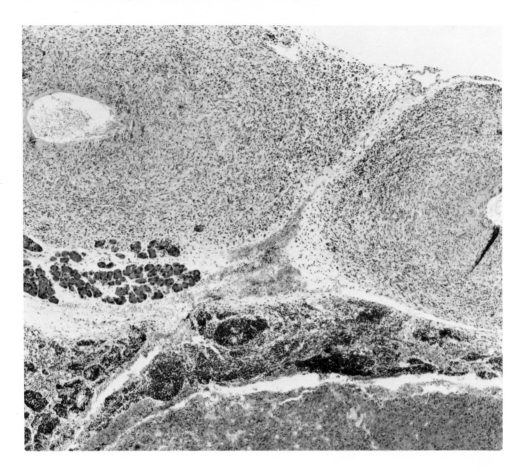

FIGURE 9.   Severe periarteritis nodosa involving branches of the mesenteric arteries in a 7-month-old female C57BL mouse. The vessel walls have become greatly thickened due to the extensive proliferative inflammatory process. Note lymph node with portion of blood-filled cyst in the lower part of the photomicrograph. HPS × 65.

number of organs including lungs, liver, kidneys, salivary glands, urinary bladder, mesentery, and reproductive organs.

Specific mention should be made of the histological changes observed in lymphoid tissues unaffected by lymphoreticular tumors, which were not discussed previously. Although detailed quantitative morphological studies were not performed, the following observations may be useful in interpretation of functional tests.

An increased number of plasma cells was found in lymph nodes of aged mice as compared to those of young mice. NZB mice, however, often showed an excessive increase in the numbers of plasma cells as compared to the other strains. Another characteristic of lymph nodes of the NZB strain was cystic dilatation of sinuses, which was not classifiable as "mesenteric disease" (see above). The structure of lymph nodes of aged C57BL mice frequently showed a somewhat expanded paracortical area but with a moderate lymphocytic depletion. Germinal centers were found infrequently in aged C57BL mice, in contrast to the situation in CBA and especially NZB mice. CBA mice showed the least severe changes in lymphoid tissues with age as compared to C57BL and NZB mice.

Age-related thymic atrophy was common to all three strains. Specific differences in

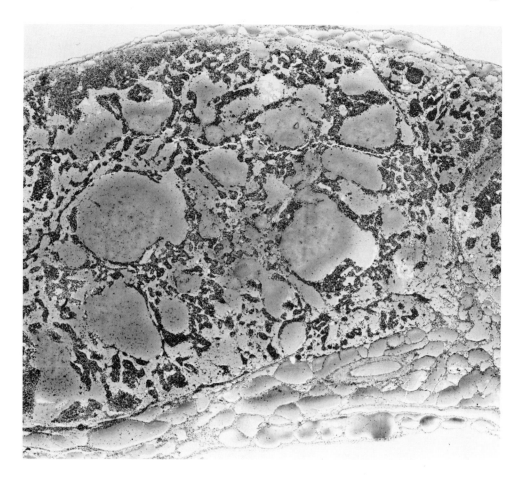

FIGURE 10. Mesenteric lymph node from a 23-month-old female C57BL mouse showing dilated blood-filled sinuses compatible with "mesenteric disease". HPS × 32.

thymus morphology among the strains, with the exception of cyst formation in CBA mice, were not noted on routine histological examination, although decreased numbers of epithelial cells have been reported to occur in thymuses of NZB mice.[40]

The types and frequencies of lesions observed in the three strains of mice discussed above can be seen to differ considerably from one another. In general terms, it can be stated that the age-related pathological changes of the C57BL mice were dominated by lymphoreticular neoplasia and amyloidosis, the NZB by immune complex mediated lesions, autoimmune hemolytic anemia, and thrombovascular disease, and the CBA by lesions in the endocrine and reproductive systems. Whether the variety of lesions seen within a specific strain are interrelated, and, more specifically, whether the lesions observed have a direct influence on the functional changes in the immune system with age, must still be determined. It is clear, however, that one must be cognizant of the various pathological changes within a particular strain in order to make valid interpretations of functional experiments.

2. Rats

Data on the survival characteristics and age-related pathological changes for several rat strains have been reported by a number of investigators, many of whose studies have been referred to in previous sections. We will not attempt a review of these find-

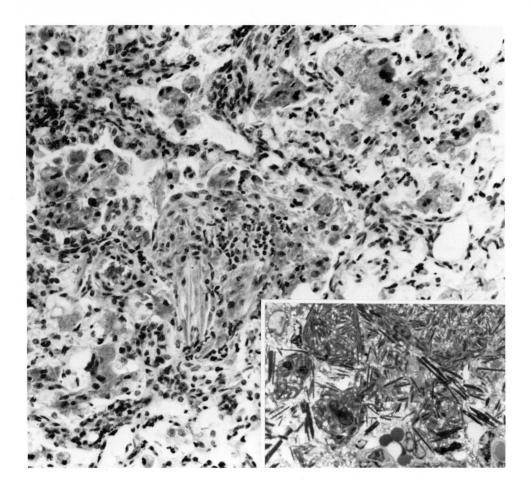

FIGURE 11.   Acidophilic macrophage pneumonia in a 4-month-old male C57BL mouse. Numerous large macrophages with intracytoplasmic crystalline structures fill the alveolar spaces and the lumen of a bronchiole (upper center). Note several multinucleated giant cells adjacent to large extracellular crystals. HPS × 260. Inset: Epon-embedded 0.5 μm section showing detail of alveolar macrophages and crystals. Toluidine blue × 800.

ings with speculations on their possible effect on immunological studies in this section, but instead we will limit our discussion to a brief outline of the nonneoplastic age-related changes observed in the thymus and lymph nodes of rats used for aging studies at our institute.

The rat strains maintained for aging studies at the Institute for Experimental Gerontology TNO are the WAG/Rij, the BN/BiRij and their F₁ hybrid. Details on the longevity, pathology, and husbandry conditions of these rats have been published[7,30] and will not be further mentioned here.

a. Thymus

Although the thymuses of rats showed a predictable atrophy with age, the degree of atrophy and the time of onset varied with the strain and sex. In general, all thymuses of aged rats were characterized by a depletion of cortical lymphocytes.

In female WAG/Rij and (WAG×BN)F₁ rats, the loss of cortical lymphocytes was accompanied by a mild proliferation and cystic dilatation of epithelial structures in the medulla. The female BN/BiRij rat exhibited some significant differences in this

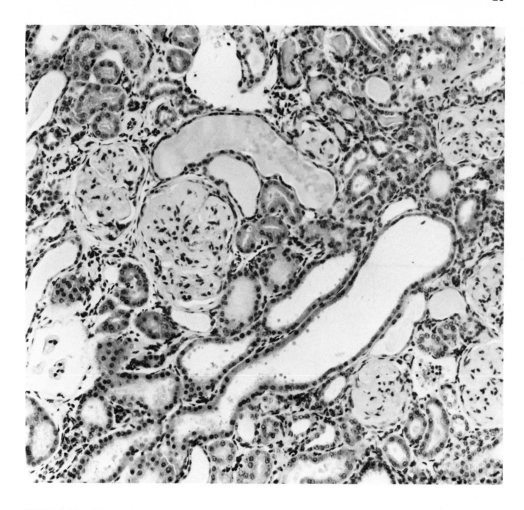

FIGURE 12. Severe glomerulonephritis in a 17-month-old female NZB mouse characterized by extensive thickening and hyalinization of capillary walls with focal fibrinoid necrosis of glomerular tufts. Note accompanying dilatation and atrophy of tubules, tubular cast formation, and mild interstitial inflammation. HPS × 210.

respect, however, in that after the age of approximately 24 months, an often quite massive proliferation of epithelial cords and tubules (Figure 16) in an otherwise atrophic thymus had taken place.[7,41] Moreover, evidence was obtained by electron microscopic and autoradiographic studies that the epithelium in these thymuses was capable of active protein synthesis and secretion. More work is needed, however, before a relation can be postulated between these epithelial structures and thymic hormone-like factors, as well as their possible significance in aged rats of this strain.

The degree of thymic atrophy tended to be greater in male rats of these strains than in females. The WAG/Rij male (which, interestingly, also had a 50% survival age which was approximately 9 months less than that of the female), however, showed the earliest and most severe atrophy, with only occasional lymphocytes and fibrovascular remnants remaining.[7] The difference in degree of thymic atrophy between males and females was studied by Kruisbeek,[42] who showed a correlation between thymic morphology and T-cell functions in 18-month-old WAG/Rij rats.

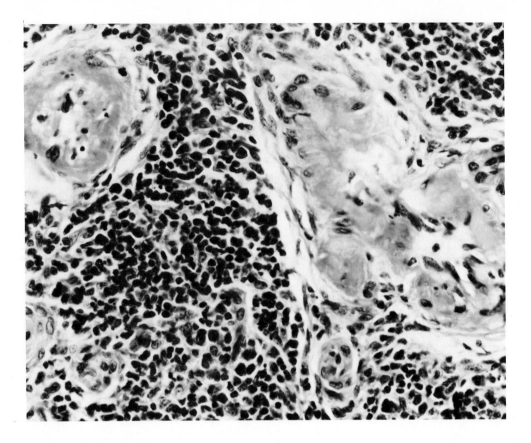

FIGURE 13.   Hyalinization and fibrinoid necrosis of central arterioles of spleen from a 6-month-old female
NZB mouse. HPS × 500.

b. Lymph Nodes

The changes observed in lymph nodes from our aging rats consisted primarily of a
decrease in the number of germinal centers and an increase in the number of plasma
cells residing in the medullary cords. Hemosiderin-laden macrophages appeared to increase in frequency in the lymph nodes with age. In addition, collections of large acidophilic macrophages with foamy or granular cytoplasm were frequently seen in both
the cortex and medulla of lymph nodes from old rats. Others[43,44] have shown that these
cells contained stored mucosubstances and phospholipids in their cytoplasm, presumably indigestible residues of phagocytized material. The significance of these macrophages is unclear at present.

The occurrence of cystic sinusoids in lymph nodes appeared to increase in frequency
with age, but specific incidence data are lacking. The lesion was observed in a number
of lymph nodes, although it appeared to occur more frequently in anterior mediastinal
lymph nodes. Grossly, these lymph nodes were enlarged, but they should not be mis-
taken for neoplastic processes since generally the cysts were readily appreciated upon
cutting. The cysts were filled with proteinaceous fluid and appeared to arise from dilated sinusoids (Figure 17). They were lined by flattened, endothelial-like cells. The
etiology and significance of this lesion is unknown.

Finally, brief mention should be made at this point that in view of the relatively
frequent occurrence of neoplastic lesions of certain types in aging rats of various
strains, it is quite likely that in many situations aging rats harboring tumors may be

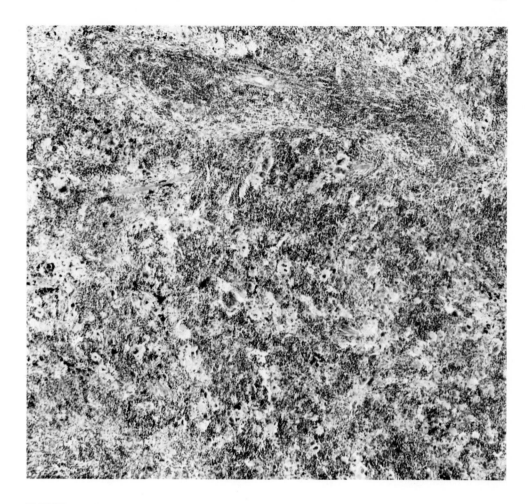

FIGURE 14. Extensive hematopoiesis in spleen of an 18-month-old male NZB mouse. Note the numerous megakaryocytes in the red pulp, a common finding in this strain. HPS × 100.

used for a variety of in vivo or in vitro immunological studies. In this connection, the investigator should be cognizant of possible influences that the presence of a tumor in the test animal may have on immunological functions. It was recently shown, for example, that four different types of transplantable spontaneous rat tumors were capable of severely impairing T cell responsiveness in the recipients.[45,46] This effect was shown to be due not to intrinsic lymphocyte defects, but rather to changes in macrophage-lymphocyte ratios.[46] This type of data again demonstrate the necessity of having available complete information on the various lesions present in one's laboratory animals in order to interpret experimental data.

B. Selected Diseases and Conditions Not Directly Related to Aging

The purpose of the following is to briefly bring to the attention of the investigator some non-age-related conditions which may affect the results of a number of immunological studies.

1. Infectious Diseases

One of the most prevalent and serious viral infections of rodents is Sendai virus infection caused by paramyxovirus type 1. Infection rates of 66% in mouse colonies

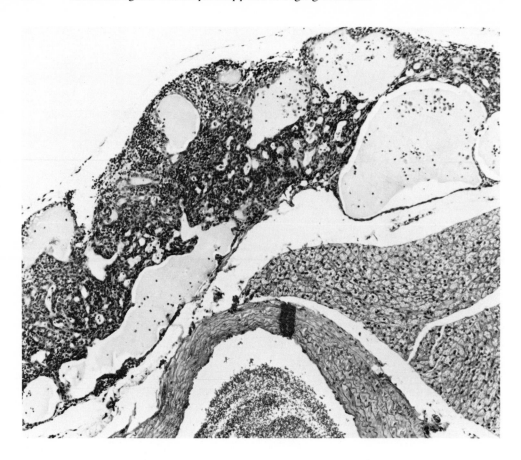

FIGURE 15.   Atrophic thymus from a 30-month-old male CBA mouse showing numerous cysts and proliferation of tubular epithelial structures. HPS × 96.

and 63% of rat colonies have been reported.[47] In addition to acute interstitial pneumonia, important effects of an acute infection caused by this virus are the development
of residual chronic lung lesions, high mortality among preweaning and juvenile mice,
and an approximate doubling of the mortality rate for older age groups,[48] and a syn-
ergistic effect with certain other respiratory disease pathogens[49] presumably related to
an inhibitory effect of the virus on phagocytic cells.[50] The long-term effects of subclinical Sendai virus infection on several immune functions can be profound, and are characterized by increased fragility of T and B cells, decreased T and B cell proliferative
capacities,[51] and the apparent initiation of autoimmune diseases in immunologically
immature and immunodeficient aging mice.[52] Evidence for the suppression of the immune response has also been obtained in Sendai virus infected rats.[53]

An important cause of hepatitis in mice is mouse hepatitis virus (MHV), which is a
coronavirus. The disease is highly transmissible and probably worldwide in distribution. There appears to be a genetically determined strain susceptibility, and certain
strains (e.g., C3H) are reported to be resistant. The most important clinical signs are
diarrhea and high mortality in susceptible infant mice up to about 10 days of age, and
chronic wasting disease with active necrotizing hepatitis in nude mice which is usually
fatal in 1 to 4 weeks. A similar course of the disease is seen in genetically resistant
strains following a number of procedures which depress the cell-mediated immune response, such as neonatal thymectomy.[54] Nude mice infected with MHV showed altered

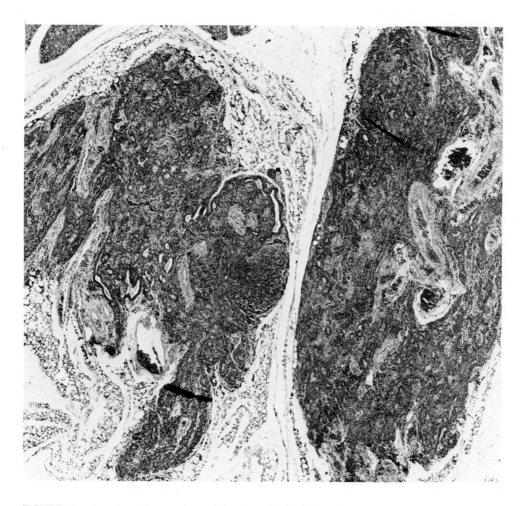

FIGURE 16. Atrophy with extensive proliferation of epithelial cords and tubules in thymus from a 28-month-old female BN/Bi rat. HPS × 43.

immune responsiveness to sheep red blood cells in that the number of splenic plaque-forming cells was increased as compared to controls, and in addition, increased numbers of theta-positive lymphocytes were detected in spleens of infected mice.[55] It has also been reported that the growth of transplanted tumors in nude mice infected with MHV is diminished or absent.[56]

Lactic dehydrogenase virus (LDH) causes a clinically silent infection in mice which is characterized by increased activity of a number of serum enzymes. The importance of this viral infection, for which reliable diagnostic tests are not available, is its effects on the immune system. In addition to stimulation of splenic plaque-forming cells, antibody responses to certain antigens are often increased apparently as the result of increased retention of membrane-bound antigen by macrophages from LDH virus-infected mice.[57]

Murine respiratory mycoplasmosis (MRM), caused by *Mycoplasma pulmonis,* is probably one of the most important diseases of rats and mice in terms of its widespread nature and high morbidity within an experimental animal colony. The clinical and pathological features of this disease have been described in detail.[58] This disease, which varies in severity from animal to animal, is primarily an upper respiratory disease,

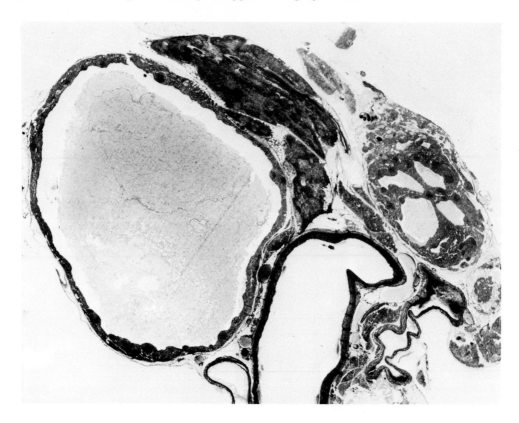

FIGURE 17.   Mediastinal lymph node from a 26-month-old female Sprague-Dawley rat with sinusoidal cysts of varying sizes. The cysts contain proteinaceous fluid. The thymus is at the upper center, and the aorta at the lower center. HPS × 10.

with purulent rhinitis, laryngitis, tracheitis, and otitis media. Bronchitis with bronchiectasis and severe peribronchial lymphoid hyperplasia are commonly seen in infected animals, and the disease characteristically runs a chronic course. In addition to the devastating effect this respiratory disease can have on long term experiments, *M. pulmonis* also has specific effects on the immune system. Recently, it has been shown that *M. pulmonis* possesses nonspecific mitogenic activity for both rat B and T lymphocytes,[59] although the response of B cells was much stronger than that of T cells. It has also been shown that the mitogenic activity resides in the organism's outer surface membrane proteins.[60] Using other mycoplasma species, others have reported that large doses of organisms depressed lymphocyte reactivity to mitogens, while small doses increased the response.[61] These investigators also showed that mycoplasmas inhibited the phagocytic capacity of neutrophils in vitro and in vivo. An apparent correlation between mycoplasma capping and blast transformation of infected lymphocytes was shown.[62] Appropriately, these authors warned ''investigators using lymphocytes as model systems to investigate mitogenicity, lymphocyte triggering, surface antigens, and viral pathology'' to beware of mycoplasma contamination in their cultured cells.

2. Parasitic Diseases

Although infections with the intestinal flagellates *Giardia muris* and *Spironucleus (Hexamita) muris,* which are commonly present in conventional mouse colonies, are known to cause wasting disease and increased mortality in nude mice,[63] very little is known about the specific effects of these parasites on the host immune system. Recently, however, it was shown that levels of lgG1, lgG2a and lgG2b were elevated in nu/nu and nu/ + mice with spironucleosis as compared to non-infected controls.[64]

Similarly, pinworm (*Aspiculuris tetraptera, Syphacia obvelata,* and *S. muris*) infestations of mice and rats maintained conventionally are extremely common, and even, at times, in so-called barrier facilities. Many consider these nematodes to have a negligible effect on the host, while others have reported a number of effects on the host's immune system as a result of pinworm infestation, including increased or decreased humoral antibody response to heterologous antigens, and enhancement or suppression of growth of certain neoplasms.[65]

A common parasitic disease of conventionally maintained mice which, based on our observations, can be expected to influence the lymphoid tissues of the host to some extent, is infestation by the dwarf tapeworm *Hymenolepis nana.* This cestode has either a direct or indirect life cycle. The direct cycle can occur in the absence of an intermediate host (e.g., cockroach), and thus autoinfection is possible in the usual laboratory setting.

In the usual situation, when ova are ingested the larvae develop in the small intestine and invade the tunica propria of intestinal villi where they give rise to cysticercoid forms. After a few days, the cysticercoids migrate into the intestinal lumen where they develop into adult tapeworms. Migration of larvae to other organs is exceptional.

During a survey of histopathological lesions in aging mice of several inbred strains which were maintained under conventional conditions at our institute a number of years ago, it appeared that one of these strains showed a high frequency of aberrant larval migration. In 14 or 42 male RFM mice examined, aberrant *H. nana* larvae were found in the mesenteric lymph node, and in four cases larvae were also identified in sections of lung. In only 3 or 47 female RFM mice were larval forms found in the mesenteric lymph node, as was the case in 1 of 29 female C57BL mice. No larvae of *H. nana* were found histologically in 43 male and 42 female CBA, 105 male C57BL, and 21 male and 20 female NZB mice.

In the mesenteric lymph node, larvae were located preferentially near or in the subcapsular sinus (Figure 18) and they were surrounded by granulomatous inflammation, with many giant cells and varying degrees of fibrosis. In the cases with lung involvement, pulmonary nodules were seen grossly[66] which contained massive numbers of larvae in alveolar spaces and airways accompanied by chronic inflammation and hyperplasia of alveolar epithelial cells.

The cause for the apparent susceptibility of male RFM mice to aberrant migration by the parasitic larvae is not clear. Aging RFM mice were also found to have a high incidence of lymphoreticular malignancies (74% in males, and 91% in females; unpublished data), involving especially the mesenteric lymph node, and one can speculate whether an accompanying disturbance of lymph drainage from the intestine with resultant lymphangiectasia may have facilitated the migration of larvae to the mesenteric lymph node and elsewhere. Larvae were indeed identified within extranodal dilated lymph vessels in some cases, but in 3 of 10 cases with mesenteric lymph node involvement, no lymphoreticular tumor was found. In addition, female RFM mice, which had a lower incidence of aberrant larval migration, had a somewhat higher incidence of lymphoreticular tumors than males.

Another possible explanation might be that the aberrant migration of the cestode larvae in this mouse strain is facilitated by a severe form of immunodeficiency. Several lines of circumstantial evidence, which are based primarily on the similarity of certain pathological findings in RFM to those in nude mice, suggest that the RFM may indeed be immunodeficient (unpublished data).

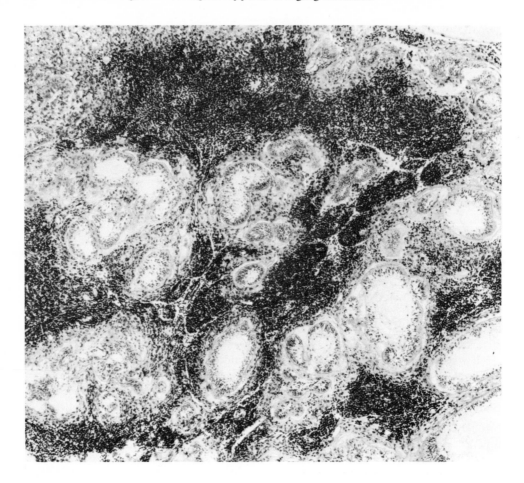

FIGURE 18.   Larvae of *Hymenolepis nana* in mesenteric lymph node of a 12-month-old male RFM mouse. Note accompanying chronic inflammation and disruption of lymph node architecture. HPS × 96.

In any event, it is important to recognize that in certain conventionally maintained mouse strains lymph nodes may harbor parasites. Such tissues will generally be enlarged and may therefore possibly be misinterpreted as being neoplastic, and they will contain numerous inflammatory cells which may yield spurious results when used for immunological tests.

3. Environmental and Nutritional Conditions

Only brief mention will be made of a condition which may be encountered in laboratories using lethally irradiated mice. A common practice to prevent the early death syndrome (i.e., pseudomonas infection) in such mice is to provide them with chlorinated (12 to 16 ppm chlorine) or acidified (pH3) water. A recent study revealed that the number of peritoneal macrophages harvestable from mice drinking hyperchlorinated water (i.e., 25 to 30 ppm chlorine) was significantly reduced as compared to that from mice drinking tap water.[67] In addition, the macrophage-mediated cytotoxicity against several tumor cell lines was markedly suppressed in macrophages from mice receiving hyperchlorinated water.

It is well known that nutrition profoundly affects the immune system, and no attempt will be made to review the voluminous literature on the subject. It is known, for example, that dietary restriction increases the lifespan of certain rodent strains, and it was shown that early in life, restricted mice appeared immunosuppressed as judged by decreased response of T and B cells to a number of mitogens.[68] These authors postulated that dietary restriction may act to delay the maturation of the immune system. Others have shown that thymus weight and cellularity were markedly reduced, coupled with a diminished suppressor T cell activity, in mice fed a low-protein diet.[69] Even marginal deficiences of certain dietary components can lead to significant alterations in the immune response. For example, spleen cells from rats born to mothers marginally deficient in choline and methionine showed a decreased response to mitogenic stimulation and a decreased antibody response to sheep red cells.[70]

Practically speaking, most diets formulated for laboratory rodents contain the proper balance of nutrients in the quantities which are sufficient and in some cases exceed those required for reproduction, growth and maintenance. However, most investigators are not aware that concentrations of essential ingredients may vary appreciably in different batches of a formulation made with different lots of natural ingredients although the crude analysis remains the same. In addition, feeds may contain unexpected additives or biologically active components which have found their way into the food chain, many of which can introduce important variables in any experiment using laboratory animals.[71]

V. DESIRABLE HEALTH STATUS FOR RODENTS IN AGING RESEARCH

For long-term studies, including biological aging research, it is of great importance to have available animals of good quality.[2,3] It was not long ago that an investigator who initiated experiments of more than just short-term duration in relation to the potential age expectancy of the species, was almost certainly doomed to lose most of his experimental animal population or, at best, end up with disease-ridden old animals from which any experimental conclusions were of dubious value.[72] These problems have largely been overcome due to a continual refinement of germfree technology, of cesarean derivation techniques, and of techniques for rearing and maintaining animals behind physical barriers that exclude pathogenic organisms. The value of excluding pathogenic organisms in long-term studies can be illustrated by longevity data of Fischer 344 rats maintained under different conditions. Under conventional conditions, the Fischer 344 rat was reported to have a life span of 12 ± 0.1 months[74] with a maximum of 21 months,[73] but this same rat strain reared and maintained behind a barrier can live at least 33 months with a 50% survival age of more than 28 months.[13] Nowadays, specified pathogen free (SPF) animals are widely used in gerontological research. SPF animals were defined in 1964 by the nomenclature subcommittee of the International Committee on Laboratory Animals[75] as animals that are free of specified microorganisms and parasites, but not necessarily free of other unnamed contaminants. This definition already suggests that the microbiological status of such animals can differ considerably among research laboratories and this can certainly complicate comparisons of data between various institutions.[30] In addition, the definition has been frequently misused in the past, and many supposedly SPF animals are merely cesarean-derived and barrier-maintained with no quality control to ensure that they remain free of the specified pathogens.[72] One can partially compensate for these shortcomings by listing in publications specifically the microorganisms and parasites which are absent, instead of merely using the term SPF.

It must be admitted that there are some disadvantages associated with the use of SPF animals. These include: (1) the costs of producing and maintaining SPF animals which add an extra financial burden to the already expensive longevity studies[4,5,30,] and

(2) the physical barrier required is usually such that the carrying out of frequent experimental procedures on the animals is often limited or almost impossible.

In order to reduce the costs of longevity studies for aging research as well as to lower the barrier to such an extent that the investigator can handle his animals more easily without appreciably compromising their health status, the following regimen for rearing and maintaining rodents at the Institute for Experimental Gerontology TNO has been employed in the past years and is still used with minor modifications (for detailed information, see refs. 7, 30, 76). Mice and rats are born and reared under strict SPF conditions. At an age of 12 weeks for virgins and approximately 8 months for retired breeders, the animals are transferred to a clean environment and maintained behind a less rigid barrier but under high standards of hygiene. Animals reared and maintained in this way have been designated "clean conventional". "Clean conventional" must be regarded as an intermediate status between SPF and conventional, and can be applied to animals free of infectious diseases, but also free of parasites which are often present in conventionally bred animals. The conditions and standard protocols for SPF as well as "clean conventional" rooms currently employed in our institute have been published.[76] It must be emphasized that strict precautionary measures must be taken when animals or biological materials are introduced into the animal facility from elsewhere, and that appropriate quarantine procedures be available. It is our experience that with adequate management and a continual surveillance of the animals, this regimen functions well for long-term investigations.

VI. MONITORING THE HEALTH STATUS OF AN ANIMAL COLONY

As has been stated in a preceding section, the health status of experimental animals may often have profound effects on biological responses. To avoid misinterpretation of experimental data, a regular monitoring program of the animals should be an integral part of a more extensive screening program, including an evaluation of other environmental factors, such as physical and chemical factors.[77] One of the most crucial requirements in such a program is the proper sampling of each animal population or subpopulation. Jonas[78] has given some general recommendations for sample sizes and sampling frequencies.

A health monitoring program should consist of a bacteriological, parasitological, serological, and pathological examination of a number of animals in a certain time period. It must be emphasized that histopathological examination of all major organs is necessary, since a number of infectious and other diseases cannot as yet be reliably detected by other means such as serology (e.g., cytomegalovirus, sialodacryoadenitis virus, mouse hepatitis virus, and murine adenovirus infections). As an example of an animal health surveillance program for mice and rats which is based on a protocol previously proposed by Lindsey,[78a] the procedure followed by the REP-Institutes TNO is given.

Each week twenty animals are examined. This number was chosen such that each animal subpopulation is sampled and tested semiannually. Each animal is accessioned separately, anesthetized with ether or by an injection of sodium pentobarbital, and exsanguinated. Blood may be obtained from the brachial vessels,[79] jugular vein,[80] periorbital venous sinus, or heart.[81] The serum is harvested and diluted 1:5 with phosphate-buffered saline and heat-inactivated at 56°C for 30 minutes. The individual serum samples are tested for antibodies to a number of viruses and *Mycoplasma pulmonis* (Table 4) with the hemagglutination-inhibition (HI) test and/or complement fixation (CF) test. These tests are performed by a competent virology laboratory.

Table 4
ROUTINE SEROLOGICAL
SCREENING AT THE REP-
INSTITUTES TNO

Disease agent	Serological test	
	CF	HI
Sendai virus	X	X
Ectromelia virus	X	X
Reovirus type 3	X	X
K-virus		X
Polyoma virus		X
Minute virus of mice		X
Theiler's GD VII virus		X
Mengovirus		X
Pneumonia virus of mice		X
Kilham rat virus		X
Mouse adenovirus	X	
Lymphocytic choriomeningitis	X	
Mouse hepatitis virus	X	
Mycoplasma pulmonis	X	

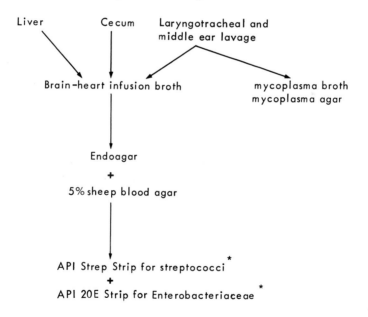

Routine Bacteriological Screening at the REP Institutes TNO

FIGURE 19.   Scheme of bacteriological screening procedures of rodents at the REP-Institutes TNO. (*API System, SA, Montalieu-Vescieu, France).

After the animals are bled, both tympanic membranes are penetrated with a sterile Pasteur pipette and the middle ear cavities are lavaged with sterile isotonic saline. The aspirated fluid is transferred to sterile test tubes and submitted to the bacteriology laboratory for culturing of mycoplasma and aerobic bacteria. In addition, a portion of a liver lobe and the tip of the cecum are removed aseptically for bacteriological examination. The culturing procedure is given in Figure 19.

After sampling for bacteriological cultures, all tissues are carefully screened for gross lesions including a thorough examination for ectoparasites. Tissues are then fixed and processed by routine procedures. A thorough microscopic examination of all major organ systems is essential to detect possible disease-causing agents. Special attention is also given to the presence of fungi and endoparasites. When all data, including the bacteriological, serological, parasitological and pathological findings, become available, evaluation of each animal subpopulation takes place. If changes in the health status are detected, their potential effects on experiments, and on the animal colony as a whole, must be quickly determined and corrective measures instituted if necessary.

One must be aware that this program still has some deficiences in that not all conceivable diseases or latent infections can be detected, but in most instances, this type of surveillance program will suffice to define the health status of an experimental animal colony.

VII. SUMMARY

In this chapter several age-related and non-age-related conditions have been described which may influence the interpretation of studies on immune function in aged animals.

Non-age-related diseases such as caused by MHV, Sendai virus, mycoplasma, and certain endoparasites may, in addition to being life-threatening conditions, also have a direct influence on immune function. The importance of monitoring the experimental animal colony to assess the health status is self evident and has been discussed in Sections V and VI.

As discussed in the section on the definition of an aged animal, one has to be sure one is dealing with an aging population before initiating investigations on the relation of immune parameters to aging. The characteristics of an aging population are a more or less rectangular survival curve and the finding of multiple pathological changes at death. The increasing interindividual variability with age, even within an inbred strain, is reflected in the histological lesions and functional parameters.

After discussing these general characteristics of aged animals which may influence functional studies, the effects of more specific age-related lesions on the immune system are mentioned. Such lesions may affect lymphoid tissues directly because these tissues are their site of origin or they may be secondarily affected (e.g., lymphoid atrophy in tumor-bearing animals). It is not known whether other age-associated diseases, which do not result in significant histological lesions in the lymphoid tissues, may directly or indirectly affect immune parameters (e.g., certain endocrine tumors), or whether they might themselves reflect a disordered immune function (e.g., periarteritis nodosa).

In any case, one must be cautious in interpreting age-related changes in immune parameters as resulting from aging phenomena of the immune system when interference by other age-associated changes cannot be excluded.

ACKNOWLEDGMENT

The authors wish to thank Dr. M. J. Blankwater and Dr. J. Radl for their critical reading of the manuscript, and Mr. A. A. Glaudemans for photomicroscopy.

REFERENCES

1. **Hollander, C. F.,** Experimental gerontological research, *Ned. T. Geront.,* 9, 125, 1978.
2. **Hollander, C. F.,** Proper use of the laboratory rats and mice in gerontological research, in *Physiology and Cell Biology of Aging,* Vol. 8, Cherkin, A., Finch, C. E., Kharasch, N., Makinodan, T., Scott, F. L., and Strehler, B., Eds., Raven Press, New York, 1979, 223.
3. **Hollander, C. F.,** Animal models for aging and cancer research, *J. Natl. Cancer Inst.,* 51, 3, 1973.
4. **Hollander, C. F. and Burek, J. D.,** Animal models in gerontology, in *Lectures on Gerontology,* Vol. 1, Viidik, A., Ed., Academic Press, London, in press, chap. 14.
5. **Burek, J. D. and Hollander, C. F.,** Experimental gerontology, in *The Laboratory Rat,* Vol. 2, Baker, H. J., Lindsey, J. R., and Weisbroth, S., Eds., Academic Press, New York, 1980, chap. 7.
6. **Cohen, B. J. and Anver, M. R.,** Pathological changes during aging in the rat, in *Special Review of Experimental Aging. Progress in Biology,* Elias, M. F., Eleftheriou, B. E., and Elias, P. K., Eds., EAR, Inc. Bar Harbor, Maine, 1976, 379.
7. **Burek, J. D.,** *Pathology of Aging Rats. A Morphological and Experimental Study of the Age-Associated Lesions in Aging BN/Bi, WAG/Rij and (WAG×BN)F₁ Rats,* CRC Press, West Palm Beach, Fla., 1978.
8. **Simms, H. S.,** Longevity studies in rats. I. Relation between life span and age of onset of specific lesions, in *Pathology of Laboratory Rats and Mice,* Cotchin, E. and Roe, F. J.C., Eds., F. A. Davis, Philadelphia, 1967, 733.
9. **Berg, B. N.,** Longevity studies in rats. II. Pathology of aging rats, in *Pathology of Laboratory Rats and Mice,* Cotchin, E. and Roe, F. J. C., Eds., F. A. Davis, Philadelphia, 1967, 749.
10. **Snell, K. C.,** Spontaneous lesions of the rat, in *The Pathology of Laboratory Animals,* Ribelin, W. E. and McCoy, J. R., Eds., Charles C Thomas, Springfield, Ill., 1965, 270.
11. **Gilbert, C. and Gillman, J.,** Spontaneous neoplasms in the albino rat, *S. Afr. J. Med. Sci.,* 23, 257, 1958.
12. **Thompson, S. W., Huseby, R. A., Fox, M. A., Davis, C. L., and Hunt, R. D.,** Spontaneous tumors in the Sprague-Dawley rat, *J. Natl. Cancer Inst.,* 27, 1037, 1961.
13. **Coleman, G. L., Barthold, S. W., Osbaldiston, G. W., Foster, S. J., and Jonas, A. M.,** Pathological changes during aging in barrier-reared Fischer 344 male rats, *J. Gerontol.,* 32, 258, 1977.
14. **Goodman, D. G., Ward, J. M., Squire, R. A., Chu, K. C., and Linhart, M. S.,** Neoplastic and nonneoplastic lesions in aging F 344 rats, *Toxicol. Appl. Pharmacol.,* 48, 237, 1979.
15. **Maekawa, A. and Odashima, S.,** Spontaneous tumors in ACI/N rats, *J. Natl. Cancer Inst.,* 55, 1437, 1975.
16. **Cohen, B. J., Anver, M. R., Ringler, D. H., and Adelman, R. C.,** Age-associated pathological changes in male rats, *Fed. Proc., Fed. Am. Soc. Exp. Biol.,* 37, 2848, 1978.
17. **Deerberg, F., Pitterman, W., and Rapp, K.,** Longevity study in HAN: Wistar rats: experience in maintaining aging rats for gerontological investigations, in *Interdisciplinary Topics in Gerontology,* Vol. 13, von Hahn, H. P., Ed., S. Karger, Basel, 1978, 66.
18. **Cosgrove, G. E., Satterfield, L. C., Bowles, N. D., and Klima, W. C.,** Diseases of aging untreated virgin female RFM and BALB/c mice, *J. Gerontol.,* 33, 178, 1978.
19. **Rabstein, L. S., Peters, R. L., and Spahn, G. T.,** Spontaneous tumors and pathologic lesions in SWR/J mice, *J. Natl. Cancer Inst.,* 50, 751, 1973.
20. **Rowlatt, C., Chesterman, F. C., and Sheriff, M. U.,** Lifespan, age changes and tumour incidence in an ageing C57BL mouse colony, *Lab Animals,* 10, 419, 1976.
21. **Smith, G. S., Walford, R. L., and Mickey, M. R.,** Lifespan and incidence of cancer and other diseases in selected long-lived inbred mice and their F₁ hybrids, *J. Natl. Cancer Inst.,* 50, 1195, 1973.
22. **Kawada, K. and Ojima, A.,** Various epithelial and non-epithelial tumors spontaneously occurring in long-lived mice of A/St, CBA, C57BL/6 and their hybrid mice, *Acta Pathol. Jpn.,* 28, 25, 1978.
23. **Holland, J. M., Mitchell, T. J., Gipson, L. C., and Whitaker, M. S.,** Survival and cause of death in aging germfree athymic nude and normal inbred C3Hf/He mice, *J. Natl. Cancer Inst.,* 61, 1357, 1978.
24. **Sharkey, F. E.,** Histopathological observations on a nude mouse colony, in *The Nude Mouse in Experimental and Clinical Research,* Fogh, J. and Giovanella, B. C., Eds., Academic Press, New York, 1978, chap. 5.
25. **Kohn, R. R.,** *Principles of Mammalian Aging,* Prentice-Hall, Englewood Cliffs, N. J., 1971, chap. 1.
26. **Mackay, I. R., Whittingham, S. F., and Mathews, J. D.,** The immunoepidemiology of aging, in *Comprehensive Immunology,* Vol. 1, *Immunology and Aging,* Makinodan, T. and Yunis, E., Eds., Plenum Press, New York, 1977, chap. 4.

27. **Adler, W. H., Jones, K. H., and Brock, M. A.,** Aging and immune function, in *The Biology of Aging,* Behnke, J. A., Finch, C. E., and Moment, G. B., Eds., Plenum Press, New York, 1978, chap. 13.

28. **Hijmans, W. and Hollander, C. F.,** The pathogenic role of age-related immune dysfunction, in *Comprehensive Immunology,* Vol. 1, *Immunology and Aging,* Makinodan, T. and Yunis, E., Eds., Plenum Press, New York, 1977, chap. 3.

29. **Blankwater, M. J.,** *Ageing and the Humoral Immune Response in Mice,* Institute for Experimental Gerontology TNO, Rijswijk, The Netherlands, 1978.

30. **Hollander, C. F.,** Current experience using the rat in aging studies, *Lab Anim. Sci.,* 26, 320, 1976.

31. **Dunn, T. B.,** Normal and pathologic anatomy of the reticular tissue in laboratory mice, with a classification and discussion of neoplasms. *J. Natl. Cancer Inst.,* 14, 1281, 1954.

31a. **Meihuizen, S. P., Personal Communication,** Institute for Experimental Gerontology TNO, Rijswijk, The Netherlands.

32. **Stewart, H. L., Deringer, M. K., Dunn, T. B., and Snell, K. C.,** Malignant schwannomas of nerve roots, uterus and epididymis in mice, *J. Natl. Cancer Inst.,* 53, 1749, 1974.

33. **Walker, A. I. T., Thorpe, E., and Stevenson, D. E.,** The toxicity of dieldrin (HEOD). I. Long-term oral toxicity studies in mice. *Food Cosmet. Toxicol.,* 11, 415, 1973.

34. **Ayers, K. M. and Jones, S. R.,** The cardiovascular system, in *Pathology of Laboratory Animals,* Vol. 1, Benirschke, K., Garner, F. M., and Jones, T. C., Eds., Springer-Verlag, New York, 1978, chap. 1.

35. **Yoshiki, T., Hayasaka, T., Fukatsu, R., Shirai, T., Itoh, T., Ikeda, H., and Katagiri, M.,** The structural proteins of murine leukemia virus and the pathogenesis of necrotizing arteritis and glomerulonephritis in SL/Ni mice, *J. Immunol.,* 122, 1812, 1979.

36. **Ward, J. M.,** Pulmonary pathology of the motheaten mouse, *Vet. Pathol.,* 15, 170, 1978.

37. **Ploemacher, R. E. and van Soest, P. L.,** Morphological investigation on ectopic erythropoiesis in experimental hemolytic anemia, *Cytobiology,* 15, 391, 1977.

38. **Talal, N. and Steinberg, A. D.,** The pathogenesis of autoimmunity in New Zealand Black mice, *Curr. Top. Microbiol. Immunol.,* 64, 79, 1974.

39. **Eaton, G. J., Custer, R. P., Johnson, F. N., and Stabenow, K. T.,** Dystrophic cardiac calcinosis in mice, *Am. J. Pathol.,* 90, 173, 1978.

40. **De Vries, M. J. and Hijmans, W.,** Pathological changes of thymic epithelial cells and autoimmune disease in NZB, NZW, and (NZB×NZW)F₁ mice, *Immunology,* 12, 179, 1967.

41. **Meihuizen, S. P. and Burek, J. D.,** The epithelial cell component of the thymuses of aged female BN/Bi rats, *Lab. Invest.,* 39, 613, 1978.

42. **Kruisbeek, A. M.,** *Thymus Dependent Immune Competence. Effects of Ageing, Tumour-Bearing and Thymic Humoral Function,* Institute for Experimental Gerontology TNO, Rijswijk, The Netherlands, 1978.

43. **Magnusson, G. and Majeed, S.,** Histochemical study of mesenteric lymph nodes in old rats, *Lab. Anim.,* 12, 99, 1978.

44. **Majeed, S. and Magnusson, G.,** Ultrastructural study of mesenteric lymph nodes in old rats, *Lab. Anim.,* 12, 103, 1978.

45. **Kruisbeek, A. M. and van Hees, M.,** Role of macrophages in the tumor-induced suppression of mitogen responses in rats, *J. Natl. Cancer Inst.,* 58, 1653, 1977.

46. **Kruisbeek, A. M., Zijlstra, J., and Zurcher, C.,** Tumor-induced changes in T cell mitogen responses in rats: suppression of spleen and blood lymphocyte responses and enhancement of thymocyte responses, *Eur. J. Immunol.,* 8, 200, 1978.

47. **Parker, J. C., Whiteman, M. D., and Richter, C. B.,** Susceptibility of inbred and outbred mouse strains to Sendai virus and prevalence of infection in laboratory rodents, *Infect. Immun.,* 19, 123, 1978.

48. **Zurcher, C., Burek, J. D., van Nunen, M. C. J., and Meihuizen, S. P.,** A naturally occurring epizootic caused by Sendai virus in breeding and aging rodent colonies. I. Infection in the mouse, *Lab. Anim. Sci.,* 27, 955, 1977.

49. **Howard, C. J., Stott, E. J., and Taylor, G.,** The effect of pneumonia induced in mice with *Mycoplasma pulmonis* on resistance to subsequent bacterial infection and the effect of a respiratory infection with Sendai virus on the resistance of mice to *Mycoplasma pulmonis, J. Gen. Microbiol.,* 109, 79, 1978.

50. **Jakab, G. J. and Green, G. M.,** Pulmonary defense mechanisms in consolidated and nonconsolidated regions of lungs infected with Sendai virus, *J. Infect. Dis.,* 129, 263, 1974.

51. **Kay, M. M. B.,** Long term subclinical effects of parainfluenza (SENDAI) infection on immune cells of aging mice, *Proc. Soc. Exp. Biol. Med.,* 158, 326, 1978.

52. **Kay, M. M.B.,** Parainfluenza infection of aged mice results in autoimmune disease, *Clin. Immunol. Immunopathol.,* 12, 301, 1979.

53. **Garlinghouse, L. E., Jr. and Van Hoosier, G. L.,** Studies on adjuvant-induced arthritis, tumor transplantability, and serologic response to bovine serum albumin in Sendai virus-infected rats, *Am. J. Vet. Res.,* 39, 297, 1978.

54. **Sheets, P., Shah, K. V., and Bang, F. B.,** Mouse hepatitis virus (MHV) infection in thymectomized C3H mice, *Proc. Soc. Exp. Biol. Med.,* 159, 34, 1978.

55. **Tamura, T., Machii, K., Ueda, K., and Fujiwara, K.,** Modification of immune response in nude mice infected with mouse hepatitis virus, *Microbiol. Immunol.,* 22, 557, 1978.

56. **Kyriazis, A. P., Di Persio, L., Michael, J. G., and Pesce, A. J.,** Influence of the mouse hepatitis virus (MHV) infection on the growth of human tumors in the athymic mouse, *Int. J. Cancer,* 23, 402, 1979.

57. **Michaelides, M. C. and Simms, E. S.,** Immune response in mice infected with lactic dehydrogenase virus. IV. Functional status of the macrophage during acute LDV infection, *Immunology,* 36, 241, 1979.

58. **Lindsey, J. R., Cassell, G. H., and Baker, J. R.,** Diseases due to mycoplasmas and rickettsias, in *Pathology of Laboratory Animals,* Vol. 2, Benirschke K., Garner, F. M., and Jones, T. C., Eds., Springer-Verlag, New York, 1978, chap. 15.

59. **Naot, Y., Merchav, S., Ben-David, E., and Ginsburg, H.,** Mitogenic activity of *Mycoplasma pulmonis.* I. Stimulation of rat B and T lymphocytes, *Immunology,* 36, 399, 1979.

60. **Naot, Y., Siman-Tov, R., and Ginsburg, H.,** Mitogenic activity of *Mycoplasma pulmonis.* II. Studies on the biochemical nature of the mitogenic factor, *Eur. J. Immunol.,* 9, 149, 1979.

61. **Thomsen, A. C. and Heron, I.,** Effect of mycoplasmas on phagocytosis and immunocompetence in rats, *Acta. Pathol. Microbiol. Scand. Sect. C,* 87, 67, 1979.

62. **Stanbridge, E. J. and Weiss, R. L.,** Mycoplasma capping on lymphocytes, *Nature (London),* 276, 583, 1978.

63. **Boorman, G. A., Lina, P. H. C., Zurcher, C., and Nieuwerkerk, H. T. M.,** *Hexamita* and *Giardia* as a cause of mortality in congenitally thymus-less (nude) mice, *Clin. Exp. Immunol.,* 15, 623, 1973.

64. **Kunstyr, I., Meyer, B., and Ammerpohl, E.,** Spironucleosis in nude mice: an animal model for immuno-parasitologic studies, in *Proceedings of the Second International Workshop on Nude Mice,* Univ. of Tokyo Press, Tokyo/Gustav Fischer Verlag, Stuttgart, 1977, 17.

65. **Taffs, L. F.,** Pinworm infections in laboratory rodents: a review, *Lab. Anim.,* 10, 1, 1976.

66. **van Zwieten, M. J. and Zurcher, C.,** Selected parasitologic, bacteriologic and virologic diseases of the mouse intestinal tract, in *Pathology Atlas of the European Late Effects Project Group,* Gössner, W., Hollander, C. F., Maisin, J. R., and Nilsson, A., Eds., 1976.

67. **Fidler, I. J.,** Depression of macrophages in mice drinking hyperchlorinated water, *Nature (London),* 270, 735, 1977.

68. **Gerbase-DeLima, M., Liu, R. K., Cheney, K. E., Mickey, R., and Walford, R. L.,** Immune function and survival in a long-lived mouse strain subjected to under-nutrition, *Gerontologia,* 21, 184, 1975.

69. **Bell, R. G. and Hazell, L. A.,** The influence of dietary protein insufficiency on the murine thymus. Evidence for an intrathymic pool of progenitor cells capable of thymus regeneration after severe atrophy, *Austr. J. Exp. Biol. Med. Sci.,* 55, 571, 1977.

70. **Gebhardt, B. M. and Newberne, P. M.,** Nutrition and immunological responsiveness. T-cell function in the offspring of lipotrope- and protein-deficient rats, *Immunology,* 26, 489, 1974.

71. **Newberne, P. M.,** Influence on pharmacological experiments of chemicals, and other factors in diets of laboratory animals, *Fed. Proc., Fed. Am. Soc. Exp. Biol.,* 34, 109, 1975.

72. **Hend, R. W.,** The concept of specific pathogen free (SPF) and its influence on laboratory animal research, *J. Inst. Anim. Tech.,* 29, 41, 1978.

73. **McBroom, J. M. and Weiss, A. K.,** A longitudinal and comparative study of the soft tissue calcium levels throughout the life span of highly inbred rats, *J. Gerontol.,* 28, 143, 1973.

74. **Jay, G. E., Jr.,** Genetic strains and stocks, in *Methodology in Mammalian Genetics,* Burdette, W. J., Ed., Holden-Day, Inc., San Francisco, 1963, 107.

75. *International Committee on Laboratory Animals, Terms and Definitions,* Bulletin, No. 14, ICLA, London, 1964.

76. **Solleveld, H. A.,** Types and quality of animals in cancer research, *Acta Zool. Pathol. Antverp.,* 72, 5, 1978.

77. **Lindsey, J. R., Conner, M. W., and Baker, H. J.,** Physical, chemical and microbial factors affecting biologic response, in *Laboratory Animal Housing,* Proc. Symp. Inst. Lab. Anim. Resources, National Academy of Sciences, Washington, D. C., 1978, 31.

78. **Jonas, A. M.,** Long-term holding of laboratory rodents, in *ILAR News,* 19, 4, 1976.

78a. **Lindsey, J. R.,** Personal Communication, University of Alabama, Birmingham.

79. **Young, L. and Chambers, T. R.,** A mouse bleeding technique yielding consistent volume with minimal hemolysis, *Lab. Anim. Sci.,* 23, 428, 1973.

80. **Parker, J. C., Tennant, R. W., Ward, T. G., and Rowe, W. P.,** Virus studies with germfree mice. I. Preparation of serologic reagents and survey of germfree and monocontaminated mice for indigenous murine viruses, *J. Natl. Cancer Inst.,* 34, 371, 1965.

81. **Riley, V.,** Adaptation of an orbital bleeding technique to rapid serial blood studies, *Proc. Soc. Exp. Biol. Med.,* 104, 751, 1960.

Chapter 2

MEASURING THE FUNCTIONAL ABILITIES OF STEM CELL LINES

David E. Harrison

TABLE OF CONTENTS

I.STEM CELLS

A. Cell Types Assayed

Stem cells in the immune and hemopoietic system form the precursor cell lines that can multiply to produce more of themselves and differentiate to form functional cell types. Unfortunately, in many publications, any precursor cell types for which assays were available have been referred to as stem cells. This practice fails to distinguish between cell types of widely proliferative and functional capacities. Ideally only the earliest precursor cell types that have the maximal ability to reproduce themselves should be referred to as stem cells. However, neither the earliest precursor cell types nor the maximal reproductive ability are easy to define in theory or in practice. It is possible that later cell types are not detectably different from their immediate precursors, having only slightly less ability to reproduce themselves and only slightly more tendency to differentiate further. Thus an immunohemopoietic differentiation pathway may approximate a continuum, and a cell type identified along that pathway is actually a range of cell types from the portion of the continuum in which cells meet the criteria used for identification.

B. Functional Measures

All commonly used assays for precursor cells measure hemopoietic cells, and none is specific for the earliest precursors. Of commonly used assays, the closest one to a genuine stem cell assay measures the number of macroscopically visible spleen colonies in lethally irradiated recipients.[1] Each colony is produced by a CFU-S (colony forming unit-spleen), a single cell capable of proliferating to produce 10^5 to 10^6 cells in 9 to 10 days[2,3] that produces one or more of the following cell types: erythrocytes, granulocytes, and megakarocytes.[4] Two later stages of erythropoietic cell precursors are measured in vitro as BFU-E (burst form unit - erythroid) and CFU-E (colony forming unit - erythroid). The BFU-E is the earlier precursor because it does not produce colonies until after 7 to 9 days in vitro of exposure to high levels of erythropoietin, and it forms colonies of several thousand cells; the CFU-E responds to 10 to 100 times lower levels of erythropoietin and produces much smaller colonies in 2 to 3 days.[5,6,7] Granulocytes are produced by the CFU-C (colony forming unit — culture), the first cell type reported to form colonies in vitro.[8,9] Figure 1 outlines the cell types detected by these assays placed in the general scheme of immunohemopoietic differentiation. This figure also includes competitive repopulation assays which will be discussed in more detail later. These are a new type of assays that may measure the functional ability of the earliest precursor cell lines, although they do not give numbers of stem cells. Such assays can be used to test precursors of specific lymphoid and hemopoietic cell types (Figure 1).

In many aging studies, the maximal functional abilities of stem cell lines must be determined. Therefore, the earliest precursor cell types are of primary interest, since they have maximal abilities to renew themselves and to produce differentiated descendants. Their capacities can only be rigorously tested in vivo, because no in vitro system is available that allows immunohemopoietic precursors to proliferate as rapidly or for as long periods as they do in vivo. This means that the animal model system chosen to test the stem cell lines is of primary importance in such experiments.

II. ANIMAL MODELS

A. Genetically Defined Animals

This discussion will be limited to the mouse because it is the most commonly used, convenient, and versatile animal[11-114] available for immunohematological experiments.

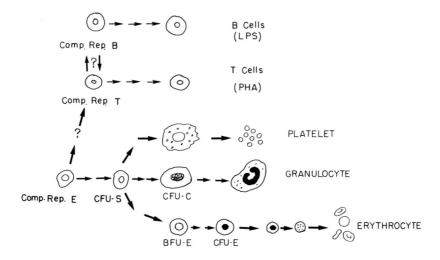

FIGURE 1.   Stem cell differentiation in the immunohemopoietic systems may begin with a single cell type, or several cell types, that multiply to replenish themselves and differentiate to populate the animal. The newly developed competitive repopulation (Comp. Rep.) assay was designed to measure the functional abilities of these earliest precursors. Comp. Rep. B, T, and E assays, respectively, test precursors of: B cells proliferating in response to lipopolysaccharide (LPS) in vitro, T cells proliferating in response to phytohemagglutinin (PHA) in vitro, and erythropoietic cells proliferating in response to severe bleeding in vivo. In these assays, chromosome markers are identified in mitotic cells following procedures detailed previously[10] and discussed later in this chapter (Table 1). Comp. Rep. E assays can also be performed using hemoglobin markers.[42]

Cells that form macroscopic colonies on spleens of irradiated mice (CFU-S) are the earliest precursors detectable as single cells; they differentiate to form platelets, granulocytes, and erythrocytes. Colony forming units in semisolid agar cultures (CFU-C) produce granulocytes. Burst forming units and colony forming units that respond to erythropoietin in vitro (BFU-E and CFU-E, respectively) are earlier and later precursor cells committed to form erythrocytes.

To avoid graft rejections and allogeneic or hybrid resistance, stem cell donors and recipients should have the same genotype, that is, they should be members of the same inbred strain or F_1 hybrids from crosses between the same two inbred strains. Inbred strains have been created by mating brother with sister, or younger parent with offspring, for a sufficient number of uninterrupted generations to produce mice homozygous at practically every locus.[11] At least 40 generations of brother - sister mating are required to achieve maximum homozygosity, and strains separated prior to that much inbreeding often show significant genetic differences, because all loci were not homozygous when separation occurred.[12]

The full strain and substrain designation must always be reported, because some substrains with similar names are known to have genetic differences.[12] For example, the CBA/J strain was separated from the CBA/HT6J and CBA/CaJ strains in 1932, after only 30 generations of inbreeding.[12] Both residual heterozygosity and mutation since 1932 account for the fact that CBA/J mice differ significantly from the other two strains, and rapidly reject their skin grafts. The CBA/CAJ and CBA/HT6J strains were separated in 1955 after more than 80 generations of inbreeding;[12] in 1975 they still accepted each other's skin.[13] Unfortunately, CBA/J mice are often mistakenly used as controls for CBA/HT6J mice that carry a useful cell marker, the T6 chromosome translocation. Mice of the CBA/CaJ strain, not the CBA/J strain, should be used as controls for CBA/HT6 mice.

A wide variety of mutations and genetic polymorphisms useful in immunohematology are available in lines congenic with an inbred strain. This means that such lines have essentially the same genotype as the inbred strain except for the particular genetic polymorphism. Ideally, mutations or translocations are studied segregating in the strain on which they originally occurred, but often they must be transferred by backcrossing to the genetic backgrounds of more pertinent inbred strains. To do this, mutants are bred to the animals of the desired strain for at least ten successive generations or backcrosses. Of course, genes closely linked to the mutation are also transferred into the selected strain background, but the numbers of foreign genes associated with the mutant allele decline with each backcross in proportion to how closely they are linked. After ten generations of backcrossing, the number of foreign genes is small, and for most purposes, the mutation may be considered a difference at a single locus in the new strain, forming a congenic line.

Genetic markers to distinguish donor and recipient cells unambiguously, are often necessary when the functional ability of stem cells is studied in vivo, yet donors and recipients should be of the same inbred strain to avoid graft versus host reactions and other complications. These requirements can be met by using congenic lines, differing essentially only by the genetic marker, to distinguish donor and recipient. Markers used in such experiments include: differences in hemoglobin type that may be analyzed by solubility[14,15] or quantitative electrophoresis;[15,16] The T6 chromosome translocation, developed as a hemopoietic cell marker by Ford,[17] and commonly used to identify dividing cells;[3,10,17,18] the W/W^v anemia, whose genetically defective stem cells cause the anemia, so that cure of the anemia both identifies and demonstrates the functional ability of normal stem cell lines;[16,19,20] granulocytes containing giant lysosomal granules in mice homozygous for mutant alleles at the beige locus;[19] and specific antigenic differences that can be analyzed by reactivity of antibodies against the specific antigen.[20,21] In some cases, cells from parental strain donors and F_1-hybrid recipients are quantitatively distinguished. However, care must be taken to avoid strain combinations in which parental type stem cells are affected by hybrid resistance.[22]

B. Animal Care

In addition to identifying the exact genotype, the animal models used should be maintained in a controlled environment. To the extent possible, the following factors should be optimized and should remain unchanged: food, water, caging, bedding, temperature, humidity, and the light cycle. Animals should not be stressed by overcrowding, fighting, noise, careless handling, or exposure to toxic substances. Perhaps most important, microorganisms that might interfere with experiments must be defined; if possible, they should be eliminated. Much general information on mouse care is provided by Green;[11] more recent information is found in recent ILAR reports,[23,24,25] and descriptions of pathogen control are provided by Simmons and Brice.[26]

Special care must be taken with aging animals because they often are more susceptible to environmental stress than are young or middle-aged individuals. Thus, effects that appear to be changes due specifically to age may actually be caused by environmental stress. This is especially true for pathogens, because old individuals tend to be more vulnerable to disease than young ones. A pathogen present in an animal colony may have no detectable effects on young animals, yet may cause gross effects on old animals that are mistakenly interpreted as effects of age. Even old animals maintained in an optimal environment have much higher incidences than young controls of noninfectious diseases, such as cancers and organ malfunctions. These diseases may affect the results of tests on an old animal, yet the apparent change with age is not a direct result of aging, but of the disease, the incidence of which increases with age. For this reason all old individuals should be grossly autopsied, and if possible, histopathological studies should be made. Tissues from old individuals should never be pooled, because different old mice may have different types of defects causing opposing effects. For example, spleen cells from different old individuals were mixed with young spleen cells; the mixture showed all three possible results from the interactions of old and young cells in immune responses: above, below, or the same as the responses calculated from the sum of individual old and young cell responses.[27]

III. DETAILS OF STEM CELL ASSAYS

A. Intravenous (i.v.) Injections

Although large numbers of cells may be injected intraperitoneally into a mouse, most of these fail to function normally in the CFU-S assay, producing only 0.002 times the number of macroscopic spleen colonies per injected marrow cell that would have been observed after i.v. injection.[28] To inject mice conveniently i.v., they are warmed slightly. This causes increased circulation in the lateral tail veins, used by the mice for cooling. A short (3/8 in) 26 g or smaller needle is carefully inserted in the tail vein, and the cells are injected smoothly during 2 to 10 seconds. As much as 0.5 to 1.0 mℓ of suspension may usually be injected without harming a mouse. However, it is essential that the suspension contain no clumps of cells or stroma. These may be removed from marrow or fetal liver cell suspensions by filtering the cell suspensions through 100-200 mesh nylon cloth. In our experience, spleen cell suspensions must be washed by centrifugation and resuspension two to four times before being filtered.

To prepare cell suspensions, spleens or fetal livers are disrupted gently with glass homogenizers. Marrow is vigorously washed out of dissected femors and tibias by cutting off the ends and flushing rapidly with at least 2 mℓ of media through a 22- to 23-g needle. We used CMRL 1066 medium in early experiments, but found equally good CFU-S preservation using a HEPES buffered-salt solution at a pH of 7.4.[10] If the suspended cells are cooled on ice, they may be held for several hours before they are injected into recipients. A portion of the suspension is counted, for example, by an electronic cell counter, and if necessary, the suspensions are diluted so that convenient amounts provide the correct number of cells per innoculum. Recipients are usually lethally irradiated 1 to 24 hr before cells are injected. We have stopped using dye - exclusion techniques to assess percentages of dead cells, because less than one in 10,000 marrow cells is a stem cell, and the survival of the stem cells may not be related to overall percentages of cells that survive.

B. Serial Transplantation

In many experiments, stem cell lines from individual donors are passed on to one or more successive recipients. Marrow cells are suspended and transplanted, as previously described, from each successive donor. Spleen cells have less lifesparing capacity per CFU-S[29] and appear therefore not to contain such early precursor cells as marrow; circulating blood cells contain CFU-S with extremely deficient capacities to repopulate irradiated recipients.[30] If the earliest precursor cells available in adults are desired, it is more reliable to use marrow cells.

All stem cells in recipients should be removed by lethal irradiation, or, even better, recipients with geneticlly defective stem cells may be used.[16,19,20,28] Lethal irradiation is usually provided by high-energy X-rays (produced, for example, by 250 kVp at 20 Ma using 1 mm each of lead and copper filtration or by gamma irradiation from Cs-137 or Co-60 irradiators). The maximum amount of irradiation that recipients of stem cell lines can survive should be used to minimize regeneration of recipient cells; this amount usually ranges between about 700 and 1200 R. The higher levels of irradiation may be required with Cs-137 irradiators and large, healthy mice. Nevertheless, regeneration of stem cells may occur; it is necessary to use genetic markers to identify stem cell lines from the original donor unambiguously.[28] The functional abilities of stem cell lines appear to decline with each successive serial transplantation.[10,18,28,31] This effect makes it likely that regenerating recipient cells will replace donor cells after several serial transfers, and makes the use of genetic markers to identify donor cells imperative in such experiments.[18,28,31]

Marrow cell grafts from aging donors may contain partially transformed cancer cells, even when donors are used that show no gross or micropathologic sign of cancer. This probably explains why all recipients of stem cell lines from certain old C57BL/6J donors died within a few weeks of each other with similar cancer-like lesions, even after as long as 15 to 18 months and as many as two serial transplantations.[31,32] In our experiments, such results have been most commonly observed when the old donors were of genotypes in which such cancers often appeared late in life. The types of cancers common to aging mice should be determined when characterizing the donor strains used.

C. CFU-S

The cells forming macroscopic colonies in spleens of lethally irradiated recipients are the earliest precursors that can be assayed as single cells, and often are considered stem cells.[28,32A] For each recipient, 5 to 10×10^4 marrow cells should be used, because this is the number of i.v.-injected cells that produces 5 to 15 macroscopic colonies per spleen. Larger numbers of injected cells appear to contain a lower concentration of CFU-S, probably because colonies become confluent and difficult to count, and possibly also because higher cell doses cause recipients to recover faster, so that there is less stimulus for colony growth. If donors and recipients of different genotypes are used, there may be reductions in colony numbers due to allogenic and F_1-hybrid resistance.[22] Cell markers are not usually necessary in these short-term (8- to 12-day) experiments; however, the numbers of colonies in irradiated control recipients that received the cell suspending medium should be determined. If sufficient irradiation was used, their numbers should be insignificant (less than 0.1 to 0.2). If they are significant but low (less than 1 to 2) they should be subtracted from the numbers of colonies in experimental groups. If an average of more than one to two colonies is found, the experiment should be repeated using recipients of higher doses of irradiation.

Colonies vary greatly in size, and attempts have been made to estimate numbers of cells per colony.[10,33] Unfortunately, such experiments are tedious, and the examples cited produced conflicting results. Spleens of lethally irradiated recipients may be sectioned and microscopic colonies scored;[34] much additional information can thus be made available about colony types, if sufficient time and skill is available.[35]

Because enumerating macroscopic bumps on a spleen is so easy, this technique is usually employed, although it oversimplifies by not accounting for colony size or type. Whether a CFU-S produces erythrocytes, granulocytes, or megakaryocytes may be regulated by the microenvironment in which it grows.[3] The size of a colony is affected by external stimuli such as the bearer's hematocrit and by how many serial transplantations the cell line has undergone.[10]

When marrow cells are injected into a lethally irradiated recipient, only about 17% of the CFU-S implant or seed in the spleen, as determined by retransplantation experiments a few hours after the cells are injected.[36] The seeding efficiency in the spleen may change in certain experimental treatments; therefore it is wise to be sure that the fraction of CFU-S actually forming spleen colonies remains constant. It is possible that only 8% of injected CFU-S remain in the spleen after 24 hr for example.[36A]

Recently techniques have been reported for growing CFU-S in vitro for as long as several months. An adherent cell layer was formed by an initial marrow culture, then a second marrow culture was introduced, and unattached CFU-S were harvested when the culture medium was changed.[37] Numbers of CFU-S produced varied widely among cultures, and dependable production of several times the numbers of CFU-S used to produce the cultures was not demonstrated. No measures of long-term function, such as lifesparing or repopulating abilities, have been reported using CFU-S produced in vitro.

Although CFU-S assays are commonly considered to measure function of stem cells, they are not specific for the earliest stem cells with the maximum proliferative capacities. Instead, every cell capable of forming a macroscopic colony is scored as a CFU-S, regardless of how much proliferative capacity remains after the colony has been produced. Early workers showed that the number of CFU-S per colony varied greatly;[36] probably the colonies containing the most CFU-S were formed by the earliest precursors. Measurements of CFU-S numbers sometimes fail to correlate with long-term functional capacities. This might be expected, because colony numbers are measured after only a short time (8 to 10 days) and because neither the cell types produced by the spleen colonies nor their remaining proliferative ability is assessed.

When long-term stem cell functions are measured by the ability to maintain the lives of lethally irradiated recipients, or to repopulate them, these measurements do not correlate with CFU-S numbers in certain systems. For example, numbers of CFU-S grossly underestimate life sparing ability when they are reduced by hybrid resistance[38] or by the W/W^v genetic anemia.[39] The life-sparing capacity associated with a given number of CFU-S from spleen is about one third that of the same number of CFU-S from marrow.[29] When equal numbers of CFU-S from circulating blood and marrow are mixed in irradiated recipients, after three weeks essentially all the proliferating cells have the karyotype of the marrow donor.[30] In similar experiments, fetal liver cells eventually almost completely repopulate irradiated recipients, even when mixed with numbers of adult marrow cells that contain five to ten times as many CFU-S.[40] A single serial transplantation reduces CFU-S numbers very little, but the ability to repopulate irradiated recipients with precursors of erythropoietic and immune competent cells is only one half to one fifth that of untransplanted marrow cells.[10]

D. Life-Sparing Ability

The simplest assay for long-term function of stem cell lines takes advantage of the fact that lethally irradiated animals will die in 8 to 15 days unless they are repopulated by grafted stem cells. The recipients used to measure life-sparing ability must be of a constant age and genotype, and must be maintained in a constant environment, because these factors affect the sensitivity to irradiation. The amount of irradiation required for a lethal dose varies significantly with genotype, and increases with age until the mice are fully grown (usually 5 to 15 months of age, depending on genotype and conditions). It often decreases greatly if a pathogen is introduced, and may decrease in warm, humid weather if the animal's environment is not controlled.

To measure the life-sparing ability of a stem cell population, varying doses are i.v. injected into lethally irradiated recipients. The recipients are examined every day from 5 to 20 days after the irradiation and marrow injection, and less often thereafter. For example, using adult marrow cells of one type, five to ten doses over the range of 2×10^4 to 5×10^5 cells are injected i.v. into at least five to ten recipients for each dose. Controls given no cells are always used to be sure that the irradiation was lethal. In long-term experiments with pigmented animals, a greying of the fur after several months is caused by the loss of irradiated melanoblasts and demonstrates that the individual had been irradiated.

Unfortunately these techniques do not readily provide quantitative data about stem cell function. Although the endpoint, death, is clear-cut, the exact cause of death is not. It is necessary to use 25 to 50 mice for each marrow type tested in each experiment, and experiments should be repeated several times to make quantitative comparisons of life-sparing abilities. When recipients live for more than 2 weeks, it is possible that their regenerated cells are maintaining some of their functions. This possibility can only be eliminated by quantitative experiments using cell markers, and if these are available, I recommend that the easier and more accurate competitive repopulation procedures should be used rather than life-sparing assays.

E. Competitive Repopulation

Measurements of stem cell functional ability by competitive repopulation were first made by Ford,[17] who injected irradiated recipients with mixtures of cells from two donors with distinguishable chromosome markers; the repopulating ability of cells from one donor was proportional to the percentage of cells of that donor's type growing in the recipient. In such experiments, fetal liver cells repopulated much better,[40] and circulating nucleated cells much less successfully,[30] when mixed with marrow cells, than would be expected from the numbers of CFU-S observed in these tissues. Cells from the first old donor tested repopulated less well than young cells,[41] but marrow from the second old donor had better repopulating ability than that of the young cells with which it was mixed.[18]

It is likely that the functional ability of the earliest stem cells is rigorously tested in repopulating lethally irradiated recipients, because the grafts are subjected to maximal stimuli in vivo, both to proliferate and to differentiate. Furthermore, the grafted cell lines continue to function throughout the recipients' lives and even may be serially transplanted to test long-term function.[18,41] However, these experiments have two defects: (1) cells from the two donors or pools that are mixed are only compared relative to each other and (2) chromosomes are scored in mitotic cells, and histological types are not easily identified in dividing cells prepared for chromosome identification. Therefore, the types of differentiated cells that are being produced remain unknown.

These defects have been partially alleviated in subsequent experiments. To compare many different stem cell donors, identical preparations from each of them must compete with cells from a standard pool of competitors, C. Suspensions containing constant numbers of marrow cells from each donor are mixed with identical portions from pool C. These mixtures are transplanted into lethally irradiated recipients. The relative repopulating and proliferative abilities of each donor's cells are determined by measuring how completely they repopulate the recipients in competition with the same type C cells. An example of such an experiment[10] is outlined in Table 1.

Stem cell lines that produce a particular type of differentiated cell can be assessed using differentiated cell markers characteristic of, or specific stimuli acting on, that cell type. For example, erythropoietic stem cells can be assessed using hemoglobin markers.[42] When chromosome markers are used to identify descendents of stem cells, stimuli causing specific cell types to proliferate may be used to produce mitosis of those cell types; for example, severe bleeding in vivo stimulates erythropoietic cells, and phytohemagglutinin (PHA) or lipopolysaccharide (LPS) in vitro stimulates specific T and B cell populations respectively (Figure 1). Chromosome markers were used to identify cells stimulated by bleeding and PHA in the example[10] outlined in Table 1. There was a significant amount of variability between recipients of identical cell mix-

Table 1
A MITOTIC COMPETITION EXPERIMENT

Genotype	Marker	Use in experiment
CBA/HT6J	2 T6 Chromosomes	Donor type: Individual old or young donor cell lines, transplanted for the first or second time. Call D_1, D_2,...D_i,...D_n.
(CBA/HT6Jx CBA/CaJ) F_1	1 T6 Chromosome	Competitor type: pooled young cells transplanted for the first time. Call C.
CBA/CaJ	None	Recipient type: lethally irradiated.

Note: Procedure: 1. Mix 3×10^6 marrow cells from each Donor D_i with 3×10^6 marrow cells from pool C. 2. Inject mixtures i.v. into recipients. 3. Determine the percentages of mitotic cells having 0, 1, or 2 T6 chromosome translocations after bleeding in vivo or PHA in vitro.

After Harrison, D. E., Astle, C. M., and DeLaittre, J. A., *J. Exp. Med.,* 147, 1526, 1978.

tures in these experiments, therefore, at least five recipients should be scored using identical mixtures (Di + C) from each donor Di in Table 1.

When chromosome markers are used, all mitotic cells are scored. These may include significant numbers of mitoses from cells proliferating independently from the specific stimuli. Using stimulation in vitro, several cultures can be prepared from the same recipient cells, and those stimulated by the specific mitogen used can be compared with those not stimulated. If both the percentages of mitotic cells and the percentages having each chromosome marker are determined, corrections can be made for nonspecifically proliferating cells. This correction is not possible in vivo; therefore, the quantitative measurement of differing hemoglobin types[42] is more specific for erythropoietic precursor cells than is stimulation by bleeding.

Using hemoglobin markers in recent experiments, the decline in repopulating ability of erythropoietic precursor cell lines after a single transplantation appeared to be much greater[43] than that shown using chromosome markers after stimulation by bleeding.[10] Probably nonerythropoietic cell lines that proliferate nonspecifically in the marrow were much less affected by transplantation than were erythropoietic stem cell lines. However, it is also possible that transplanted stem cells produced erythrocytes with a shorter lifetime in the circulation, causing decreased representation of their hemoglobin types.

If many experiments are to be compared, it is essential that cells used as competitors (C) be from identical donors in each experiment. Even better would be a very large pool of donor type cells frozen in liquid nitrogen in many identical portions that could be used to directly compare the competitor pools used in the different experiments.

Competitive repopulation assays do not measure the number of stem cells, but compare the functional abilities of the samples tested. This may be all that is possible in practical functional tests, if precursor cells form a continuum from early to late types with decreasing capacities for self-renewal, and increasing probability of differentiation and faster proliferation,[44] so that measurements of precursor cell numbers would be misleading without also knowing their place along the continuum.

IV. STEM CELLS: AGING AND TRANSPLANTATION

A. Limitations in Functional Capacity

A fundamental question about stem cell lines is whether their functional capacities are unlimited. This question has not yet been definitively answered. Evidence that they are unlimited comes from studies demonstrating that stem cell lines from old and young donors have similar functional capacities (recently reviewed[28]). If only an insignificant amount of functional capacity is lost after a lifetime of normal functioning, it is unlimited for most practical purposes.[28,32A] However, evidence from studies in which functional capacities declined when stem cells were serially transplanted or forced to recover from irradiation or from drug-induced damage, suggests that functional capacities are limited.[10,28,32A,44,45] It is widely believed that stem cells have a limited proliferative capacity, but exhaust insignificant amounts of it during a lifetime of normal function, because of their numbers and the mechanisms by which they proliferate in vivo.[28,32A,44,45] However, the evidence for this possibility is not so overwhelming that it should be accepted as true without further verification.[28] It is also possible that the procedures of transplantation or poisoning by irradiation and drugs, damage the earliest stem cell lines and cause functional declines.

In preliminary studies, the decline in repopulating ability caused by a single serial transplantation was not changed by transplanting 10^5 cells instead of 10^7 or by joining the intact donor and irradiated recipient in a parabiosis and allowing stem cells to populate the recipient through their connected circulatory systems during 4 months.[46] Furthermore, a similar decline was caused by sublethal irradiation.[46] Apparently, the deleterious effects of procedures that transfer or stress the stem cells may be similar over a 100 - fold range of cell numbers transplanted, at least if several months are allowed for the transplanted cells to repopulate the recipient. Thus the simple explanation that proliferative capacity is exhausted by the proliferation required to repopulate the irradiated recipient may be inadequate.

B. Causes of Their Decline

Possibly the earliest stem cells present in adults do have unlimited functional and proliferative capacities, however, the stimulus to differentiate into precursor cell lines committed to produce particular cell types is so strong in irradiated, drug-treated or W-anemic mice, that essentially all the stem cells are forced to differentiate. They may form committed precursor cell lines capable of producing differentiated cells over several years of normal functioning, but eventually such lines would be exhausted.[31,32] Furthermore, the earliest stem cells appear incapable of passing into the circulation, otherwise they would have been transplanted by parabiosis. A set of accurate kinetic models for such differentiation cannot be constructed without knowing how rapidly stem cells and committed precursor cells at various stages of differentiation proliferate, and how this is affected by the various natural stimuli, feedback, or by stimuli introduced in experimental manipulations. Although it is complex, hemopoietic cell differentiation is one of the best defined and most easily studied systems of mammalian cell differentiation (Figure 1); experiments to address these questions can be designed.[5,10,18,28,32A,42,44,45] The possibility of well-defined experiments makes this system a useful one to use for testing theories of cell differentiation and aging.

C. An Immunohemopoietic Stem Cell

Whether the same stem cell can produce differentiated progeny that populate and function normally in both the immune and the hemopoietic systems is not known, although the bulk of evidence now suggests that it can.[47,48] This evidence is not completely convincing because often in collecting it, cells were identified in lymphoid tissues using markers that had been induced by irradiation. Such irradiated cells with abnormal karyotypes may have been transformed and therefore may have populated tissues where they otherwise would not have been found.[48] In other cases, allogeneic or xenogeneic transplantation systems were used that may have stimulated lymphoid cell growth by graft versus host reactions.[47] Therefore, it remains possible that some parts of the immune system are populated by stem cell lines independent of those that can populate the hemopoietic system. In this case, all types of immunohemopoietic stem cells would not be represented by the easily testable hemopoietic precursor cell types. The question of whether lymphoid stem cell lines are intrinsically changed with age is not settled.[10,28,33,49] It has enormous practical importance in designing therapies to alleviate the effects of declining immune responses in aging individuals.[49]

Studies of hemopoietic cells have figured prominently in this review because much information is available on them, not because they should be studied to the exclusion of lymphoid stem cells. More originality will be required to study the latter, but they may prove particularly interesting. Clones of cells already differentiated to produce a particular antibody had enormous proliferative capacity, passing through 7 serial transplantations and an estimated 90 doublings.[50] It will be interesting to learn how much proliferative capacity their precursor cells have, and to define how they are related to hemopoietic precursor cells.

REFERENCES

1. **Till, J. E. and McCulloch, E. A.,** A direct measure of the radiation sensitivity of normal mouse marrow cells, *Radiat. Res.,* 14, 213, 1961.
2. **Becker, A. J., McCulloch, E. A., and Till, J. E.,** Cytological demonstration of the clonal nature of spleen colonies derived from transplanted mouse marrow cells, *Nature (London),* 197, 452, 1963.
3. **Trentin, J. J.,** Determination of bone marrow stem cell differentiation by stromal hemopoietic inductive microenvironments (HIM), *Am. J. Pathol.,* 65, 621, 1971.
4. **Wu, A. M., Till, J. E., Siminovitch, L., and McCulloch, E. A.,** A cytological study of the capacity for differentiation of normal hemopoietic colony-forming cells, *J. Cell Physiol.,* 69, 177, 1967.
5. **Gregory, C. J. and Eaves, A. C.,** Three stages of erythropoietic progenitor cell differentiation distinguished by a number of physical and biological properties, *Blood,* 51, 527, 1978.
6. **Chui, D. H. K., Liao, S. K., and Walker, K.,** Fetal erythropoiesis in steel mutant mice. III. Defect in differentiation from BFU-E to CFU-E during early development, *Blood,* 51, 539, 1978.
7. **Adamson, J. W. and Brown, J. E.,** Aspects of erythroid differentiation and proliferation, in *Molecular Control of Proliferation and Differentiation,* Papaconstantinou, J. and Rutter, W. J., Eds., 35th Symp. Soc. Devel. Biol., Academic Press, New York, 1978, 161.
8. **Metcalf, D., Bradley, T. R., and Robinson, W.,** Analysis of colonies developing in vitro from mouse bone marrow cells stimulated by kidney feeder layers or leukemic serum, *J. Cell. Physiol.,* 69, 93, 1967.
9. **Metcalf, D. and Moore, M. A.,** *Haemopoietic Cells. Their Origin, Migration and Differentiation,* North-Holland, New York, 1971.
10. **Harrison, D. E., Astle, C. M., and DeLaittre, J. A.,** Loss of proliferative capacity in immunohemopoietic stem cells caused by serial transplantation rather than aging, *J. Exp. Med.,* 147, 1526, 1978.
11. **Green, E. L.,** *The Biology of the Laboratory Mouse,* 2nd ed., McGraw-Hill, New York, 1966.
11A. **Harrison, D. E.,** Use of genetic anemias in mice as tools for hematological research, in *Cellular Dynamics of Haemopoiesis,* Lajtha, L. J., Ed., *Clinics in Haematology,* Vol. 8, W. B. Saunders, London, 1979, 239.

12. **Bailey, D. W.,** Sources of subline divergence: relative importance for the sublines of six major inbred strains of mice, in *The Origin of Inbred Strains,* Morse, H. C., II, Ed., Academic Press, New York, 1978, 197.

13. **Harrison, D. E. and Cherry, C.,** Unpublished data, 1975.

14. **Popp, R. A.,** Competence of retransplanted homologous marrow cells in relation to time after original transplantation into irradiated mice, *Int. J. Radiat. Biol.,* 4, 155, 1961.

15. **Russell, E. S. and McFarland, E. C.,** Genetics of mouse hemoglobin, *Ann. N. Y. Acad. Sci.,* 241, 25, 1974.

16. **Harrison, D. E.,** Normal production of erythrocytes by mouse marrow continuous for 73 months, *Proc. Nat. Acad. Sci. U.S.A.,* 70, 3184, 1973.

17. **Ford, C. E.,** The use of chromosome markers, in *Tissue Grafting and Radiation,* Micklem, H. S. and Loutit, J. F., Eds., Academic Press, New York, 1966, 197.

18. **Ogden, D. A. and Micklem, H. S.,** The fate of serially transplanted bone marrow cell populations from young and old donors, *Transplantation,* 22, 287, 1976.

19. **Murphy, E. D., Harrison, D. E., and Roths, J. B.,** Giant granules of beige mice, *Transplantation,* 15, 526, 1973.

20. **Harrison, D. E. and Cherry, M.,** Survival of marrow allografts in *W/ W* anemic mice: effect of disparity at the Ea-2 locus, *Immunogenetics,* 2, 219, 1976.

21. **Van Bekkum, D. W. and Weyzen, W. W. H.,** Serial transfer of isologous and homologous hematopoietic cells in irradiated host, *Pathol. Biol.,* 9, 888, 1967.

22. **Cudkowicz, G. and Bennett, M.,** Peculiar immunology of bone marrow allografts, *J. Exp. Med.,* 134, 1513, 1971.

23. **Newberne, P. M.,** (Committee Chairman), Control of diets in laboratory animal experimentation, *ILAR News Report,* National Academy of Science, Washington, D. C., 1978.

24. **Jones, A. M.,** (Committee Chairman), Long-term holding of laboratory rodents, *ILAR News* XIX:L1-L25, National Academy of Sciences, Washington, D. C., 1978.

25. **Lang, C. M.,** (Committee Chairman), Laboratory animal management: rodents, *ILAR News,* XX (3):L1-L15, National Academy of Sciences, Washington, D. C., 1977.

26. **Simmons, M. L. and Brick, J. O.,** *The Laboratory Mouse. Selection and Management,* Prentice-Hall, Englewood Cliffs, N. J., 1970.

27. **Makinodan, T., Albright, J. W., Good, P. I., Peter, C. P., and Heidrick, M. L.,** Reduced humoral immune activity in long-lived old mice: an approach to elucidating its mechanism, *Immunology,* 31, 903, 1976.

28. **Harrison, D. E.,** Proliferative capacity of erythropoietic stem cell lines and aging: an overview, *Mech. Ageing Dev.,* 9, 409, 1979.

29. **Kretchmar, A. L. and Conover, W. R.,** A difference between spleen-derived and bone marrow derived colony-forming units in ability to protect lethally irradiated mice, *Blood,* 36, 772, 1970.

30. **Micklem, H. S., Anderson, N., and Ross, E.,** Limited potential of circulating haemopoietic stem cells, *Nature (London),* 256, 41, 1975.

31. **Harrison, D. E.,** Mouse erythropoietic stem cell lines function normally 100 months: loss related to number of transplantations, *Mech. Ageing Dev.,* 9, 427, 1979.

32. **Harrison, D. E.,** Normal function of transplanted marrow cell lines from aged mice, *J. Gerontol.,* 30, 279, 1975.

32A. **Schofield, R.,** The pluripotent stem cell, in *Cellular Dynamics of Haemopoiesis, Clinics in Haematology,* Vol. 8, Lajtha, L. J., Ed., W. B. Saunders, London, 1979, 221.

33. **Albright, J. W. and Makinodan, T.,** Decline in the growth potential of spleen-colonizing bone marrow stem cells of long-lived aging mice, *J. Exp. Med.,* 144, 1204, 1976.

34. **Davis, M. L., Upton, A. C., and Satterfield, L. C.,** Growth and senescence of the bone marrow stem cell pool in RFM/Un mice, *Proc. Soc. Exp. Biol. Med.,* 137, 1453, 1971.

35. **Lewis, J. P., O'Grady, L. F., Bernstein, S. E., Russell, E. S., and Trobough, F.,** Growth and differentiation of *W/ W* marrow, *Blood,* 601, 1967.

36. **Siminovitch, L., McCulloch, E. H., and Till, J. E.,** The distribution of colony-forming cells among spleen colonies, *J. Cell. Comp. Physiol.,* 62, 327, 1963.

36A. **Playfair, J. H. L. and Cole, L. J.,** Quantitative studies on colony-forming units in isogenic radiation chimeras, *J. Cell. Comp. Physiol.,* 65, 7, 1965.

37. **Dexter, T. M., Allen, T. D., and Lajtha, L. G.,** Conditions controlling the proliferation of haemopoietic stem cells in vitro, *J. Cell. Physiol.,* 91, 335, 1977.

38. **McCulloch, E. A. and Till, J. E.,** Repression of colony-forming ability of C57BL hematopoietic cells transplanted into non-isologous hosts, *J. Cell. Comp. Physiol.,* 61, 301, 1963.

39. **Harrison, D. E.,** Lifesparing ability (in lethally irradiated mice) of *W/ W* mouse marrow with no macroscopic colonies, *Radiat. Res.,* 52, 553, 1972.

40. **Micklem, H. S., Ford, C. E., Evans, E. P., Ogden, D. A., and Papworth, D. S.,** Competitive in vivo proliferative of foetal and adult haematopoietic cells in lethally irradiated mice, *J. Cell. Physiol.,* 79, 293, 1972.

41. **Micklem, H. S., Ogden, D. A., and Payne, A. C.,** Aging, Haemopoietic stem cells and immunity, in *Haemopoietic Stem Cells,* Vol. 13, Ciba Found. Symp., Solstenholme, G. E. W. and O'Conner, M., Eds., Elsevier/North-Holland, Amsterdam 1973, 285.

42. **Harrison, D. E.,** Competitive repopulation: a new assay for long-term stem cell functional capacity, *Blood,* 55, 77, 1980.

43. **Harrison, D. E.,** Unpublished data, 1979.

44. **Hellman, S., Botnick, L. E., Hannon, E. C., and Vigneullel, R. M.,** Proliferative capacity of murine hematopoietic stem cells, *Proc. Natl. Acad. Sci., U.S.A.,* 75, 490, 1978.

45. **Reincke, U. Brookoff, D., Burlington, H., Cronkite, E. P., Pappas, N., and Zanjani, E.,** Susceptibility of hematopoietic stem cells (CFU-S) to ^{55}Fe radiation damage, *Radiat. Res.,* 74, 66, 1978.

46. **Harrison, D. E.,** Immunopoietic stem cell lines: effects of aging and transplantation, *Proceedings of 1979 NIH Conference on Immunological Aspects of Aging,* Segre, D., Ed., in press, 1980.

47. **Nowell, P. C., Hirsch, B. E., Fox, D. E., and Wilson, D. B.,** Evidence for the existence of multipotential lympho-hematopoietic stem cells in the adult rat, *J. Cell. Physiol.,* 75, 151, 1970.

48. **Abramson, S., Miller, R. G., and Philipps, R. A.,** The identification in adult bone marrow of pluripotent and restricted stem cells of the myeloid and lymphoid systems, *J. Exp. Med.,* 145, 1567, 1977.

49. **Makinodan, T.,** Mechanism, prevention, and restoration of immunologic aging, in Birth Defects: Original Article Series Vol. XIV, 197, 1978.

50. **Williamson, A. R. and Askonas, B. A.,** Senesence of an antibody-forming cell clone, *Nature (London),* 238, 1972.

Chapter 3

THYMUS DEPENDENT IMMUNE COMPETENCE AND AGING

Ada M. Kruisbeek

TABLE OF CONTENTS

I. INTRODUCTION — GENERAL REMARKS

A considerable amount of data seems to indicate a causal relationship between the age-related decline in normal immune functions and predisposition for several diseases. (For a recent review, see Reference 1.) Hence, retardation, reversal, or prevention of immunosenescence could perhaps delay the onset and/or minimize the severity of certain diseases of the elderly. However, a proper understanding of the basic mechanism(s) responsible for immunosenescence is lacking. Many studies on aging have revealed that the most striking changes occur in the functions of thymus-dependent lymphocytes (T cells) (reviewed in References 1 and 2), but the causes of such changes remain unclear.

Before any attempt is made to intervene with deficiencies in T-cell function, more detailed information will be required on how normal thymus-dependent immune competence is achieved and maintained. Since the thymus is necessary for the maturation of precursor cells into various types of T cells, it appears that the process(es) influencing involution of the thymus may be "the key to aging of the immune system," as suggested by Makinodan.[1] Although the mechanism(s) by which the thymus affects T-cell differentiation processes are still not fully understood, there seems to be sufficient evidence to assume that thymic humoral factors are required for T-cell maturation (reviewed in References 3 to 5). As soon as the thymus begins to show involution with age, the level of serum thymic factor(s) decreases in both mice[6,7] and man[7-9]. One might postulate that this could lead to a deficiency in T-cell functions. However, possible therapeutic application of thymic hormones to compensate for such deficiencies is still unwarranted, since only marginal in vivo effects have been reported in experimental animals up to now. Another complicating situation is that several factors have been described,[3-5] and it is unknown whether different steps of the T-cell differentiation pathway (a putative model is schematically shown in Figure 1) are controlled by different thymic factors. Furthermore, it seems highly unlikely that, in a complex differentiation pattern such as that shown in Figure 1, the only age-related abnormality would be a deficit in thymic factor production. Thus, in studies concerned with causes of age-related defects in T-cell immunocompetence, it is essential not only to place emphasis on more fundamental studies of the humoral function of the thymus, but also on studies of the T-cell differentiation pathway. Obviously, further knowledge of the normal T-cell differentiation process will also yield information concerning the theoretically possible defects in this process and thus provide a better rationale for studies on the causes of age-related defects in cellular immune functions. Therefore, a major part of this review will be devoted to current views on T-cell differentiation and on the possible effects of aging on several steps of the proposed scheme of the T-cell differentiation pathway (Figure 1).

II. T CELL UNDER NORMAL CONDITIONS AND IN AGING

In order to better understand the causes of the age-related decrease in T-cell functions[10-15] (or, in fact, of any presumably thymus-related immune deficiency), the following questions must be answered:

1.   Are precursor T cells which still have to undergo various differentiation steps present in normal numbers?
2.   Are thymic factors which induce this differentiation process present in normal concentrations?

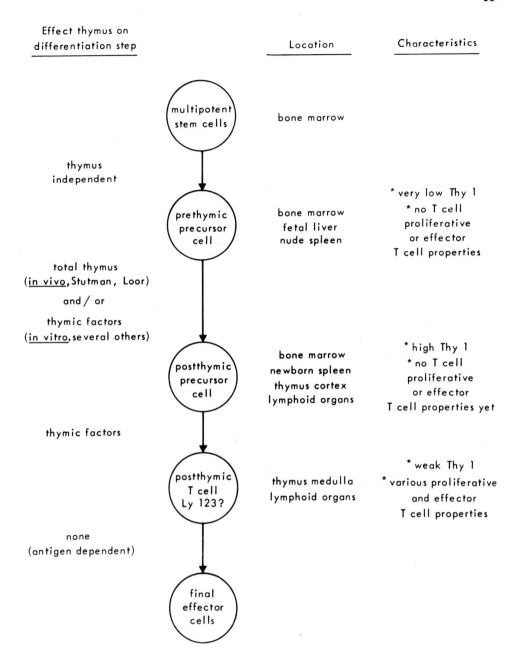

Effect thymus on
differentiation step

Location

Characteristics

multipotent
stem cells

bone marrow

thymus
independent

prethymic
precursor
cell

bone marrow
fetal liver
nude spleen

* very low Thy 1
* no T cell
proliferative
or effector
T cell properties

total thymus
(in vivo, Stutman, Loor)

and / or

thymic factors
(in vitro, several others)

postthymic
precursor
cell

bone marrow
newborn spleen
thymus cortex
lymphoid organs

* high Thy 1
* no T cell
proliferative
or effector
T cell properties yet

thymic factors

postthymic
T cell
Ly 123?

thymus medulla
lymphoid organs

* weak Thy 1
* various proliferative
and effector
T cell properties

none
(antigen dependent)

final
effector
cells

FIGURE 1.   Model for the T-cell-differentiation pathway.

3.   Are T cells (as recognized by typical membrane antigens) present in normal num-
     bers in the peripheral lymphoid organs?
4.   Can these cells proliferate upon stimulation with well-defined T-cell activators?
5.   Can these activated cells proceed to terminal differentiation into effector cells
     (T-helper, T-suppressor, and T-killer function)?

Possible approaches to answer the first two questions, and the findings reported so
far, will be dealt with separately in more detail in Sections A and B. Answers to questions three to five, i.e., "What is the effect of aging on T cell numbers, proliferative
capacity, and function?" will be summarized in Section C.

Because most of our knowledge on T-cell differentiation and its possible age-related aberrations has been obtained through studies in mice, this review is mostly concentrated on studies in those animals. Possible changes in other features of T cells such as humoral T-cell-derived products, tolerance, memory, and genetic restriction will not be discussed, as these phenomena have not been investigated in detail in aging mice.

A. Availability of Precursor T Cells

The development of T cells can be considered as taking place in two steps: 1. differentiation of immigrant stem cells (in the adult, mainly present in the bone marrow but also in the spleen)[16,17] into immature thymocytes within the thymus; and 2. the subsequent progress from immature thymocytes to immunocompetent T cells, either in or outside the thymus.[18]

1. Precursor T Cells in the Bone Marrow and the Spleen

One of the possible causes for the age-related decrease in T-cell functions could be a deficiency in bone marrow progenitors of T cells. A few investigators have found that, given sufficient time (3 to 10 months), marrow from old donors can restore immune functions in young irradiated recipients.[19,20] Approaching the problem from the other direction, it was found[20,21] that the poor response of old, sublethally irradiated mice to SRBC (sheep red blood cells) could not be restored by marrow grafts from young recipients. Both types of studies seem to indicate that availability of T-lymphocyte progenitor cells is not the only limiting factor in aging mice. In the reconstitution attempts in old mice, the old recipient's thymus might have prevented young bone marrow from further differentiation. When a young marrow graft was combined with a young thymus graft,[21] the low response of sublethally irradiated old mice to SRBC and T-cell mitogens could be elevated.

Recently, a different picture of precursor T cells in the bone marrow has emerged from the studies of Tyan,[22,23] who found that the capacity of bone marrow from old donors to repopulate thymuses in young irradiated mice is strongly reduced. In those experiments, there was a much shorter observation period (i.e., 21 days) than used by others,[19,20] and the defects could be attributed to both an absolute decrease in the number of progenitor T cells and a diminished proliferative capacity in part of these cells.

The degree of repopulation of thymuses from young irradiated mice was also dependent on the age of the donor when spleen cells were injected.[24] The relative precursor cell content of the spleen sharply decreases during the early postpartum period and reaches exceedingly low levels in 42-week-old mice.[24]

2. Precursor T Cells in the Thymus and Lymphoid Organs

The thymus also contains precursor T cells. These cells are considered to be more differentiated than the precursors found in bone marrow, since they have acquired the Thy 1-membrane antigen, a specific characteristic of T cells. "Immature" thymocytes present in the cortex of the thymus are characterized by a high density of Thy 1 and TL antigens,[25,26] corticosteroid sensitivity,[27-29] and minimal immune competence.[27,28] Another population of thymocytes (present primarily in the medulla) includes the immunocompetent T cells of the thymus[25,29] and represents approximately 10% of the organ. These cells are characterized by the absence of TL and a lesser amount of Thy 1-antigens on their surface,[25,29] increased density of H-2 antigen,[25,29] and relative resistance to corticosteroids.[27] Thus, the majority (i.e., the corticosteroid-sensitive cells) of cells in the thymus possibly still has to undergo further differentiation steps before becoming fully competent T cells.

It has been questioned whether all of these cells represent precursors of peripheral T cells. Nevertheless, the thymus does contain precursor cells which, in cooperation with humoral thymic function (provided by thymus transplants in a Millipore® chamber), can differentiate in vivo into cells exhibiting properties of competent T cells (graft versus host reactivity [GvH] skin graft rejection, and delayed-type hypersensitivity[18,30]).

It also has been shown[18,31] that precursor cells from the thymus migrate to the peripheral lymphoid organs where they undergo further differentiation; therefore, these precursor cells are termed "postthymic" precursor cells. This raises the possibility that a decrease or defect in precursor cells in the thymus or periphery also contributes to immunosenescence with increasing age.

Age-related changes in intrathymic or postthymic precursor cells have not been reported so far. Obviously, age-related thymus involution leads to a decrease in the absolute number of thymic cells with increasing age, but whether this phenomenon also represents a decrease in precursor cells is unknown. The functional capacity of the aged thymus has been investigated[32-34] by implanting one thymic lobe from donor mice (ranging in age from 1 day to 33 months) under the kidney capsule of T-cell-deprived syngeneic young recipients (thymectomized, lethally X-irradiated, and bone-marrow-reconstituted). Recovery of splenic Thy 1-positive cells and repopulation of splenic thymus-dependent areas were not distinctly different in the various groups, although newborn thymuses induced the appearance of Thy 1-positive cells in the spleen more rapidly.[32,33] In contrast, with advancing age, thymic tissue lost the capacity to restore T-cell mitogen reactivity, mixed lymphocyte reactivity, and T-helper cell function in the spleens of recipient mice.[32-34] These results may indicate that a reduction in the number of precursors capable of differentiating into functional T cells occurs with advancing age. However, since total thymuses were grafted, the contribution of diminished thymic humoral function and/or the thymic microenvironment (to be discussed in Section B) to the observed reduction in restorative capacity cannot be determined.

3. Concluding Remarks

What emerges from all of the above-mentioned studies is that aging probably results in both a decrease in the number of precursor T cells in the bone marrow and development of defects in the regulation of differentiation by the thymus. The latter conclusion is substantiated by the studies of Hirokawa, et. al.,[32-34] which indicated that, even in combination with young bone marrow (i.e., when transplanted into young recipients), old thymuses fail to reconstitute T-cell functions in thymectomized recipients. It should be realized that changes in thymic influence and in hemopoietic cells during aging might be interrelated. In thymectomized mice, hemopoietic bone marrow cells show reduced numbers of colony-forming cells (CFU-S) and a lower proliferative rate,[35-37] although these results could not be confirmed with nu/nu mice, using other strain combinations.[38] The reduced CFU- content of thymectomized mice can be restored by thymic transplantation or in vitro thymus hormone treatment.[37] Thus, the thymus might also provide a feedback mechanism for the regulation of lymphopoiesis;[39] however, a direct effect of thymus deprivation on T-lymphocyte precursors in the bone marrow has not yet been demonstrated. Such a feedback mechanism also could explain why old bone marrow in combination with young thymus (i.e., when transplanted into young irradiated recipients) succeeds in restoring various immune functions, while young bone marrow in combination with old thymus (i.e., when transplanted into old irradiated recipients) does not.[20,21] On the basis of these assumptions, the relationship between the thymus and bone marrow during aging appears to be a promising area for future investigation.

B. Influence of Thymic Factors on T Cell Differentiation

Although the mechanism(s) by which the thymus affects T-cell differentiation are not fully understood, it seems reasonable to assume that humoral thymic factor(s) is(are) required for T-cell maturation.[3-5,18] Most of the present knowledge of the biological effects of thymic factors comes from in vitro studies which have indicated that several T-cell marker and functional properties can be induced in distinct types of the precursor T cells of the scheme shown in Figure 1. Instead of summarizing the effects exerted by thymic factors here, attention will be focused on their possible sites of action and on the evidence showing that reduced thymic factor production contributes to age-related defects in immune competence.

1. Putative Target Cells for the Action of Thymic Factors (Figure 1)

The target cell(s) for the action of thymic factors have not yet been precisely identified, but three types of target cells can be postulated on the basis of in vivo studies performed in mice in which thymus transplants in Millipore® chambers were used as a source of thymic factors: prethymic precursor cells, intrathymic and postthymic precursor cells. The scheme representing their possible interrelationships (Figure 1) is based on the following observations in mice.

Step A — (From stem cell to prethymic precursor cell): The fact that weakly Thy 1-positive cells are found in the spleen of nude mice,[40-42] even in nude mice born from homozygous nu/nu parents,[43] indicates that the generation of this cell type is thymus-independent. It can be regarded as being under a negative thymic influence, i.e., it is not present in normal mice and disappears under thymic humoral influence.[40]

Step B — (From prethymic precursor cell to postthymic precursor cell): The in vivo studies of Stutman (reviewed in Reference 18) and others[44,45] indicate that humoral thymic influence is *not* sufficient to induce maturation of prethymic precursor cells to competent T cells. In contrast, traffic through an intact thymus is a prerequisite for further differentiation.

These prethymic precursor cells are found in the bone marrow, in fetal liver before day 14 to 16 of embryonic life, and in the nude mouse spleen.[18] The prethymic precursor cell in the nude mouse spleen is identified by the presence of low amounts of Thy 1 antigen which can be detected only with sandwich immunofluorescence techniques,[40-43] or with rabbit antimouse brain antiserum,[46] and not with cytotoxicity or direct immunofluorescence techniques.

Step C — (From postthymic precursor cell to postthymic T cell): Many data from in vivo experiments indicate that humoral thymic influence (as provided by thymus transplants in cell-impermeable Millipore® chambers) can confer upon postthymic precursor cells several proliferative and functional properties associated with mature T cells (see References 18, 47, and 48). These postthymic precursor cells are found in different quantities in spleen, blood, bone marrow, lymph nodes, and neonatal spleen and can be easily killed by treatment with anti-Thy 1 antiserum and complement,[49] thus being distinguishable from the prethymic precursor.

Cortical thymocytes (i.e., most of the corticosteroid-sensitive cells) can also be regarded as belonging to the category of postthymic precursor cells on an operational basis.[48] These intrathymic, corticosteroid-sensitive precursor T cells are, however, different from the peripheral, postthymic precursor cells in that they express the TL surface antigens,[26,29] whereas peripheral precursor cells do not. The relevance of TL antigens as differentiation markers is questionable, however, as they do not occur in all mouse strains. It has been shown[18,31] that at least some of these immature corticosteroid-sensitive thymocytes migrate to the periphery where they undergo further maturation. Hence, the majority of peripheral T cells would be derived from cortical thymocytes.[18,31] These migrating thymocytes have already lost the TL antigens before leaving the thymus.[25] Peripheral postthymic precursors disappear within 30 to 60 days after neonatal thymectomy (neoTx),[47,48] which explains why thymus grafts in Millipore® chambers at 30 days or later after neoTx are no longer effective in restoring immune functions.[47,48]

In summary, the above data are in accord with the concept of Stutman[18] which states that a subpopulation of T-cell precursors, termed *postthymic,* is present in the lymphoid and hemopoietic tissues of adult and newborn mice. These cells are defined by their thymus dependency for renewal and represent the most likely candidates for the action of the humoral influence of the thymus. On the other hand, the early embryonic hemopoietic tissue and the nude mouse spleen contain a population of cells, termed *prethymic,* that is "insensitive" to the humoral function of the thymus and requires contact with the thymus microenvironment for its further differentiation. The current findings in thymic factor studies in which thymic extracts or serum factors are employed (reviewed in References 3-5) do not yet provide conclusive evidence concerning the site of action of these factors.

2. Possible Contribution of Depressed Thymic Factor Production to Age-Related Immunological Dysfunctions

Thymus-dependent factors possibly exhibiting the capacity to induce T-cell differentiation can be found in the serum of normal young individuals.[3] Evidence is accumulating that a decrease in circulating thymic factors occurs with increasing age. Firstly, in man, serum thymosin-like activity, as measured with the rosette-inhibition assay,[6] rapidly decreases from the age of 25 onwards.[9] Secondly, the level of a human thymus-dependent serum factor, measured by a cyclic AMP assay,[50] is also decreased with advancing age.[8] Thirdly, the serum thymic factor level, as measured with the mouse rosette-inhibition assay, is decreased in both man (from the age of 20 onwards) and mice (from the age of 6 months onwards).[6,7]

NZB and (NZB × NZW)F_1 hybrid mice have a normal level of serum thymic factor at birth, but this level decreases prematurely between the third and sixth week of life.[6,7] As the serum thymic factor seems to be of thymic epithelial origin,[7,51] these findings are in accord with the early abnormalities reported in NZB thymic epithelial cells.[52] In this respect, it is of interest that NZB mice show an earlier onset of decline in thymus-dependent immune functions[53] than many other mouse strains and are often regarded as a model for a premature age-related decrease in immune capacity.

The reduction in serum thymic factor level in normal-aged mice and man[7-9] parallels the decrease in thymus weight which starts in young adults.[32,54] Though this weight loss largely represents loss of cortical lymphocytes, the number of epithelial cells also decreases with advancing age.[32,54] In addition, distinct structural changes occur in the thymus epithelium. In aged mice, formation of small clusters of membrane-bordered epithelial cells devoid of thymocytes and containing cysts is observed, in contrast to young thymuses, in which the epithelial cells form a network densely packed with thymocytes.[32]

All of these findings seem to indicate that thymic secretory activity is diminished with increasing age. On the basis of the expected role of thymic factors in T cell differentiation, this could lead to a deficit in T-cell functions, but whether depressed thymic factor production plays a role in the pathogenesis of age-related T cell-function deficiencies remains to be proven. Suggestions have been made that there is a correlation between the premature decrease in thymic factor level in NZB mice and the early onset of T-cell function deficiencies observed in these animals.[53] Treatment of NZB mice with thymic extracts restores their depressed serum thymic factor level[6,7] and the number of Thy 1-positive cells in their spleens and lymph nodes,[6] delays the formation of antinucleic acid antibodies if treatment is started early in life,[55] restores Con A responsiveness[56] and mixed lymphocyte reactivity[57] in lymph node cells and the anti-SRBC response of spleen cells.[57] Unfortunately, no long term follow-up study on the effect of thymic extract treatment on T cell abnormalities has been performed.

3. Concluding Remarks

In summary, the above data indicate that the extent of the contribution of, and the mechanism by which depressed thymic factor production affect the age-related decrease in cellular immune functions are still unknown.

There are indications that reconstitution of depressed thymic factor production in old age[6,7] by thymic factor treatment might restore T-cell dysfunctions. It seems appropriate at this point to emphasize that thymic humoral factors should not be considered too much as a panacea for the reconstitution of T-cell functions in old age. A prerequisite for a beneficial effect of these factors is that the target cells for their action still be present. For reasons outlined in Section A.3, one could question whether this is indeed always the case. Furthermore, it should be realized that the exact role of thymic factors in the T-cell differentiation process, especially with regard to their site of action, is still uncertain (see Section B.1). Thus, besides more research into the causes of age-related dysfunction of T cells, more basic research into T-cell differentiation processes is required before correction of the defects can be envisaged. It is anticipated that elucidation of these processes may also reveal at which stages defects can occur and thus provide a better rationale for attempts at reconstitution.

C. Influence of Aging on T-Cell Numbers, Proliferative Capacity and Function

Demonstration of fully developed specific cellular immune reactions is complicated by the fact that many features of this manifestation of immunity are still not well established. It is known that T cells are the essential elements involved in host defense against viruses, fungi, and mycobacteria. In addition, T cells are involved in graft rejection, GvH reactivity, delayed-type hypersensitivity, and possibly tumor resistance. However, the exact functions and interactions of the various fully differentiated T cell subsets participating in these phenomena are not clear.

In vivo studies on cellular immune competence in aging rodents have revealed that delayed type skin reactivity,[10] capacity to reject allogeneic skin grafts,[11-13] and GvH reactivity[10,14] generally show a decrease, although some exceptions have been reported.[10,13,15] Most of our present knowledge of the consequences of aging on cellular immune competence, however, has been gained through in vitro studies of lymphocyte function. Obviously, the limited availability of old animals does not permit extensive in vivo evaluation of several forms of immune competence. In addition, the various compartments of the immune system can be studied separately in in vitro experiments. These then offer possibilities for determining the contribution of these separate compartments to the observed aberrations in immune competence. Therefore, this summary of changes in T-cell functions during aging will be limited to reports in which in vitro techniques were employed.

1. Effects of Aging on T-Cell Numbers

T-cell numbers in peripheral lymphoid organs of aging mice, as recognized by the presence of Thy 1 antigen, generally remain at the normal level[11,20,58-61] when determined by cytotoxicity assays. Confusing in this respect is that a few authors using immunofluorescence rather than cytotoxicity tests reported a definite decrease in the relative number of splenic T cells.[62,63] Also a decrease in the relative number of peripheral T cells was found in aging NZB mice,[61,64,65] which display an earlier onset of decline in thymus-dependent immune functions.[53] Thus, no conclusive answer to the question of whether T cells are still present in normal numbers can yet be given.

Age-related changes in the proportion of T-cell subsets identified by other markers (e.g., Lyt alloantigens, Fc-receptors, Qa-1 antigens) have not been reported so far. Since the presence of these markers is associated with distinct T-cell functions (for a recent review, see Reference 66), information on variations with age would contribute to an understanding of the causes of functional changes in T-cell subpopulations.

2. Effects of Aging on T-Cell Proliferative Capacity

T-cell proliferation of peripheral lymphocytes induced by mitogens[11,20,59,67-71] or by allogeneic stimulation[11,60,69,72-76] decreases with advancing age. This phenomenon has been attributed to a relative decrease in the number of responsive cells.[75,77-79] It seems that this deficiency occurs *despite* the fact that the relative *number* of T cells (i.e., Thy 1-positive cells) remains the same (see above). Thus, one would conclude that the T-cell differentiation pathway *does* proceed to the stage of acquiring the Thy 1 marker, but disturbances occur in the acquisition of the capacity to proliferate. Other possibilities are (1) the determination of the number of Thy 1-positive cells was incorrectly performed or by methods not sufficiently sensitive; it should be noted in this respect that *only* when immunofluorescence techniques were used was a decline in the relative number of Thy 1-positive cells found[62,63]; (2) the subpopulation of Thy 1-positive cells which responds to mitogens or alloantigens is decreased while a simultaneous increase in the number of Thy 1-positive nonresponder cells occurs; (3) T-cell proliferation is inhibited by suppressor T-cell function which seems to increase during aging.[80-83] So far, however, such increased suppressor T-cell function was been shown to exhibit effects only in humoral immune functions.[80-83]

3. Effects of Aging on Effector Functions of T Cells in Cellular Immune Competence

With regard to the effects of aging on differentiation of antigen-activated cells into final effector T cells, a somewhat confusing picture emerges. This is mainly due to the fact that both suppressor and killer T cell function are augmented by, or (in certain situations) even completely dependent on, helper T cells (for a recent review, see Reference 66). It is therefore difficult to obtain direct evidence for changes in these T-cell functions. A few authors have reported that the in vitro generation of splenic killer T cells after allogeneic stimulation in mixed lymphocyte cultures is depressed with increasing age,[64,84,85] but no conclusion can be reached as to whether this is due to a decrease in the number of antigen-sensitive precursor killer cells or to a loss of T-helper and T-killer cell synergism.

In vivo immunization with allogeneic cells also leads to induction of specific killer cells[86] whose activity can be tested in vitro. Production of splenic killer cells has been found to be decreased with advancing age[15,87,88] and could be attributed to both a reduction in the number of precursor killer cells and a decrease in proliferative capacity.[88]

Direct estimates of possible changes in suppressor T cells involved in cellular immune functions have not yet been made. It is clear that our scant knowledge of cellular effector T-cell functions warrants a wide expansion of efforts in this area.

4. Concluding Remarks

A summary of the influence of senescence on thymus-dependent immune parameters involved in cellular immune competence has been presented. The indications are that T cells with the capacity to proliferate and further differentiate efficiently into effector cells are gradually lost with increasing age. Most authors have reported that these defects cannot be attributed to an overt loss of Thy 1-positive cells.[11,20,58-61] The observed functional defects may be explained by either shifts in the proportion of Thy 1-positive responder and nonresponder T cells or, alternatively, by defects in interactions between the different T-cell subpopulations rather than by intrinsic defects in particular subpopulations only.[89]

The loss of the regulatory role of the thymus in T-cell differentiation is considered to be one of the keys, if not the only key, to T-cell aging.[1,2] However, in view of recent findings indicating a loss of T-cell progenitor cells from bone marrow and spleen of aged mice,[16,22,23] it would appear that not just the thymus affects T-cell aging. Apart from directing attention to the bone marrow, these findings also negate the picture of the aging T-cell system as sketched above, since, theoretically, a decrease in bone marrow precursors should also lead to a quantitative decrease in peripheral T cells. This hypothesis is in contradiction with the generally observed normal level of T cells.[11,20,58-61] Perhaps the exceptions provide a clue to this controversy, i.e., by using immunofluorescence rather than cytotoxicity techniques, a few authors noted a definite decrease in the relative number of splenic T cells.[62,63] Alternatively, the Thy 1-positive cells still found in aging mice represent long-lived T cells which are no longer fully competent. Attention should also be paid to the possibility that, in conventional environments, viral infections might cause differentiation of T cells. Recent reports[90,91] indicate that, even in nu/nu mice (i.e., with no thymic influence), significant numbers of Thy 1-positive cells appear in the spleen after infection with mouse hepatitis virus.

III. DISCUSSION

More questions than answers emerge from the above review; nevertheless, a few conclusions can be drawn concerning the role of the thymus in immunosenescence.

It has been demonstrated that intrinsic changes occur in the thymus, which render it incapable of restoring thymus-dependent immune functions after transplantation into young thymectomized recipients.[32-34] One possible reason for this might be a decrease in the number of intrathymic precursor T cells, which, under the influence of thymic humoral factors, still have to differentiate into mature T cells. Employing thymic epithelial culture supernatants (TES) as a source of humoral thymic factors,[92-94] we found that several properties of mature T cells can be induced by TES in thymocytes from young mice and rats in vitro (i.e., T cell proliferative capacity induced by mitogens and alloantigens, T-helper and T-killer cell function, decreased Thy 1-antigen density, and sensitivity to corticosteroids). Surprisingly, TES does *not* influence thymocytes from old donors,[95] suggesting that a loss of cells sensitive to the action of thymic factors occurs with increasing age. This would fit in with the finding that with increasing age a loss of thymocyte precursors in the bone marrow or a decrease in the proliferative capacity of these cells occurs.[22,23] However, a decrease in prethymic precursor T-cell numbers in the bone marrow cannot be the only explanation for age-related immune defects, since grafting old mice with young bone marrow was not found to restore their depressed immune functions,[20,21] whereas a combination of young thymus and bone marrow does.[21] In other words, future research should be directed to the question of why the old thymus no longer provides a suitable environment for the influx of bone-marrow-derived precursor T cells. In addition, more basic research is needed to reveal whether there is a direct relation between diminished thymus function and a decrease in prethymic precursor T cells in the bone marrow, as suggested by some authors[35-37,39] though disputed by others.[28]

In summary, the thymus seems to influence immunosenescence by several different mechanisms, among which are

1. A decline in the production of thymic humoral factors,[7-9] probably due to a decrease in the number of epithelial cells.[32,54] Possible intrinsic changes in the epithelial cells remain to be investigated.

2. A decrease in the relative number of intrathymic precursor T cells[95] which give rise to peripheral postthymic precursor T cells, the potential target cells for the action of thymic factors. It is clear that the general atrophy of the thymus during aging also results in an absolute decrease in the number of precursor T cells.

3. A loss of the capacity to be repopulated by bone marrow-derived precursor T cells.[20,21]

Obviously, the defect mentioned in number two might be the consequence of that mentioned in number three and/or the reported decrease in thymocyte precursor cells in the bone marrow[22,23] However, these statements are based on suggestive and incomplete data only and serve merely to direct attention to areas which need further investigation.

Among other areas deserving further attention in attempts to elucidate the causes of the age-related decline in cellular immune competence are the following.

1. Further inventory of the changes in several effector T-cell functions is warranted. Insufficient information on changes in helper, killer, and suppressor T-cell functions is available (see Section C. 3). The possible contribution of defects in cell-cell interactions to deficiencies in these effector T-cell functions is also still unclear.

2. Investigations of the mechanisms of T-T cell interactions have shown soluble products of T cells to play a regulatory role. Both helper and suppressive T-cell-derived factors have been described (see, e.g., Reference 96). It seems timely that the effects of aging on the production of these important regulatory products be investigated, also because the possibility of correcting defects with such factors seems feasible.

3. By using cell populations which (at least in young animals) have been shown to be induced to maturation by certain thymic factors, one could investigate the sensitivity of these same populations from old donors to the action of thymic factors and thus attempt to localize the defects in the T-cell differentiation pathway.

4. It has been known for some time that killer T cells developing in mice infected with certain viruses kill only virus-infected target cells sharing H-2K or H-2D antigen with the infected host, but not cells infected with the same virus but sharing neither H-2K nor H-2D with the host.[97] This phenomenon of "H-2 restriction" has also been found by others in the T-cell-mediated lysis of hapten-modified target cells and target cells differing from the immunized donor by minor (non-H-2) transplantation antigens (reviewed in References 97 and 98). Zinkernagel et al.[98-100] recently provided evidence that this H-2 restriction is acquired during differentiation of prethymic precursor T cells within the thymus. During this differentiation process, the cells acquire the capacity to recognize those H-2 antigens which are expressed on radioresistant cells in the thymus, independent of the lymphocytes' own H-2 specificity and independent of antigenic stimulation. These findings indicate that the specificity of certain cellular immune reactions is determined by the H-2 antigens of (possibly) the thymic epithelial cells. The capacity of T cells to recognize H-2 self antigens is a crucial requirement for protection against viral infections. Thus, in order to assess T-cell functions which are highly relevant for the host's immune protection, it seems necessary to deter-

mine in aging mice antigen-specific responses for which H-2 restriction has been demonstrated.

It will be interesting to discover whether the thymus from aged donors is still capable of "teaching" precursor T cells to recognize those H-2 antigens expressed on the radioresistant portion of the thymus. In other words, to investigate whether this important aspect of the repertoire of T cell immunocompetence, i.e., capacity to recognize H-2 self-antigens, is maintained during aging.

This brief set of statements can clearly serve as a summary of how many gaps in the present knowledge of aging and cellular immunocompetence still have to be filled. It can be expected that the information derived from further studies will be of help in designing models for in vivo reconstitution in a more meaningful way. This last statement also implies that the present knowledge in this field by no means justifies reconstitution attempts, which await a better rationale. Another conclusion from the present state of knowledge in immunosenescence is that, with so many theoretically possible defects in the T-cell differentiation pathway, and in the expression of effector functions by mature T cells, immunosenescence will be expressed differently among aging individuals. This speculative possibility may be the reason for the increased variability among aging individuals[1,2,95] and certainly delays rapid developments in the understanding of immunosenescence.

ACKNOWLEDGMENTS

The author wishes to thank Germaine van Deursen for her expert secretarial help in the preparation of the manuscript.

REFERENCES

1. **Makinodan, T.,** The thymus in aging, in *Geriatric Endocrinology,* Greenblat, R. B., Ed., Raven Press, New York, 1978, 217.
2. **Kay, M. M. B. and Makinodan, T.,** Immunobiology of aging: evaluation of current status, *Clin. Immunol. Immunopathol.,* 6, 394, 1976.
3. **Bach, J. F. and Carnaud, C.,** Thymic factors, *Prog. Allergy,* 21, 342, 1976.
4. **Goldstein, A. L., Thurman, G. B., Cohen, G. H., and Hooper, J. A.,** Thymosin: chemistry, biology and clinical applications, in *The Biological Activity of Thymic Hormones,* van Bekkum, D. W., Ed., Kooyker Scientific Publications, Rotterdam, The Netherlands, 1975, 173.
5. **Stutman, O.,** Two main features of T cell development: thymus traffic and postthymic in *Contemporary Topics in Immunobiology,* Vol. 7, Stutman, O., Ed., Plenum Press, New York, 1977, 1.
6. **Bach, J. F., Dardenne, M., and Salomon, J. C.,** Studies on thymus products. IV. Absence of serum thymic activity in adult NZB and (NZB×NZW)F₁ mice, *Clin. Exp. Immunol.* 14, 247, 1973.
7. **Bach, J. F., Dardenne, M., Pleau, J. M., and Bach, M. A.,** Isolation, biochemical characteristics and biological activity of a circulating thymic hormone in the mouse and in the human, *Ann. N. Y. Acad. Sci.,* 249, 186, 1975.
8. **Astaldi, A., Astaldi, G. C. B., Wijermans, P., Groenewoud, M., Schellekens, P. Th. A. and Eijsvoogel, V. P.,** Thymus dependent factor in human serum, *J. Reticuloendoth. Soc.,* 22, (Abstr.), 84, 1977.
9. **Hooper, J. A., McDaniel, M. C., Thurman, G. B., Cohen, G. H., Schulof, R. S., and Goldstein, A. L.,** Purification and properties of bovine thymosin, *Ann. N. Y. Acad. Sci.,* 249, 125, 1975.

10. **Walters, C. S. and Claman, H. N.,** Age-related changes in cell-mediated immunity in Balb/c mice, *J. Immunol.,* 115, 1438, 1975.

11. **Menon, M., Jaroslow, B. N., and Koesterer, R.,** The decline of cell-mediated immunity in aging mice, *J. Gerontol.,* 29, 499, 1974.

12. **Teller, M. N.,** Interrelationships among aging immunity and cancer, in *Tolerance, Autoimmunity and Aging,* Siegel, M. M. and Good, R. A., Eds., Charles C Thomas, Springfield, Ill., 11, 18, 1972.

13. **Teller, M. N.,** Age changes and immune resistance to cancer, *Adv. Gerontol. Res.,* 4, 25, 1972.

14. **Kishimoto, S., Shigemoto, S., and Yamamura, Y.,** Immune response in aged mice. Change of cell-mediated immunity with ageing, *Transplantation,* 15, 455, 1973.

15. **Stutman, O., Yunis, E. J., and Good, R. A.,** Studies on thymus function. III. Duration of thymic function, *J. Exp. Med.,* 135, 339, 1972.

16. **Basch, R. S. and Kadish, J. L.,** Hematopoietic thymocyte precursors. II. Properties of the precursors, *J. Exp. Med.,* 145, 405, 1977.

17. **El-Arini, M. O. and Osoba, D.,** Differentiation of thymus-derived cells from precursors in mouse bone marrow, *J. Exp. Med.,* 137, 821, 1973.

18. **Stutman, O.,** Intrathymic and extrathymic T cell maturation, *Immunol. Rev.,* 42, 138, 1978.

19. **Harrison, D. E. and Doubleday, J. W.,** Normal function of immunologic stem cells from aged mice, *J. Immunol.,* 114, 1314, 1975.

20. **Micklem, H. S., Ogden, D. A., and Payne, A. C.,** Ageing, haemopoietic stem cells and immunity, in *Haemopoietic stem cells,* Vol. 13, CIBA Found. Symp., Elsevier, Amsterdam, 1973, 285.

21. **Hirokawa, K., Albright, J. W., and Makinodan, T.,** Restoration of impaired immune functions in aging animals. Effect of syngeneic thymus and bone marrow grafts, *Clin. Immunol. Immunopathol.,* 5, 371, 1976.

22. **Tyan, M. L.,** Impaired thymic regeneration in lethally irradiated mice given bone marrow from aged donors, *Proc. Soc. Exp. Biol. Med.,* 152, 33, 1976.

23. **Tyan, M. L.,** Age-related decrease in mouse T cell progenitors, *J. Immunol.,* 118, 846, 1977.

24. **Bach, M. A. and Bach, J. F.,** Studies on thymus products. VI. The effects of cyclic nucleotides and prostaglandins on rosette-forming cells. Interactions with thymic factor, *Eur. J. Immunol.,* 3, 778, 1973.

25. **Raff, M. C.,** Evidence for subpopulation of mature lymphocytes within the mouse thymus, *Nature (London),* 229, 182, 1971.

26. **Raff, M. C.,** Surface antigens for distinguishing T and B lymphocytes in mice, *Transplant. Rev.,* 6, 52, 1971.

27. **Jacobsson, H. and Blomgren, H.,** Changes of the PHA-responding pool of cells in the thymus after cortisone or X-ray treatment of mice. Evidence for an inverse relation between the production of cortical and medullary thymocytes, *Cell. Immunol.,* 4, 93, 1972.

28. **Jacobsson, H. and Blomgren, H.,** Studies on the recirculating cells in the mouse thymus, *Cell. Immunol.,* 5, 107, 1972.

29. **Konda, S., Stockert, E., and Smith, R. T.,** Immunologic properties of mouse thymus cells: membrane antigen patterns associated with various cell subpopulations, *Cell. Immunol.,* 7, 275, 1973.

30. **Stutman, O., Yunis, E. J. and Good, R. A.,** Studies on thymus function. I. Cooperative effects of thymic function and lymphohemopoietic cells in restoration of neonatally thymectomized mice, *J. Exp. Med.,* 132, 583, 1970.

31. **Weissman, I. L., Masuda, T., Olive, C., and Friedberg, S. H.,** Differentiation and migration of T lymphocytes, *Isr. J. Med. Sci.,* 11, 1267, 1975.

32. **Hirokawa, K.,** The thymus and ageing, in *Comprehensive Immunology,* Vol. 1, Good, R. A. and Day, S. B., Eds., Immunology and Ageing, Makinodan, T. and Yunis, E., Eds., Plenum Press New York 1977, 51.

33. **Hirokawa, K. and Makinodan, T.,** Thymus involution: Effect on T cell differentiation, *J. Immunol.,* 114, 1659, 1975.

34. **Hirokawa, K. and Sado, T.,** Early decline of thymic effect on T cell differentiation, *Mech. Ageing Dev.,* 7, 89, 1978.

35. **Zipori, D. and Trainin, N.,** Defective capacity of bone marrow from nude mice to restore lethally irradiated recipients, *Blood,* 42, 671, 1973.

36. **Zipori, D. and Trainin, N.,** Impaired radioprotective capacity and reduced proliferative rate of bone marrow from neonatally thymectomized mice. *Exp. Hematol.,* 3, 1, 1975.

37. **Zipori, D. and Trainin, N.,** The role of a thymus humoral factor in the proliferation of bone marrow CFU-S from thymectomized mice, *Exp. Hematol.,* 3, 389, 1975.

38. **Pritchard, H. and Micklem, H. S.,** Haemopoietic stem cells and progenitors of functional T lymphocytes in the bone marrow of ''nude'' mice, *Clin. Exp. Immunol.,* 14, 597, 1973.

39. **Van Bekkum, D. W.,** Pathways and control of lymphocytopoiesis, in *Leukemia and asplastic anemia,* Proc. Int. Conf. on Leukemia and Aplastic Anemia, Il Pensiero Scientifico, 1976, 31.

40. **Roelants, G. E. and Mayor-Whitney, K. S.,** The regulation of the T-lymphocytes precursor pool by a humoral factor released by the thymus, *Cell. Immunol.,* 34, 420, 1977.

41. **Roelants, G. E., Mayor, K.S., Hägg, L. B., and Loor, F.,** Immature T lineage lymphocytes in athymic mice. Presence of TL, lifespan and homeostatic regulation, *Eur. J. Immunol.,* 6, 75, 1976.

42. **Roelants, G. E., Loor, F., von Boehmer, H., Sprent, J., Hägg, L. B., Mayor, K. S. and Ryden, A.,** Five types of lymphocytes (Ig⁻O⁻, Ig⁺O⁺ weak, Ig⁻O⁺ strong, Ig⁺O⁻ and Ig⁺O⁺) characterized by double immunofluorescence and electroforetic mobility. Organ distribution in normal and nude mice, *Eur. J. Immunol.,* 5, 127, 1975.

43. **Loor, F., Amstutz, H., Hägg, L. B., Mayor, K. S., and Roelants, G. E.,** T lineage lymphocytes in nude mice born from homozygous nu/nu parents, *Eur. J. Immunol.,* 6, 663, 1976.

44. **Loor, F. and Hägg, L. B.,** The restoration of the T-lymphoid system of nude mice: Lower efficiency of nonlymphoid, epithelial thymus grafts, *Cell. Immunol.,* 29, 200, 1977.

45. **Pierpaoli, W. and Besedovsky, H. O.,** Failure of "thymus factor" to restore transplantation immunity in athymic mice, *Br. J. Exp. Pathol.,* 56, 180, 1975.

46. **Sato, V. L., Waksal, S. D., and Herzenberg, L. A.,** Identification and separation of pre T cells from nu/nu mice: differentiation by preculture with thymic reticuloepithelial cells, *Cell. Immunol.,* 24, 173, 1976.

47. **Stutman, O., Yunis, E. J., and Good, R. A.,** Carcinogen-induced tumors of the thymus. IV. Humoral influence of normal thymus and functional thymomas and influence of postthymectomy period on restoration, *J. Exp. Med.,* 130, 809, 1969.

48. **Stutman, O., Yunis, E. J., and Good, R. A.,** Carcinogen-induced tumors of the thymus. III. Restoration of neonatally thymectomized mice with thymomas in cell impermeable chambers, *J. Natl. Cancer Inst.,* 43, 499, 1969.

49. **Stutman, O.,** Humoral thymic factors influencing postthymic cells, *Ann. N. Y. Acad. Sci.,* 249, 89, 1975.

50. **Astaldi, A., Astaldi, G. C. B., Schellekens, P. Th. A., and Eijsvoogel, V. P.,** A thymic factor in human sera demonstrated by a cAMP assay, *Nature (London),* 260, 713, 1976.

51. **Dardenne, M., Papiernik, M., Bach, J. F., and Stutman, O.,** Studies on thymus products. III. Epithelial origin of the serum thymic factor, *Immunology,* 27, 299, 1974.

52. **De Vries, M. J. and Hijmans, W.,** Pathological changes of thymic epithelial cells and autoimmune disease in NZB, NZW and (NZB/NZW)F₁ mice, *Immunology,* 12, 179, 1967.

53. **Talal, N.,** Disordered immunologic regulation and autoimmunity, *Transplant. Rev.,* 31, 240, 1976.

54. **Burek, J.,** *Pathology of Aging Rats: A Morphological and Experimental Study of the Age-Associated Lesions in Aging BN/Bi, WAG/Rij and (WAG × BN) F₁ Rats,* CRC Press, West Palm Beach, Florida, 1978.

55. **Talal, N., Dauphinee, M., Pillarisetty, R., and Goldblum, R.,** Effect of thymosin on thymocyte proliferation and autoimmunity in NZB mice, *Ann. N. Y. Acad. Sci.,* 249, 438, 1975.

56. **Thurman, G. B., Ahmed, A., Strong, D. M., Gershwin, M. E., Steinberg, A. D., and Goldstein, A. L.,** Thymosin-induced increase in mitogenic responsiveness of lymphocytes of C57BL/6J, NZB/W and nude mice, *Transplant. Proc.,* 7, 299, 1975.

57. **Gershwin, M. E., Ahmed, A., Steinberg, A. D., Thurman, G. B. and Goldstein, A. L.,** Correction of T cell function by thymosin in New Zealand mice, *J. Immunol.,* 113, 1068, 1974.

58. **Gerbase-De Lima, M., Wilkinson, J., Smith, G. S., and Walford, R. L.,** Age-related decline in thymic-independent immune functions in a long-lived mouse strain, *J. Gerontol.,* 29, 261, 1974.

59. **Hori, Y., Perkins, E. H., and Halsall, M. K.,** Decline in phytohaemagglutinin responsiveness of spleen cells from ageing mice, *Proc. Soc. Exp. Biol. Med.,* 144, 48, 1973.

60. **Stutman, O.,** Lymphocyte subpopulations in NZB mice: deficit of thymus dependent lymphocytes, *J. Immunol.,* 109, 602, 1972.

61. **Stutman, O.,** Cell-mediated immunity and aging, *Fed. Proc., Fed Am. Soc. Exp. Biol.,* 33, 2028, 1974.

62. **Brennan, P. C. and Jaroslow, B. N.,** Age-associated decline in theta antigen on spleen thymus-derived lymphocytes of B6CF₁ mice, *Cell. Immunol.,* 15, 51, 1975.

63. **Callard, R. E. and Basten, A.,** Immune function in aged mice. I. T cell responsiveness using phytohaemagglutinin as a functional probe, *Cell Immunol.,* 31, 13, 1975.

64. **Hirano, T. and Nordin, A. A.,** Age-associated decline in the in vitro development of cytotoxic lymphocytes in NZB mice, *J. Immunol.,* 117, 1093, 1976.

65. **Stobo, J. D., Talal, N., and Paul, W. E.,** Lymphocyte classes in New Zealand mice. I. Ontogeny and mitogen responsiveness of thymocytes and thymus-derived lymphocytes, *J. Immunol.,* 109, 692, 1972.

66. **Cantor, H. and Boyse, E. A.,** Lymphocytes as models for the study of mammalian cellular differentiation, *Immunol. Rev.,* 33, 105, 1977.

67. Hung, C.-Y., Perkins, E. H., and Yang, W. K., Age-related refractoriness of PHA-induced lympho-cyte transformation II. ^{125}I-PHA binding to spleen cells from young and old mice, *Mech. Ageing Develop.*, 4, 103, 1975.

68. Meredith, P., Gerbase-de Lima, M., and Walford, R. L., Age-related changes in the PHA: ConA stimulatory ratios of cells from spleens of a long-lived mouse strain, *Exp. Gerontol.*, 10, 247, 1975.

69. Rodey, G. E., Good, R. A., and Yunis, E. J., Progressive loss in vitro of cellular immunity with ageing in strains of mice susceptible to autoimmune disease, *Clin. Exp. Immunol.*, 9, 305, 1971.

70. Lawton, J. W. M. and Murphy, W. H., Characterization of the blastogenic response of C58 spleen cells: age-dependent changes, *Immunology*, 26, 1093, 1974.

71. Mathies, M., Lipps, L., Smith, G. S., and Walford, R. L., Age-related decline in response to phyto-haemagglutinin and poke-weed mitogen by spleen cells from hamsters and a long-lived mouse strain, *J. Gerontol.*, 28, 425, 1973.

72. Adler, W. H., Takiguchi, T., and Smith, R. T., Effect of age upon primary alloantigen recognition by mouse spleen cells, *J. Immunol.*, 107, 1357, 1971.

73. Konen, T. G., Smith, G. S., and Walford, R. L., Decline in mixed lymphocyte reactivity of spleen cells from aged mice of a long-lived strain, *J. Immunol.*, 110, 1216, 1973.

74. Meredith, P., Tittor, W., Gerbase-De Lima, M., and Walford, R. L., Age-related changes in the cellular immune response of lymph node and thymus cells in long-lived mice, *Cell Immunol.*, 18, 324, 1975.

75. Merhav, S. and Gershon, H., The mixed lymphocyte reaction of senescent mice: sensitivity to alloan-tigen and cell replication time, *Cell Immunol.*, 34, 354, 1977.

76. Nielsen, H. E., The effect of age on the response of rat lymphocytes in mixed lymphocyte culture to PHA and in the GvH reaction, *J. Immunol.*, 112, 1194, 1974.

77. Abraham, C., Tal, Y., and Gershon, H., Reduced in vitro response to concanavalin A and lipopoly-saccharide in senescent mice: a function of reduced number of responding cells, *Eur. J. Immunol.*, 7, 301, 1977.

78. Hung, C.-Y., Perkins, E. H. and Yang, W. K., Age-related refractoriness of PHA-induced lympho-cyte transformation. I. Comparable sensitivity of spleen cells from young and old mice to culture conditions, *Mech. Ageing Develop.*, 4, 29, 1975.

79. Kruisbeek, A. M., Age-related changes in Con A and LPS-induced lymphocyte transformation. I. Effect of culture conditions on mitogen responses of blood and spleen lymphocytes from young and aged rats, *Mech. Ageing Develop.*, 5, 125, 1976.

80. Goidl, E. A., Iunes, J., and Weksler, M. E., Immune response of aged mice, *Fed. Proc., Fed. Am. Soc. Exp. Biol.*, 35, 321, 1976.

81. Makinodan, T., Albright, J. W., Good, P. I., Peter, C. P., and Heidrich, M. L., Reduced humoral immune activity in long-lived old mice: An approach to elucidating its mechanisms, *Immunology*, 31, 903, 1976.

82. Segre, D. and Segre, M., Humoral immunity in aged mice. II. Increased suppressor T cell activity in immunologically deficient old mice, *J. Immunol.*, 116, 735, 1976.

83. Segre, D. and Segre, M., Age-related changes in B and T lymphocytes and decline of humoral immune responsiveness in aged mice, *Mech. Ageing Develop.*, 6, 115, 197.

84. Gelfland, M. C. and Steinberg, A. D., Mechanism of allograft rejection in New Zealand mice. I. Cell synergy and its age-dependent loss, *J. Immunol.*, 110, 1652, 1973.

85. Shigemoto, S., Kishimoto, S., and Yamamura, Y., Change of cell-mediated cytotoxicity with ageing, *J. Immunol.*, 115, 307, 1975.

86. Brunner, K. T., Manuel, J., Rudolf, M., and Chapuis, B., Studies of allograft immunity. I. Produc-tion, development and in vitro assay of cellular immunity, *Immunology*, 18, 501, 1970.

87. Bach, M. A., Lymphocyte-mediated cytotoxicity: effects of ageing, adult thymectomy and thymic factor, *J. Immunol.*, 119, 641, 1977.

88. Goodman, S. A. and Makinodan, T., Effect of age on cell-mediated immunity in long-lived mice, *Clin. Exp. Immunol.*, 19, 533, 1975.

89. Gershon, R. K. and Metzler, C. M., Suppressor cells in aging, in *Immunology and Aging*, Makino-dan, T., and Yunis, J., Eds., *Comprehensive Immunology*, Vol. I., Good, R. A. and Day, J. B., Eds., Plenum Press, New York, 1977, 103.

90. Scheid, M. P., Goldstein, G., and Boyse, E. A., Differentiation of T cells in nude mice, *Science*, 190, 1211, 1975.

91. Tamura, T., Machii, K., Ueda, K., and Fujiwara, K., Modification of immune response in nude mice infected with mouse hepatitis virus, *Microbiol. Immunol.*, 22, 557, 1978.

92. Kruisbeek, A. M. and Astaldi, G. C. B., Distinct effect of thymic epithelial culture supernatant on T cell properties of mouse thymocytes separated by the use of peanut agglutinin, *J. Immunol.*, 123, 984, 1979.

93. **Kruisbeek, A. M., Zijlstra, J. J., and Kröse, C. J. M.,** Increase in T cell mitogen responsiveness in rat thymocytes by thymic epithelial culture supernatants, *Eur. J. Immunol.,* 7, 375, 1977.

94. **Kruisbeek, A. M., Astaldi, G. C. B., Blankwater, M. J., Zijlstra, J. J., Levert, L. A., and Astaldi, A.,** The in vitro effect of a thymic epithelial culture supernatant on mixed lymphocyte reactivity and intracellular cAMP levels of thymocytes and on antibody production to SRBC by nu/nu spleen cells, *Cell. Immunol.,* 35, 134, 1978.

95. **Kruisbeek, A. M. and Meihuizen, S. P.,** Ageing and the thymus-dependent immune system, *Ned. T. Geront.,* 9, 220, 1978.

96. **Tokuhisa, T., Taniguchi, M., Okumura, K., and Tada, I.,** An antigen-specific I region gene product that augments the antibody response, *J. Immunol.,* 120, 414, 1978.

97. **Doherty, P. C., Blanden, R. V., and Zinkernagel, R. M.,** Specificity of virus-immune effector T cells for H-2K or H-2D compatible interactions: implications for H-antigen diversity, *Transplant. Rev.,* 29, 89, 1976.

98. **Zinkernagel, R. M., Callahan, G. M., Althage, A., Cooper, S., Klein, P. A., and Klein, J.,** On the thymus in the differentiation of "H-2 self-recognition" by T cells: evidence for dual recognition? *J. Exp. Med.,* 147, 882, 1978.

99. **Zinkernagel, R. M., Callahan, G. N., Klein, J., and Dennert, G.,** Cytotoxic T cells learn specificity for self H-2 during differentiation in the thymus, *Nature (London),* 271, 251, 1978.

100. **Zinkernagel, R. M., Callahan, G. N., Althage, A., Cooper, S., Streilein, J. W., and Klein, J.,** The lymphoreticular system in triggering virus plus self-specific cytotoxic T cells: evidence fo T help, *J. Exp. Med.,* 147, 897, 1978.

Chapter 4

QUANTITATION OF MURINE CYTOLYTIC T LYMPHOCYTES AND THEIR IMMEDIATE PRECURSORS

K. T. Brunner, H. R. MacDonald, and C. Taswell

TABLE OF CONTENTS

I. INTRODUCTION*

Early attempts to quantitate lymphocyte-mediated destruction of target cells were hampered by the lack of reliability of tests assessing cell death by morphological critera. With the introduction of the procedure of incorporating radioisotopically labeled markers into target cells, assay systems measuring cell-mediated cytotoxicity have gained much objectivity and accuracy. The most widely used radioisotope has been ^{51}Cr. When added to target cells in the form of ^{51}Cr-labeled sodium chromate, it is retained in the cytoplasm for a relatively extended period of time and is not released significantly until the cell membrane is sufficiently damaged to allow efflux of intracellular molecules. Since label is not reincorporated into undamaged cells, direct target-cell lysis is the only parameter measured, and cells involved in mediating this process can be referred to as cytolytic effector cells.

Although target-cell destruction could thus be measured more quantitatively, the problem of determining the actual frequency of effector cells as a function of target cell lysis has until recently remained largely unresolved. Due to the lack of easily accessible systems measuring cytolytic effector cells at the single-cell level, cytotoxicity has usually been measured at the population level. In the widely used ^{51}Cr-release assay described in detail in Section II, the cytolytic activity of populations of lymphoid cells containing effector cells is defined by the concentration of lymphocytes required to obtain 50% specific ^{51}Cr release. The relative frequency of effector cells contained in different lymphoid cell populations may then be estimated by comparing the numbers of lymphocytes needed to induce 50% lysis. Although it has yielded valuable results in selected systems, this technique has serious limitations.

One objection which imposes severe limitations on the interpretation of results concerns the absence of parallel dose-response curves. If results from different lymphoid cell populations containing relatively high frequencies of CTL (such as MLC populations or MLC subpopulations obtained by velocity sedimentation fractionation) are compared, then families of parallel dose-response curves are observed (as shown in Figure 1), and direct comparisons of cytolytic activities can be made. On the other hand, if results from populations containing high and low frequencies of CTL (such as immune lymphoid-cell populations diluted by the addition of various numbers of normal cells) are compared, then the observed dose-response curves may no longer be parallel (as shown in Figure 2), and direct comparisons of cytolytic activities cannot be made. Lack of parallel curves therefore precludes any conclusions concerning relative effector-cell frequencies in these different populations. Another objection to this and similar techniques of estimating relative effector-cell frequencies at the population level concerns the fact that the cytolytic activity of lymphoid cell populations may not only be a function of the frequency, but also of the efficiency of potential effector-cell subpopulations contained within the total lymphocyte population. Therefore, even if parallel curves are obtained, no reliable direct information concerning either frequency or efficiency of effector cells can be obtained by this assay method. (See also Sections II, A1, and II,A,3). In response to these deficiencies and problems, several attempts have been made to establish mathematical models for the kinetics of lymphocyte-mediated cytolysis with the hope that such investigations would reveal a better and more informative method of data analysis for cytolytic activity. These models will be discussed in Section II, A,3.

---

* Abbreviations: CTL, cytolytic T lymphocyte; CTL-P, cytolytic T-lymphocyte precursor; MLC, mixed leukocyte culture; MLTC, mixed leukocyte-tumor cell culture; K cell, killer cell; NK cell, natural killer cell; LU, lytic unit; HEPES, N-hydroxyethylpiperazine-N- 2-ethanesulfonic acid; FDA, fluorescein diacetate; FCS, fetal calf serum; EGTA, ethyleneglycol-bis-β-aminoethylether; DMEM, Dulbecco's modified Eagle's medium; LDA, limiting dilution analysis.

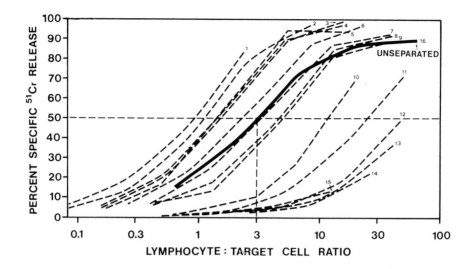

FIGURE 1. Cytolytic activity of MLC cells fractionated by velocity sedimentation. Primary cultures of C57BL/6 spleen cells and irradiated DBA/2 spleen cells were established. On day 5, 50×10^6 recovered MLC cells were separated by velocity sedimentation at 1 g.[44] Fractions of 15 ml were collected, concentrated to 1 ml by centrifugation, and tested for cytolytic activity against ^{51}Cr-labeled P-815 (DBA/2) target cells at the various lymphoid cell-to-target cell radios indicated, using a 3-hr assay. Fractions 1 to 15 contain cells with decreasing sedimentation velocity, a parameter which depends primarily on cell size.

In view of the problems related to assays of cytolytic activities at the population level, considerable efforts have in recent years been devoted to the development of assay systems allowing the enumeration of CTL and their immediate precursors at the single-cell level. Since some of these systems have met with considerable success, they will be described in further detail below. The systems are based on two different approaches. One takes advantage of the fact that, as a first step in target cell lysis, CTL attach firmly to target cells via specific receptors leading, under appropriate conditions, to the formation of stable conjugates (Section III, B). Since most of these conjugates were shown to lead to lysis, their enumeration allows the direct estimation of the frequency of CTL. The other system is based on the "limiting dilution analysis" of effector and/ or precursor cell frequencies (Sections III, A and III, C). This new and powerful technique not only allows the direct establishment of minimal CTL or CTL-P frequencies, but can also be applied to the analysis of the specificity of individual CTL-P and their clonal progeny.

II. ENUMERATION OF CYTOLYTIC T LYMPHOCYTES AT THE POPULATION LEVEL

A. ^{51}Cr–Release Assay
1. General Considerations
There have been numerous assay systems proposed for the estimation of the cytolytic potential of lymphoid cell populations containing cytolytic effector cells, including: cell counting, inhibition of antibody plaque formation, cloning efficiency, release of radioactive label, and the microcytotoxicity assay. (For references, see 1.) Of these various methods, the ^{51}Cr-release assay appears to provide the most convenient measure of cytolytic effector cell activity. It is simple to use, sensitive, quantitative, and independent of target cell multiplication. It has been useful in the detection of target cell lysis by cytolytic T lymphocytes (CTL), K cells, NK cells, and activated macro-

phages. The assay is, however, limited by the availability of appropriate target cells, i.e., target cells which release a relatively low proportion of label spontaneously, but which then release a high proportion of label when lysed. High spontaneous ^{51}Cr release may be a problem, particularly if low cytolytic activities make it necessary to prolong incubation of reaction mixtures. In general, long term assays (>24 hr) are not feasible, and best results are obtained in short-term (3- to 6-hr) assays. (If effector cell frequencies are too low, it may be possible to partially purify the lymphoid cell population to be tested, or to activate and/or expand effector cell [CTL] precursors by specific stimulation with antigen.) Another limitation is the relatively large number of target cells (up to 10^4 per tube or well) which may be required to obtain measurable reactions, although with sufficiently high specific activities of ^{51}Cr, as few as 100 to 200 target cells per microwell have been used successfully. (See Section III-A.) Variations in sensitivity of target cells to lysis may also influence results of the ^{51}Cr-release assay considerably. Generally, adherent cells, such as fibroblasts and non-lymphoid tumor cells are less sensitive than nonadherent cells, such as lymphoblasts and lymphoma cells, with the exception of macrophages, which were found to be quite sensitive. Red blood cells are not lysed by either CTL, K, or NK cells. Differences in sensitivity should be considered when cytolytic activities of different lymphoid cell populations are compared using different target cells.

Since the test has been introduced for the assay of CTL[2] various modifications have been proposed. Most of them concern the reduction of cell numbers by optimizing the geometry of the culture vessels, but none appears to provide any fundamental improvements. Usually, the cells are placed into round or V-bottomed wells of stationary microplates. V-shaped cells wells allow smaller numbers of target and lymphoid cells to be tested with greater efficiency, but also lead to overcrowding conditions when the number of lymphoid cells is above a certain upper limit.

Although ^{51}Cr-release assay does not detect effector cell activity at the single cell level, it is frequently used to estimate relative effector cell frequencies. Such estimates are based upon the establishment of dose-response curves for each lymphoid-cell population to be assayed. Usually, various numbers of immune lymphoid cells of a given population are incubated with a fixed number of target cells for 3 hr. When the percent of specific lysis (corrected for the spontaneous-release values) is plotted vs. the logarithm of the corresponding lymphocyte-target cell ratio, a series of curves which are parallel over a range of approximately 20 to 80% ^{51}Cr release may be obtained. If this is the case, as in the example presented in Figure 1, it is possible to compare directly the relative cytolytic potential of the different lymphoid-cell populations by comparing the number of cells required to give a fixed-lysis value. The number of cells required to lyse 50% of the 10,000 target cells in a standard 3-hr ^{51}Cr-release assay has been arbitrarily defined as 1 lytic unit (LU).[3] In this manner, LU per 10^6 cells and LU per culture can be used as relative measures of the frequency and total number of CTL, respectively, in any given immune-cell population. When CTL are assayed, immunological specificity is usually tested by using "control" target cells which, in theory, should not be recognized and killed by specifically sensitized CTL. Examples of such controls are target cells syngeneic with the responding strain, or if available, appropriately chosen unrelated allogeneic (third party) target cells. Usually, at least a 100-fold difference in relative activities exists between lysis of specific (allogeneic) and control (syngeneic) target cells.

Figure 2 serves to illustrate a major limitation of the methods (see Section I). In this example, increasing numbers of normal spleen cells were added to a standard number of immune spleen cells, and each of the populations obtained was tested for cytolytic activity at various lymphoid cell to target cell ratios. As shown by the results, the slopes

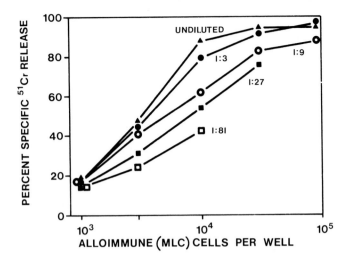

FIGURE 2. Cytolytic activity of MLC cells tested in the presence of increasing numbers of normal spleen cells. Secondary C57BL/6 anti-DBA/2 MLC cells were diluted with a suspension of normal C57BL/6 spleen cells to yield the various ratios of MLC : normal spleen cells indicated. The mixed cell populations were tested for cytolytic activity against ^{51}Cr-labeled P-815 cells at the various alloimmune (MLC) cell numbers per well indicated, using a 3 hr assay.

of the dose-response curves decrease with the presence of increasing numbers of normal spleen cells. Excess numbers of normal lymphoid cells may thus inhibit effector cell activity sufficiently to change the slope of the dose-response curves, and therefore direct comparisons of effector cell frequencies are no longer possible.

2. Methods*

a. Source of CTL

Since CTL appear only transiently in response to antigenic stimulation, it may be useful to establish the kinetics of CTL responses both in vivo and in vitro for each source of lymphoid cells. For in vivo stimulations, each route and form of antigen administration should be investigated, while, for in vitro stimulation, different culture conditions should be compared. High cytolytic activities may be observed in the following lymphoid-cell populations (listed in order of decreasing activity): secondary and primary MLC and MLTC,[5,6] in vivo populations (obtained following secondary or primary immunization) from the peritoneal cavity (obtained following i.p. immunization), from regional lymph nodes, spleen, thoracic duct, and peripheral blood.[7] Increased CTL activities are observed when phagocytic and adherent cells are removed from immune peritoneal cells,[8] when immune lymphoid cells are preincubated,[9] or when 2° MLC or MLTC population are stimulated, specifically or nonspecifically with T-cell mitogens or culture supernatants from 2° MLC.[10-13] Alloreactive CTL may also be obtained by transfer of lymphoid cells into lethally irradiated allogeneic recipients.[14]

b. Target Cells

Cells maintained in culture, as well as freshly isolated cells, show considerable variation in sensitivity to lysis and in amount of spontaneous ^{51}Cr release. However, even cells with a high spontaneous ^{51}Cr release (such as lymphocytes and thymocytes) can

* For additional details, see Reference 4.

be used as targets, provided the cytolytic activitiy of the cells to be assayed is sufficiently high to allow a short-term assay. Nonadherent cells such as lymphoblasts and lymphoma cells are not only more convenient targets, but also generally more sensitive than adherent cells. Adherent target cells can either be trypsinized, labeled in suspension and directly dispensed in the assay like nonadherent target cells, or, if spontaneous release of label becomes too high, they may be established as monolayers in individual assay tubes or microplate wells and labeled *in situ*.

c. ^{51}Cr Labeling of Target Cells

Target cells in suspension are washed with culture medium and the supernatant aspirated to leave 0.1 to 0.2 mℓ of medium. To this pellet, 0.1 mℓ of Tris-phosphate buffer-5% FBS and 0.1 mℓ or more (up to an equal volume for maximum labeling) $Na_2{}^{51}CrO_4$ solution (1 mCi/mℓ; specific activity 200 or more mCi/mg) per 2 × 10^6 target cells are added, and the cells incubated at 37°C for 45 to 60 min with occasional gentle shaking. The labeled cells are then washed three times with assay medium containing 5 to 10% FCS—10mM HEPES with a minimum of pipetting, and finally adjusted to 10,000 viable cells per mℓ. Adherent target cells established as monolayers in individual tubes or wells are labeled by adding $Na_2{}^{51}CrO_4$ solution (1 μCi in 0.1 mℓ per well) for up to 24 hr, followed by careful washing of tubes or wells.

d. Assay Procedure

Aliquots of serial 3.3-fold dilutions of lymphoid cells are added in 0.2-mℓ volumes to round-bottomed plastic tubes or in 0.1 mℓ volumes to U- or V-shaped microplate wells containing a fixed number of target cells (usually 10^4) in suspension (0.2 mℓ per tube) or cell ratios of 100, 30, 10, 3, and 1. For short-term (e.g., 3 hr) assays, the tubes or plates may be centrifuged at 200 g for 60 sec before incubation at 37°C in a CO_2 incubator (tubes may be gassed individually with 5% CO_2 in air, stoppered, and incubated in a water bath or ordinary incubator). After the chosen incubation period (generally 3 hr), 0.6 mℓ volumes of PBS are added to the tubes, and 0.5 mℓ volumes of the supernatant are collected for counting after centrifugation of the tubes at 600 g for 5 min. Samples of supernatants (100 $\mu\ell$) from microplate wells are removed directly by automatic eight-channel pipette. The amount of ^{51}Cr released is determined using liquid scintillation counting techniques with a five-fold enhancement of counting efficiency.)[15] For a standard 3-hr test, spontaneous release values (target cells incubated without effector cells) usually range from 5 to 15% while maximal release values range from 75 to 90% of the total isotope incorporated. Maximal release using the tube method is defined either by freeze-thawing three times (0.2 mℓ of target cells and 1.8 mℓ of H_2O), or if available, the plateau value observed at an excess of effector cells. Maximal release from target cells placed in microplate wells is determined by adding a given volume of detergent (for instance, NP-40*) and removing a sample for counting after 1 hr of incubation. For adherent target cells established as monolayers, it may be necessary to count both the supernatants and the cell pellets to obtain an accurate measurement of total ^{51}Cr activity present per individual assay tube or well.

e. Quantitation of Results

The method for calculation of specific cytolysis found by most investigators to be adequate for short-term assay conditions (where spontaneous release is less than 30%)

---

*   Nonidet P-40. Particle Data Laboratories.

is based on calculation of specific lysis for each lymphocyte to target cell ratio using the formula:

$$\% \text{ specific lysis } = \frac{\text{c.p.m. (exp.)} - \text{c.p.m. (spont.)}}{\text{c.p.m. (max.)} - \text{c.p.m. (spont.)}} \times 100$$

where spontaneous release is determined with or without lymphocytes present, and experimental release is that seen in the presence of immune lymphocytes. Maximal release is the plateau value observed in the presence of an excess of immune lymphoid cells, or the value observed after either freeze-thawing or detergent treatment of control target cells.

The specific ^{51}Cr-release values thus obtained are then plotted versus the $\log_{10}$ of the lymphocyte-to-target cell ratio using semilog graph paper. A curve linear between 20 and 80% lysis is usually observed, with one lytic unit (LU) arbitrarily defined as that number of lymphocytes required to yield 50% lysis of the given number of target cells in the chosen incubation time. Using this value, the number of LU present in 10^6 cells or per culture (or organ) can then be calculated.

f. Comments

Several comments concerning the technique of the ^{51}Cr-release assay should be made. (1) The geometry of the assay vessel is important. While round-bottomed tubes or wells appear to be optimal, over-crowing conditions with high effector cell concentrations are reached earlier than in the flat-bottomed tubes originally described. V-bottomed microplate wells may yield higher cytolytic values than U-bottomed wells under conditions where cell-to-cell contact is limited by low target cell numbers. (2) Labeled cells are generally more fragile than unlabeled cells, and should be manipulated as gently as possible (e.g., it may be advantageous to use centrifugation through a 50 to 100% FCS step gradient to wash the cells instead of repeated centrifugations. (3) If the test requires use of small numbers of target cells, labeling can be increased by mixing equal volumes of cells suspended in 5% FCS-Tris-phosphate buffer and Na$_2$^{51}CrO$_4$ solution and extending the incubation period to 75 min. This may yield 1 to 5 cpm per cell, and does not appear to lead to increased spontaneous release of ^{51}Cr (see also Section III). Use of 5% FBS-Tris-phosphate buffer permits more rapid, increased ^{51}Cr uptake as compared to conventional culture media. Target cells are generally considered satisfactory for the ^{51}Cr-release assay if they incorporate between 0.1 and 1.0 cpm per cell (hence permitting the routine use of between 1,000 and 10,000 target cells per individual assay). In addition, they should exhibit a spontaneous release value of less than 30% over the chosen test interval. Generally, control spontaneous release values are measured with target cells and assay medium only, yielding results identical to those where normal lymphoid cells are included. However, in some systems, high concentrations of nonimmune lymphoid cells may have a protective or a cytolytic effect. In systems where spontaneous release values are too high (greater than 30% for example), it may be more appropriate (in order to avoid overcompensating for high spontaneous release values) to use the formula:

$$\frac{\text{c.p.m. (exp.)} - \text{c.p.m. (spont.)}}{\text{c.p.m. (total)}} \times 100$$

or simply

$$\frac{\text{c.p.m. (exp.) or c.p.m. (spont.)}}{\text{c.p.m. (total)}} \times 100$$

For systems where nonimmune lymphoid cells are lytic or protective, as well as in other undefined systems, it is recommended that the actual experimental values be presented.

3. Mathematical Models

The cytolytic actvity of immune lymphoid cell populations is a function of both the frequencies and efficiences of effector cell subpopulations within the total lymphoid-cell population. Current data analysis methods for the ^{51}Cr-release assay now in widespread use do not, however, provide sufficient information concerning these two parameters of frequency and efficiency, nor do they always determine reliable values for the resultant function of cytolytic activity (see Section I). In an effort to define equations with coefficients related to these parameters, several attempts have been made to establish mathematical models for the kinetics of lymphocyte-mediated cytolysis.

Mathematical models for the kinetics of cytolysis can be classified into two groups: saturation models and collision models. Saturation models are based on reaction rates and assume that cytolysis is a steady-state process, while collision models are based on interaction probabilities and assume that effector- target-cell interactions occur randomly. In essence, saturation models employ enzyme-kinetics theory, while collision models employ Poisson-statistics theory. The saturation model was first investigated by Thorn and Henney.[16] They analyzed the kinetics of cytolysis by the direct application of the Michaelis-Menten enzyme-kinetics equation to killing and inhibition experiments, with the use of Eadie-Hofstee and Lineweaver-Burke plots. Thoma et al.[17] continued this analysis by examining the validity of predictions based on this model for the expected appearance and behavior of "traditional" cytolysis plots (fraction-specific release vs. logarithm-lymphocyte concentration). The collision model was also first investigated by Henney.[18] He assumed that Poisson statistics applied to the interactions beween effector and target cells, that each interaction led to lysis, and that each effector cell could lyse only one target. Miller and Dunkley extended Henney's first assumption and corrected the third.[19] Thus, they assumed that effector-target cell interactions were analogous to collisions between ideal gas molecules, and that an effector cell could lyse more than one target cell. Chu further revised these assumptions.[20] Since effector and target cells must be bound together for a finite period of time in order for lysis to occur, effector- target cell interactions are not analgous to ideal gas collisions. In addition, any interaction which does occur does not necessarily lead to lysis. Thus, the most recent collision model (Chu[20]) incorporated a probability term for interactions based on binding times and a probability term for lysis following each interaction, whereas the previous collision model (Miller and Dunkley[19]) incorporated only a probability term for interactions based on effector cell speed and cell and container size. Both collision and saturation models have been presented with supporting evidence. Both provide equations which linearize ^{51}Cr-release data and therefore determine coefficients related to the frequency and efficiency of effector cells. Neither, however, has yet been adequately substantiated to enable its use as a routine investigative tool.

Validation of a model for routine use must be accomplished by establishing: (1) the reproducibility of frequency- and efficiency-related parameters (slope and intercept coefficients), (2) the range of conditions (lymphocyte, target cell, and inhibitor cell concentrations) valid for the determination of these parameters, (3) high r^2 (coefficient of determination) values for linear regression curves, and (4) the range of data values (fraction specific release) valid for linear regression analysis with regard to both theoretical assumptions of the model and statistical considerations of the least square method. Deviations from linearity and discrepancies between experimental observations and theoretical predictions may be the result of faults of either the assay or the model: (1) the fraction of specific ^{51}Cr release may not equal the fraction of target cells lysed (assay), (2) cytolysis may not be a steady-state process (saturation model), (3) effector-target-cell interactions may not occur randomly (collision model), and (4) a single subpopulation of homogeneous effector cells may not approximate the behavior of what may in fact be many subpopulations of heterogeneous effector cells (both models). The verification of assumptions by direct means (e.g., observation of effector cell movement, effector-target-cell binding times, and target-cell lysis by microcinematography [Rothstein et al.[21]]) will be indispensable to the formal proof of any model ultimately established.

III. ENUMERATION OF CYTOLYTIC T LYMPHOCYTES AT THE SINGLE CELL LEVEL

A. "Micro" ^{51}Cr-Release Assay Under Limiting Dilution Conditions

1. General Considerations

The "micro" ^{51}Cr-release assay has been developed in an attempt to measure minimal frequencies of CTL in immune lymphoid-cell populations under "limiting dilution" conditions, i.e., under conditions where the lowest number of lymphocytes required to yield a positive cytolysis is determined.[22] The advantage of such a system resides in the fact that CTL frequencies so obtained are independent of any assumptions concerning the efficiency of killing (i.e., concerning for instance the number of target cells one CTL can lyse within a given time interval). Frequencies depend, however, on the sensitivity of the assay; results can only be considered as minimal estimates because they give no information concerning the killing efficiency of the CTL detected. In addition, results show that the sensitivity of the system is apparently not sufficient to detect a single lytic event, i.e., Poisson statistics are not applicable, as they are in the case of the limiting dilution assay for CTL precursors described under Section V. On the other hand, sensitivity is high enough to detect, under optimal conditions, frequencies of CTL which are of the same order of magnitude as those reported by several authors using a similar microassay,[23] a plaque assay,[24] or conjugate formation[25] for enumeration.

2. Methods*

Target cells, preferably highly sensitive lymphoma cells obtained either in the ascitic form or cultured and harvested when in logarithmic growth phase, are strongly labeled with $Na^{51}CrO_4$ (as described under II, A, 2, c), resulting in 1 to 5 c.p.m. per cell. Using either polyethylene microfuge tubes (Milian, Geneva) or V-bottomed microplates (Cook microtiter or equivalent) 100 to 200 target cells are placed into replicate tubes or wells (20 per lymphocyte to target cell ratio), in a total volume of 400 μl (tubes) or 150 μl (wells). To initiate the assay, tubes or plates are centrifuged (tubes in a Beckman microfuge, 13,000 × g for 1 min.) (plates at 200 × g for 1 min), and incubated for 6 hr at 37°C in a CO_2 incubator. Tubes or plates are then recentrifuged (tubes at 13,000 × g for 5 min) (plates at 200 × g for 5 min). To collect supernatants from microfuge tubes, the tubes are frozen at −90°C, the tips containing the cell pellet severed from the supernatants with a razor blade, and both portions counted in a gamma counter. This method was found to yield more reproducible results, since both portions of each assay tube can be counted, and the quantity of ^{51}Cr released into the supernatants calculated as a percentage of the total c.p.m. present in each tube. Supernatants from the microplates are withdrawn for counting using an automatic pipette. In this microplate modification of the assay, a mean value for the total c.p.m. added to each well

* For additional details, see Reference 22.

is determined by measuring 20 samples of target cells pipetted directly into the counting tubes. Significant lysis is considered to be three standard deviations greater than the spontaneous release values observed.

B. Enumeration of Cytolytic T Lymphocyte-Target-Cell Conjugates
1. General Considerations

The initial stages of cell-mediated cytolysis involve binding of effector cells to relevant target cells.[26-28] Evidence for such binding had first been provided by the observation that cytolytic activity could be depleted by selective immunoadsorption of CTL onto specific target cell monolayers. More recently, conjugate formation between CTL and allogeneic tumor target cells in suspension has been reported after low-speed centrifugation.[25,29,30] Such binding is energy- and temperature-dependendent, and requires the presence of Mg ions. In the presence of Ca ions, binding may induce lysis in a second independent step, which in turn leads to dissociation of conjugates. Since lysis is dependent on Ca ions, dissociation of conjugates can be inhibited (and conjugates stabilized) with EGTA, a Ca^{++} chelating agent. To facilitate microscopic counting of conjugates, the lymphoid cells containing effector cells are usually stained with a vital dye (fluorescein diacetate) before mixing with target cells. Studies of conjugates by direct observation or following isolation by micromanipulation confirmed that a majority (60 to 80%) of cells forming conjugates induce lysis. This suggested that quantitation of conjugates can be used to estimate frequencies of cytolytic cells.

When frequencies of conjugate-forming cells in various immune lymphoid cell populations were determined with this technique and compared to cytolytic activities as measured in a standard 3.5 hr ^{51}Cr-release assay, a lack of correlation was ocasionally observed.[31, 32] For instance, similar numbers of conjugate-forming cells were found in 1° CTL (generated in vivo or in MLC in vitro) and in 2° CTL (generated in vitro from immune spleen or from 1° MLC cells), but 2° CTL showed considerably higher cytolytic activity than 1° CTL.[32] Further studies revealed a correlation between rate rather than degree of conjugate formation and cytolytic activity, and suggested that 2° CTL were cytolytically more active because of their higher efficiency of binding and/or their ability to cycle, i.e., to repetitively kill target cells.

These results thus demonstrate that the determination of conjugates may give a more realistic estimate of actual CTL frequencies than the standard ^{51}Cr-release assay, which may overestimate CTL frequencies in populations containing CTL with high killing efficiency. On the other hand, the question of specificity of conjugate formation has not been entirely resolved. Although most of the conjugates formed appear to be specific, i.e., to be formed with target cells carrying the appropriate antigens, a low, but not negligible fraction (5 to 10%) of lymphoid cells was found to form conjugates with syngeneic (tumor) target cells.[32] Furthermore, the question of whether alloreactive T cells other than CTL (including helper T cells) form conjugates with appropriate target cells has not been resolved. Thus, the routine quantitation of CTL by this method awaits further studies of the specificity of conjugate formation.

2. Methods

The method follows essentially the one described by Glasebrook.[32]

a. Effector Cells

Conjugate-forming cells are readily detected in immune lymphoid cell populations highly enriched in CTL. Such populations are obtained either in vivo (for instance as peritoneal cells following intraperitoneal injection of allogeneic tumor cells), or in vitro (as primary- or secondary-MLC cells). The cells are first purified by removal of phagocytic cells, dead cells, and erythrocytes by carbonyl-Fe treatment and centrifugation over Ficoll®-Hypaque® (δ = 1.09), then stained with vital dye, for instance, fluorescein diacetate (FDA, Eastman Kodak, Rochester, N.Y.). For staining, 10 $\mu\ell$ of a 5 mg/mℓ solution of FDA in acetone is added to a suspension of up to 5 × 10^7 cells in 5 mℓ assay medium (DMEM containing 5% FCS and 1% HEPES). After 5 min at room temperature, the cells are washed twice and resuspended in assay medium containing 5mMEGTA to a concentration of 7.5 × 10^6 cells per mℓ.

b. Target Cells

In the allogeneic systems so far described, target cells were obtained as lymphoma or mastocytoma tumor cells (allogeneic or syngeneic to effector cells) cultured in vitro or maintained in vivo in the ascitic form. Ascitic tumor cells are first purified by removal of phagocytic cells by carbonyl-Fe treatment. Washed cells are suspended in assay medium containing 5 mMEGTA to a concentration of 7.5 × 10^6 cells/mℓ.

c. Conjugate Formation

FDA-stained lymphoid cells are mixed in round-bottomed plastic tubes or microplate wells with syngeneic or allogeneic target cells at a ratio of 1:1 and briefly centrifuged (250 × G for 3.5 min). After 20- to 30-min incubation at 37° C, the pellets are resuspended by means of a 100-$\mu\ell$ automatic pipette and the percentage of stained lymphoid cells attached to target cells is determined in a fluorescence microscope.

C. Enumeration of Cytolytic T-Lymphocyte Precursors (CTL-P) by Limiting Dilution Analysis

1. General Considerations

Since the immediate precursors of CTL (CTL-P) cannot at present be identified on the basis of unique surface markers or other physical characteristics, direct enumeration of these cells by conventional morphological or immunochemical techniques is not feasible. Recent developments in tissue-culture methodology have, however, provided an indirect means of estimating the frequency of CTL-P responding against alloantigens in a given cell population. In particular, it has been shown by several groups that the progeny derived, at least theoretically, from single CTL precursor cells can be detected in mixed-leukocyte microcultures (micro MLC) established under limiting dilution conditions.[33-37] By applying Poisson statistical analysis to the distribution of cytolytically positive and negative microcultures, it is thus possible to obtain a minimal estimate of the frequency of CTL-P in the population tested. An example of such an analysis for C57BL/6 thymus or spleen cells responding against DBA/2 alloantigens is shown in Figure 3. In this experiment, groups of 24 microwells containing various numbers of thymus or spleen cells were cultured in round-bottomed wells of microplates with 1 × 10^6 irradiated DBA/2 stimulating cells and supernatant from secondary MLC as a nonspecific stimulus. After 7 days, individual microwells were assayed for cytolytic activity against ^{51}Cr- labeled P-815 (DBA/2) mastocytoma cells. Positive wells were defined as those in which ^{51}Cr release exceeded the mean value in a parallel group of control microcultures (established in the absence of responding cells) by at least three standard deviations. In accordance with Poisson statistics, the percentage of negative cultures (on a logarithmic scale) was plotted against the dose of responding spleen cells. The frequency of the limiting cell type (in this case CTL-P) can be determined from the slope of such a plot. In the present example, a minimal CTL-P frequency of 1/926 for thymocytes and 1/312 for spleen cells can be inferred from the data. The same analysis can be applied to other tissues and allogeneic strain combinations, as well as to other responses in which CTL-P are generated (see also Sections C, 2 and C, 3, b).

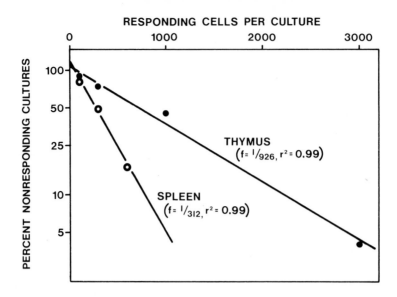

FIGURE 3.   Frequency of CTL-P directed against DBA/2 alloantigens in normal C57BL/6 spleen and thymus cell populations. Limiting numbers of normal C57BL/6 responding spleen and thymus cells were cultured in micro-MLC with 10^6 irradiated DBA/2 spleen cells and 2° MLC supernatant. 24 replicate cultures per number of responding cells were incubated for 7 days and assayed for cytotoxcity against ^{51}Cr-labeled P-815 (DBA/2) target cells. Microcultures were scored as responding when ^{51}Cr release values exceeded the mean spontaneous release (seen in control microcultures without responding cells) by more than three standard deviations. The frequency (f) of CTL-P was calculated by linear regression analysis of the data. The coefficient of determination (r^2) is indicated for each responding cell population (for details, see Section C 3).

Two important general considerations should be kept in mind for the quantitative analysis of CTL-P frequencies by limiting- dilution techniques. First, it must be established that CTL-P are the only limiting cell type under the assay conditions employed and therefore that Poisson statistical laws can legitimately be applied to the distribution of cytolytically positive and negative micro MLC. Second, even if the above condition has been satisfied, it should be noted that frequency estimates determined in this fashion are minimal estimates which do not (and usually cannot) take into account possible variations in the plating efficiency of the cell type under investigation. This latter condition can be more readily illustrated by considering the effect of plating various numbers of a homogeneous clonogenic cell population (such as tumor cells) under limiting- dilution conditions. Here again, a distribution of positive and negative wells will be observed, and a frequency of responding (i.e., growing) tumor cells can be calculated from Poisson statistics. Since the starting tumor cell population in this case is homogeneous, it can be inferred that the frequency of responding cells is, in fact, a measure of the plating efficiency. In the case of a heterogeneous population such as lymphoctyes, however, no such calculation can be performed, and the magnitude of the plating efficiency of any subpopulation (such as CTL-P) is unknown.

2. Enumeration of Cells of the CTL Lineage

Little is known of the cellular or molecular events which accompany the acquisition of differentiated function by CTL. Towards this end, it would be useful to have a quantitative assay system for the enumeration of cells which belong to the CTL lineage, irrespective of whether or not they express cytolytic function. Although such an assay has not yet been rigorously established, recent experiments in our laboratory have shown that "primed" cells isolated from unidirectional mixed-leukocyte cultures at various times can be induced to form CTL directed against the stimulating alloantigens under limiting-dilution conditions.[38, 39] Frequency estimates of these primed responding cells, which behave operationally as CTL-P, indicate that enrichments of 20 to 100-fold (as compared to unprimed cells) can be readily obtained. Furthermore, the relative frequency of such cells increases dramatically between 2 and 4 days after priming, and the physical characteristics of these cells (as assessed by velocity-sedimentation cell separation) cannot be distinguished from those of CTL.[39] Since up to 50% of the cells in separated MLC-primed populations can respond to give rise to CTL in this system, and a striking quantitative correlation was observed between CTL activity and CTL-P frequency in such separated MLC populations, it seems likely (although not formally proven) that mature CTL (or some fraction thereof) can be enumerated by such a limiting-dilution assay. In addition, the fact that changes in the physical characteristics of the responding cell population can be detected after 2 days in MLC (prior to the expression of significant cytolytic activity) raises the possibility that more immature cells of the CTL lineage may also be quantitated under limiting-dilution conditions. Figures 4 and 5 shown an example of an analysis of the frequency of CTL-P directed against DBA/2 alloantigens before, and 5 and 14 days after priming of C57BL/6 spleen cells in unidirectional mixed-leukocyte culture (MLC). Results of LDA indicate a frequency of CTL-P of 1/305 in the normal spleen, of 1/5 in the 5 day- and of 1/9 in the 14-day MLC population, i.e., of an enrichment in CTL-P of 60-fold (5-day MLC) and of 34-fold (14-day MLC) after in vitro priming. Figure 6 presents results of a comparison of the cytolytic activity of the same day-5 and day-14 MLC populations in a standard ^{51}Cr- release assay. It can be seen that the day-14 MLC population has a 17-fold lower cytolytic activity in terms of $LU/10^6$ cells than the day-5 MLC population. This result contrasts with the only two-fold lower frequency of CTL-P in the day-14 MLC population as determined by LDA. These results thus confirm previous evidence suggesting that the LDA assay detects cells of the CTL lineage irrespective of whether or not they express cytolytic function, i.e., that it detects the original CTL-P, CTL, and "memory" CTL-P derived from CTL.[37-39]

3. Methods

The method is the one originally described by Ryser and MacDonald.[37]

a. Mixed Leukocyte Microcultures (Micro-MLC)

Cultures are established in Dulbecco's modified Eagles's medium supplemented as described previously with additional amino acids and 5×10^{-5} M 2-mercaptoethanol.[2] This culture medium is further supplemented with 10% (v/v) FCS and 33% (v/v) 2° MLC supernatant as a nonspecific stimulant.[12] Micro-MLC (24 per group) are established by mixing limiting numbers of responding leukocytes with 1×10^6 irradiated (2,000 rads) allogeneic spleen cells in a final volume of 0.2 mℓ in round-bottomed microwells (Greiner, Nurtingen, West Germany). Primed responding cells (obtained as 1° MLC populations) respond as well upon addition of either irradiated allogeneic or irradiated syngeneic spleen cells. [39] Culture plates are wrapped in aluminum foil to minimize evaporation and maintained at 37°C in a water-saturated atmosphere of 5% CO_2 in air. Cultures are generally assayed on day 7.

b. Mixed-Leukocyte Tumor-Cell Microcultures (Micro- MLTC)

The question may be asked whether CTL-P directed against virus and tumor asso-

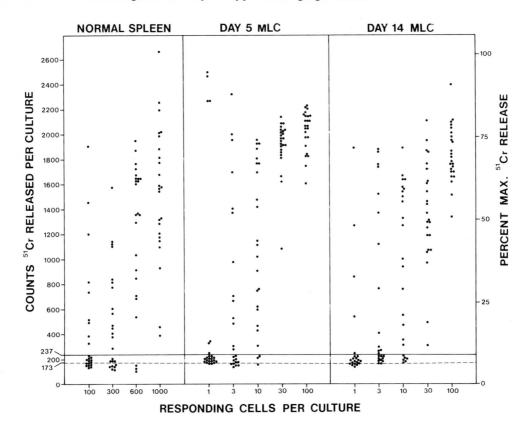

FIGURE 4.   Cytolytic activities of individual micro-MLC prepared with either normal spleen cells or day-5 and day-14 MLC cells as responding cells. Limiting numbers of normal C57B1/6 spleen cells or cells recovered after 5 and 14 days from unidirectional MLC (C57BL/6 anti-DBA/2) were cultured in micro-MLC with 10^6 irradiated DBA/2 spleen cells and 2° MLC supernatant. After 7 days all three sets of micro-cultures (containing 24 replicate cultures per number of responding cells) were assayed for cytotoxicity against ^{51}Cr- labeled P-815 (DBA/2) target cells. The dotted line represents the mean spontaneous release determined in groups of 24 control cultures containing no responding cells. The solid line represents the mean ^{51}Cr release plus three standard deviations, which defines the lower limit of positive cytolytic activity.

ciated antigens, non-H-2 linked histocompatibility determinants and chemically modified membrane constituents can also be detected by LDA. Teh et al.[36] have recently shown that CTL-P directed against TNP-modified syngeneic cells can be detected and their specificity analysed by LDA. Results in our laboratory have shown that CTL-P could also be enumerated by LDA in a syngeneic tumor system in which CTL directed against MSV-MLV associated antigens were generated.[40] Optimal micro-MLTC conditions were established by mixing limiting numbers of responding leukocytes (normal or regressor spleen cells or MLTC cells) with 3×10^4 syngeneic irradiated (5000r) lymphoma cells and 10^6 syngeneic irradiated (2000r) spleen cells in culture medium containing 33% 2° MLC supernatant.

c. Target Cells
Target cells of the appropriate haplotype are usually obtained as lymphoma or mastocytoma tumor cells maintained in culture or in ascitic form and labeled with $Na_2^{51}CrO_4$ as described in Section II,A2, c for use in cytotoxicity assays. Alternatively, especially for specificity studies, peritoneal macrophages, lectin-induced lymphoblasts or FCS-primed lymph node cells may be more adequate. The latter may be obtained by cultur-

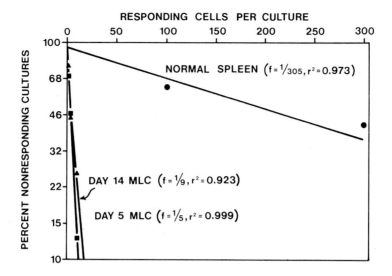

FIGURE 5. Increase in CTL-P frequency after 5 and 14 days in MLC. The frequency (f) of CTL-P directed against DBA/2 alloantigens before MLC and after 5 and 14 days in MLC was calculated by linear regression analysis of the data presented in Figure 4. Nonresponding cultures are those which were negative for cytolytic activity against ^{51}Cr-labeled P-815 target cells. The coefficient of determination (r^2) is indicated for each line.

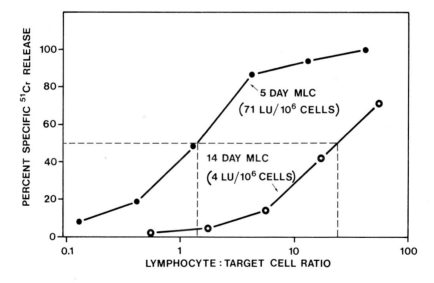

FIGURE 6. Cytolytic activity of day 5 and day 14 MLC cells. The same day 5 and day 14 C57BL/6 anti-DBA/2 MLC populations used for CTL-P frequency determinations (Figures 4 and 5) were tested for cytolytic activity against ^{51}Cr-labeled P-815 (DBA/2) target cells at the lymphocyte : target cell ratios indicated, using a 3 hr assay. Lytic units/10^6 cells were determined as indicated in Section II 2 e.).

ing inguinal and periaortic lymph node cells from mice injected 6-7 days previously at the base of the tail with FCS in complete Freund's adjuvant.[41] These FCS-primed lymph node cells are cultured with 2% FCS-supplemented medium in 16-mm diameter tissue- culture plates (Costar, Cambridge, Mass.)[44] Cultures initially containing 2×10^6 cells in 2-mℓ medium are harvested after 3- to 4-days incubation and labeled with $Na_2{}^{51}CrO_4$.

d. Assay for Cytolytic Activity

After 7 days of culture, 0.1 m of medium is removed from each microwell and replaced by 0.1 ml of ^{51}Cr labeled target cells. The plates are centrifuged and then incubated for 4 hr at 37°C. Cytolysis is assessed by counting the radioactivity of 0.1 ml of supernatant for 1 to 2 min in a well-type scintillation counter. For the determination of spontaneous release, control microcultures containing irradiated stimulating spleen leukocytes, 2° MLC SN, and FCS in the absence of responding cells, are assayed in the same manner. Micro-MLC are defined as positive for CTL activity when ^{51}Cr-release exceeds the mean spontaneous ^{51}Cr-release by at least three standard deviations. Specific lysis is calculated as described in Section II, A, 2, e.

e. Calculation of CTL-P Frequencies

Minimal estimates of CTL-P frequencies are calculated as described previously.[42] Briefly, microcultures are scored as responding or nonresponding on a statistical basis; namely, responding cultures are defined as those with ^{51}Cr-release values exceeding the mean spontaneous release by more than three standard deviations. The best fit lines describing the relationship between the number (x) of responder cells added per microculture and the fraction of nonresponding cultures per group (y) are fit by the least-squares method to the equation

$$\ln y = -fx + \ln a^{*}$$

This equation describes the zero order term of the Poisson equation. Theoretically, if the relationship between the number of responding cells and the resulting fraction of nonresponding cultures follows one-hit kinetics, the data should describe the above equation in which the y-axis intercept (a) equals 1.0 (100 percent nonresponding cultures), and the frequency (f) of the limiting event (in this case a CTL-P) is equal to the negative slope of the curve. The results of CTL-P frequency determinations are thus presented as three values determined by linear regression analysis using experimental x and y values: the frequency f, the y-axis intercept a, and the coefficient of determination r^2. A more detailed explanation of these calculations may be found in Reference 42.

IV. CONCLUSIONS

Four methods for the quantitation of CTL and/or CTL precursors are described, one operating at the population level, and three at the single-cell level. In choosing one of these four methods, its advantages and limitations should be taken into consideration. The ^{51}Cr-release assay as applied in the determination of cytolytic activities at the population level is simple to use, quantitative, and reproducible, and probably allows estimates of relative effector cell frequencies in selected systems without, however, giving information on differences in killing efficiency. A "micro" ^{51}Cr-release assay allows minimal estimates of CTL frequencies under limiting-dilution conditions. Frequencies so obtained are independent of any assumptions concerning killing efficiency, however, the assay is not sufficiently sensitive to detect individual CTL. Enumeration of lymphocyte-target cell conjugates allows the direct quantitation of a population which is highly enriched in CTL, but routine quantitation of CTL by this method awaits further studies of the specificity of conjugate formation. Finally, the enumeration of CTL precursors has become possible by limiting-dilution analysis in

---

*   A comparison of statistical methods for determining CTL-P frequencies indicates that a log likelihood maximation procedure is more valid than linear regression.

micro MLC. This method appears to provide an optimal assay system at the single-cell level, providing not only information on frequencies, but also on the specficity of individual CTL-P and their progeny. However, all precursor frequency determinations made under limiting-dilution condition must be considered as minimal estimates which are dependent on the sensitivity of the culture and/or assay system.

REFERENCES

1. **Perlmann, P. and Cerottini, J.-C.**, Cytotoxic lymphocytes, in *The Antigens*, Vol. 5, Sela, M., Ed., Academic Press, New York, 1979, 173.
2. **Brunner, K. T., Mauel, J., Cerottini, J.-C., and Chapuis, B.**, Quantitative assay of the lytic action of immune lymphoid cells on ^{51}Cr-labeled allogeneic targets in vitro ; inhibition by isoantibody and by drugs, *Immunology*, 14,181, 1968.
3. **Cerottini, J.-C., Engers, H. D., MacDonald, H. R., and Brunner, K. T.**, Generation of cytotoxic T lymphocytes in vitro. I. Response of normal and immune mouse spleen cells in mixed leukocyte culture, *J. Exp. Med.*, 140, 703, 1974.
4. **Brunner, K. T., Engers, H. D., and Cerottini, J.-C.** The ^{51}Cr release assay as used for the quantitative measurementent of cell mediated cytolysis in vitro, in *In Vitro Methods in Cell-Mediated and Tumor Immunity*, Bloom, B. R. and David, J. R., Ed., Academic Press, New York, 1976, 423.
5. **MacDonald, H. R., Engers, H. D., Cerottini, J.-C., and Brunner, K. T.**, Generation of cytotoxic T lymphocytes in vitro. II. Effect of repeated exposure to alloantigens on the cytotoxic activity of long-term mixed leukocyte cultures, *J. Exp. Med.*, 140, 718, 1974.
6. **Plata, F., Cerottini, J.-C., and Brunner, K. T.**, Primary and secondary in vitro generation of cytolytic T lymphocytes in the murine sarcoma virus system, *Eur. J. Immunol.*, 5, 227, 1975.
7. **Cerottini, J.-C., and Brunner, K. T.**, Cell- mediated cytotoxicity, allograft rejection and tumor immunity, *Adv. Immunol.*, 18, 67, 1974.
8. **Brunner, K. T. and Cerottini, J.-C.**, Cytotoxic lymphocytes as effector cells of cell- mediated immunity, in *Progress in Immunology*, Amos, B., Ed., Academic Press, New York 1971, 385.
9. **Ortiz De Landazuri, M., and Herberman, R. B.**, In vitro activation of cellular immune response to Gross virus-induced lymphoma, *J. Exp. Med.*, 136, 969, 1972.
10. **Heininger, D., Touton, M., Chakravarty, A. K., and Clark, W. R.**, Activation of cytotoxic function in T lymphocytes, *J. Immunol.*, 117, 2175, 1976.
11. **Bonavida, B.**, Concanavalin A-Mediated activation of antigen-primed lymphocytes into secondary cytotoxic lymphocytes, *J. Exp. Med.*, 145, 293, 1977.
12. **Ryser, J.-E., Cerottini, J.-C., and Brunner, K. T.**, Generation of cytolytic T lymphocytes in vitro. IX. Induction of secondary CTL responses in primary long-term MLC by supernatants from secondary MLC, *J. Immunol.*, 120, 370, 1978.
13. **Ryser, J.-E., Cerottini, J.-C., and Brunner, K. T.**, Cell- mediated immunity to antigens associated with murine sarcoma virus induced tumors: augmentation of cytolytic T lymphocyte activity by successive specific and nonspecific stimulation in vitro, *Eur. J. Immunol.*, 9, 179, 1979.
14. **Cerottini, J.-C , Nordin, A. A., and Brunner, K. T.**, Cellular and humoral response to transplantation antigens. I. Development of alloantibody- forming cells and cytotoxic lymphocytes in the graft-versus-host reaction, *J. Exp. Med.*, 134, 553, 1971.
15. **Herscowitz, H. B. and McKillip, T. B.**, A simple method for liquid scintillation counting of ^{125}Iodine and ^{51}Chromium used in antigen binding and cytotoxicity studies, *J. Immunol. Methods*, 4, 253, 1974.
16. **Thorn, R. M. and Henney, C. S.**, Kinetic analysis of target cell destruction by effector T cells. I. Delineation of parameters related to the frequency and lytic efficiency of killer cells, *J. Immunol.*, 17, 2213, 1976.
17. **Thoma, J. A., Touton, M. H., and Clark, W. R.**, Interpretation of ^{51}Cr-release data : A kinetic analysis, *J. Immunol.*, 120, 991, 1978.

18. **Henney, C. S.**, Quantitation of the cell-mediated immune response. I. The number of cytolytically active mouse lymphoid cells induced by immunization with allogeneic mastocytoma cells, *J. Immunol.*, 107, 1558, 1971.

19. **Miller, R. G. and Dunkley, M.**, Quantitative analysis of the ^{51}Cr release cytotoxicity assay for cytotoxic lymphocytes, *Cell. Immunol.*, 14, 284, 1974.

20. **Chu, G.**, The kinetics of target cell lysis by cytotoxic T lymphocytes : A description of Poisson statistics, *J. Immunol.*, 120, 1261, 1978.

21. **Rothstein, T. L., Mage, M., Jones, G., and McHugh, L. L.**, Cytotoxic T lymphocyte sequential killing of immobilized allogeneic tumor target cells measured by time-lapse microcinematography, *J. Immunol.*, 121, 1652, 1978.

22. **Engers, H. D. and Fitch, F. W.**, An estimate of the minimal frequency of cytolytic T lymphocyte effector cells general in allogeneic reactions, *J. Immunol. Methods*, 25, 13, 1979.

23. **Fischer-Lindahl, K. and Wilson, D. B.**, Estimates of the absolute frequency of killer cells generated in vitro, *J. Exp. Med.*, 145, 500, 1977.

24. **Bonavida, B., Ikejiri, B., and Kedar, E.**, Direct estimation of frequency of cytotoxic T lymphocytes by a modified plaque assay, *Nature (London)*, 263, 769, 1976.

25. **Berke, G., Gabison, D., and Feldman, M.**, The frequency of effector cells in populations containing cytotoxic T lymphocytes, *Eur. J. Immunol.*, 5, 813, 1975.

26. **Stulting, R. D. and Berke, G.**, Nature of lymphocyte-tumor interactions. A general method for cellular immunoadsorption, *J. Exp. Med.*, 137, 932, 1973.

27. **Martz, E.**, Mechanism of specific tumor cell lysis by alloimmune T-lymphocytes: resolution and characterization of discrete steps in the cellular interaction, *Contemp. Top. Immunobiol.*, 7, 301, 1977.

28. **Golstein, P. and Smith, E. T.**, Mechanism of T-cell-mediated cytolysis: The lethal hit stages, *Contemp. Top. Immunobiol.*, 7, 273, 1977.

29. **Martz, E.**, Early steps in specific tumor cell lysis by sensitized mouse T lymphocytes. I. Resolution and characterization, *J. Immunol.*, 115, 261, 1975.

30. **Zagury, D., Bernard, J., Thiernesse, N., Feldman, M., and Berke, G.**, Isolation and characterization of individual functionally reactive cytotoxic T lymphocytes : conjugation, killing and recycling at the single cell level, *Eur. J. Immunol.*, 5, 818, 1975.

31. **Grimm, E. A. and Bonavida, B.**, Studies on the induction and expression of T cell mediated immunity. VI. Heterogeneity of lytic efficiency exhibited by isolated cytotoxic T lymphocytes prepared from highly enriched populations of effector-target cell conjugates, *J. Immunol.*, 119, 1041, 1977.

32. **Glasebrook, A. L.**, Conjugate formation by primary and secondary populations of murine immune T lymphocytes, *J. Immunol.*, 121, 1870, 1978.

33. **Skinner, M. A. and Marbrook, J.**, An estimation of the frequency of precursor cells which generate cytotoxic lymphocytes, *J. Exp. Med.*, 143, 1562, 1976.

34. **Fischer-Lindahl, K., and Wilson, D. B.**, Histocompatibility antigen-activated cytolytic T lymphocytes. II. Estimates of the frequency and specificity of precursors, *J. Exp. Med.*, 145, 508, 1977.

35. **Teh, H.-S., Harley, E. Phillips, R. A., and Miller, R. G.**, Quantitative studies on the precursors of cytotoxic lymphocytes. I. Characterization of a clonal assay and determination of the size of clones derived from single precursors, *J. Immunol.*, 118, 1049, 1977.

36. **Teh, H.- S., Phillips, R. A., and Miller, R. G.**, Quantitative studies on the precursors of cytotoxic lymphocytes. V. The cellular basis for the cross-reactivity of TNP-specific clones, *J. Immunol.*, 121, 1711, 1978.

37. **Ryser, J.-E. and MacDonald, H. R.**, Limiting dilution analysis of alloantigen reactive T lymphocytes. I. Comparison of precursor frequencies for proliferative and cytolytic responses, *J. Immunol.*, 122, 1691, 1979.

38. **Ryser, J.-E. and MacDonald, H. R.**, Limiting dilution analysis of alloantigenreactive T lymphocytes. III. Effect of priming on precursor frequencies, *J. Immunol.*, 123, 128, 1979.

39. **Maryanski, J. L., MacDonald, H. R., and Cerottini, J.-C.**, Limiting dilution analysis of alloantigen-reactive T lymphocytes. IV. High frequency of cytolytic T lymphocyte precursor cells in MLC blasts separated by velocity sedimentation, *J. Immunol.*, 124, 42, 1980.

40. **Brunner, K. T., MacDonald, H. R., and Cerottini, J.-C.**, Antigenic specificity of the cytolytic T lymphocyte (CTL) response to murine sarcoma virus-induced tumors, *J. Immunol.*, 124, 1627, 1980.

41. **Corradin, G. and Chiller, J. M.**, Lymphocyte specificity to protein antigens. II. Fine specificity of T cell activation with cytochrome c and dervied peptides as antigenic probes, *J. Exp. Med.*, 149, 436, 1979.

42. **Taswell, C., MacDonald, H. R., and Cerottini, J.-C.**, Limiting dilution analysis of alloantigen-reactive T lymphocytes. II. Effect of cortisone and cyclophosphamide on cytolytic T lymphocyte precursor frequencies in the thymus, *Thumus*, 1979, 1, 119, 1979.

43. **Louis, J.**, personal communication.

Chapter 5

PRACTICAL ASPECTS OF MURINE B LYMPHOCYTE CLONING

Paul W. Kincade

TABLE OF CONTENTS

I. INTRODUCTION

A number of characteristics would be desirable in any functional assay for B lymphocytes. A simple and ideally linear relationship should exist between the number of effector cells present and the amount of activity measured, and this should be unaffected by number and degree of activation of other cell types. The assay should be sufficiently sensitive to permit multiple manipulations of cell suspensions from individual animals. For many purposes, it would be desirable if the system detected every viable B cell, or at least if all subpopulations of B cells responded with equal efficiency. Finally, the technique should be reasonably easy to perform and sufficiently flexible, to allow thorough characterization of the responding cells and investigation of the process of activation. Probably no existing system would satisfy all these requirements, and individual techniques differ greatly in applications, advantages, and disadvantages. At one extreme are mitogen- or antigen-stimulated bulk-culture assays where cells are held at relatively high density. Under such conditions, only a small proportion of potentially reactive cells may actually respond, and their function is subject to the regulatory influences of T-cell or macrophage-derived helper and suppressor factors, feedback antibody, and anti-idiotype antibody. No doubt such cultures are useful for reproducing complex in vivo interacting systems, but they are of limited value for enumerating and characterizing B cells. A very different situation applies in various limiting dilution-type assays that have recently been developed. Here the goal is to partition individual lymphocytes in nutritionally optimal medium with maximal enhancing and minimal inhibitory factors present. Over the last few years we have found a simple mitogen-stimulated cloning technique[1] to be both versatile and reliable for studies of murine B-cell heterogeneity and development. Practical aspects of this semisolid agar technique, its limitations, and the apparent efficiency with various B-cell subpopulations are detected, will be the focus of this chapter.

II. DETAILED DESCRIPTION OF THE METHOD

A. Medium

The recipe for complete McCoy's medium detailed below has been used by us for B-lymphocyte cloning as well as for various other semisolid agar culture assays over a four-year period. Most of the additives have been tested at above and below the concentrations given, and this formulation has been superior to several other commonly used media.

A stock solution of medium is prepared by dissolving powdered McCoy's modified 5a medium (Gibco®, Cat. #430- 1500) in triple-distilled H_2O. Unlike prepared liquid medium, powdered medium is usually sold without bicarbonate, and we add 2.2 g/ℓ $NaHCO_3$ at this stage, along with 0.1 g/ℓ streptomycin, and 105 units/mℓ of penicillin G. This stock solution is Millipore® filter-sterilized and stored for up to three months at 4°C. On the day of use, the following are mixed together for each 100 mℓ of complete medium for B-lymphocyte cloning:

- 15 mℓ fetal calf serum
- 85 mℓ McCoy's stock
- 0.6 mℓ sodium bicarbonate solution (7.5%)
- 1.0 mℓ sodium pyruvate solution (100 mM)
- 0.8 mℓ MEM essential amino acids (50×)
- 0.4 mℓ MEM nonessential amino acids (100×)
- 0.1 mℓ of 2-mercaptoethanol stock (0.175 mℓ concentrate per 50 mℓ H2O)

One frozen tube containing:

- 0.4 mℓ MEM vitamins mixture (100)
- 1.0 mℓ L-glutamine (200 mM)
- 0.16 mℓ L-asparagine (10 mg/mℓ)
- 0.04 mℓ L-serine (21 mg/mℓ)

Individual lots of calf serum can be quite different in their ability to support B-cell colonies, even when they are equivalent for other types of tissue cultures. We screen test batches from several suppliers and then reserve enough to last about one year. To date we have had more success with serum from Flow Laboratories than with serum from other sources. All lots of horse serum that we have tried are particularly toxic for murine B cells. It has been reported that serum can contain various mitogens, and indeed, some lots may contain endotoxin. For this reason and for general purposes, we also select serum on the basis of acceptably low backgrounds and good stimulation indexes in conventional, mitogen-stimulated liquid cultures. There is probably no such thing as a background-free serum since purified albumin containing medium sustains equivalent backgrounds to our best calf-serum-containing cultures.[2] Most lots of serum that we have used are optimal at 15% final concentration, but it is wise to test each lot at different concentrations. Heat inactivation slightly reduces the supportive potential of serum, and we also avoid filtering it.

Because mitogens native to laboratory-grade agar are important in stimulating B-lymphocyte clonal proliferation,[3] agarose cannot be used as a supporting matrix. Deliberate addition of mitogens to agarose or methocel allows colony formation, but this is much less efficient and more inconsistent than using Difco® Bacto® agar. We have compared various lots of Bacto® agar and found no significant differences between them. Mercaptoethanol is essential for B-lymphocyte cloning and is optimal at 5×10^{-5} M.[1,4]

B. Cell Preparation

In general, the techniques recommended by Shortman for preparation of viable cell suspensions are used.[5] Cell aggregates and clumps of tissue often persist in the cultures and while these can usually be discriminated from proliferating foci, they can be avoided by allowing them to settle out after layering the cell suspensions over fetal calf serum. To maintain neutral pH under atmospheric conditions and to sustain viability, cell washing and manipulations are done using RPMI-1640 medium containing HEPES buffer and 10% heat-inactivated fetal calf serum. On occasion, cell separation experiments have required that up to 24 hr elapse between the time of sacrifice and initiation of cultures. Satisfactory numbers of clonable B cells survived that treatment provided that they were maintained at 4°C. It was found that differences in cloning efficiency obtained by different individuals are often attributable to different cell counting procedures. Numbers of nucleated cells determined with ordinary light microscopes in the presence of acetic acid differ from counts done with phase-contrast microscopy, and these are also different from counts made with trypan blue. It is, therefore, important to be consistent. One should, of course, be careful that substances like heparin, ampholytes, and merthiolate are not present in the cell suspensions at the time of culture initiation.

C. Plating

Agar melts only when heated above boiling and we prepare a 10x stock solution in H$_2$O. Usually 1.5 g of Bacto® agar is placed in a loosely-capped Erlenmeyer flask with 50 mℓ of distilled-deionized H₂O. This is gradually melted in a boiling water bath or heated directly over an asbestos pad over a Bunsen burner. In the latter case, the flask must be continuously swirled to prevent sticking and scorching of the agar. All visible particles of agar must be melted, and this usually requires that the solution be brought to a boil several times. The agar solution is then allowed to cool to approximately 40°C and rapidly mixed 1:10 with complete McCoy's medium which has been brought to 37°C. This solution may be held for a short time at 37°C and cells may be added before or after agar addition. It should be noted that the osmolarity of the original medium is slightly reduced by addition of the agar solution but if necessary, it can be reduced a further 10% by addition of 0.1 mℓ of aqueous material to 1 mℓ cultures. B cells appear to tolerate such osmotic changes. The 35 mm tissue-culture dishes will have been arranged on incubator trays, numbered, and any necessary additives placed in them. For 1 mℓ cultures, it is best to keep the total volume of additives to 0.2 mℓ or less, so that the agar concentration will not be suboptimal. The warm solution of medium and cells is then quickly pipetted into the dishes with a 5 mℓ pipette or a repetitive pipettor. The dishes must be immediately swirled to achieve thorough mixing and allowed to stand undisturbed for 10 to 15 min at room temperature. Cultures can only be incubated after complete gelling has occurred. Otherwise, cells will settle to the bottom of the dish or there will be irregular strands of agar in the cultures. If this happens, clonal proliferation will be poor and colonies will by asymmetrical and difficult to enumerate. We have used Falcon® (Div. B. D. Co., Cockeysville, Md.) #1008 petri dishes or #3001 tissue culture dishes, as well as Lux® (Newbury, Park, Calif.) straight-sided #5221 or contour #5214 dishes with equivalent results. The contour dish offsets somewhat that extra thickness at the periphery of the dish which results from miniscus formation. The number of cells plated will, of course, depend on the incidence of B cells in the cell suspension and the potentiator(s) used. For spleen cells, 1 to 2 × 10⁴ nucleated cells per 1 mℓ culture is usually appropriate.

D. Potentiators

If semisolid agar cultures are prepared as described above, numbers and size of colonies will vary from experiment to experiment, and the assay will be nonlinear, particularly if cell suspensions are macrophage-deficient. That is, if twice as many cells are cultured, more than twice as many colonies result. This suggests that cell-cell interactions are occurring, that resulting colonies may not, in fact, be clones, and that the assay would be of little value for enumerating functional B cells. All of these problems can be avoided by use of one of three potentiators. The simplest of these to use is lipolysaccharide (LPS) of endotoxin.[3,4] We have always used *Salmonella typhosa* endotoxin WO 901 from Difco® and a final concentration of 25 μg/mℓ of our current lot is optimal. On one occasion we found purified lipoprotein to be ineffective and, as will be described later, the enhancing activity of LPS can be blocked by addition of polymyxin B or antilipid A antiserum to the cultures. This suggests that the lipid A moiety of LPS must be the active component. Washed sheep red blood cells (SRBC) can also be used to facilitate B-cell colony formation.[1] We have used 0.5 to 1.0% final concentrations of packed SRBC and these are added as 0.1 mℓ of a 5 to 10% solution in PBS. It can be shown that intimate contact between SRBC and B lymphocytes is unimportant by separation of the erythrocytes in a separate agar underlayer, or by forming a rim of SRBC in agar around the periphery of the dish before plating the lymphocytes in the center.[6,7] Neither SRBC stroma nor lysates are effective and, in fact, these may be inhibitory.[6] We have similar found that platelet suspensions or platelet lysates are inactive and RBC from sheep may be uniquely suitable. In our experience there is no consistent advantage of fresh sheep blood, and we routinely employ commercially supplied SRBC in Alsever's solution (Flow Labs.) used within 4 weeks of purchase. In studies of the effects of macrophages on B-lymphocyte function, we discovered a third means of potentiating colony formation.[8] Adherent macrophages elaborate soluble enhancing factor(s), as well as prostaglandins, which markedly affect colony formation; prostaglandin synthesis can be minimized by simply including in-domethacin in the cultures. Macrophages are obtained by injecting 1.5 mℓ thioglycol-late medium (Difco®) intraperitoneally and washing out the abdomen 4 days later with cold RPMI-1640 medium. We dissolve the powdered thioglycollate in H_2O, heat it to boiling, cool it, and replace the H_2O lost by boiling, and then store it for at least 2 days at room temperature before use. Usually 3 to 5×10^7 exudate cells are recovered from one mouse and approximately 75% of these are macrophages. These are washed twice in the cold and 10^5 nucleated cells are placed in each 35-mm tissue-culture dish in 15% FCS containing medium and incubated for 2 hours at 37°C. Nonadherent cells (mostly lymphocytes and polymorphs) are then aspirated off and the plates are thor-oughly washed three times to ensure that no clonable B cells are left. Approximately 20 to 30 % of the exudate cells remain in the dishes at this point and then 1.0 mℓ of cell-free 0.5% agar in complete McCoy's medium with 2ME and 1.4×10^{-7} M indo-methacin is allowed to gel over the adherent cells. Indomethacin (MW 357) is dissolved in absolute ethanol to make a 10^{-2} M stock which is diluted to a final concentration of 1.4×10^{-7} M. To ensure that the macrophages do not dry out during plating, only a few plates are aspirated at a time before adding the agar spacer layer. This can be conveniently done by two people. After the plates gel, they are stored at 37°C in a humidified incubator before use. The enhancing soluble factors produced by the ad-herent cells have not been characterized, but since the feeder layers must be used within 2-3 days of preparation, we assume they are important during the initial period of culture. There is a slight augmentation of colony formation with spacer layers even when no adherent cells are present. Presumably, this is due to the extra nutrients and mitogens in this underlayer. B-cell activating factor (BAF) derived from human mon-ocytes augments antibody responses of nude mice to SRBC,[9] but has no effect on B-lymphocyte cloning. Similarly, attempts to use medium from macrophage cell lines or the macrophage tumor cells themselves have so far been unsuccessful. If uninduced peritoneal cells are used rather than thioglycollate-induced exudate macrophages, the initial incubation period must be extended to 24 hr in order for sufficient numbers of cells to adhere. Careful study might reveal some correlation between the degree of macrophage activation and their effectivess as potentiators. It is noteworthy that mac-rophages from any strain can be used with B cells of different pedigree.[10]

All three of these potentiating systems optimize colony numbers and size and, most importantly, result in a linear relationship between numbers of cultured B cells and proliferating foci. As will be discussed later, the B cells which are detected under these various culture circumstances may not be completely overlapping. In addition, practi-cal considerations may dictate the choice of potentiating agents. The macrophage feeder layers release granulocyte-marcrophage colony-stimulating activities (CSA) and for this reason are inconvenient to use with fetal liver, newborn spleen, or adult bone marrow cultures. All of these tissues contain appreciable numbers of granulocyte-mac-rophage progenitors, and the B-cell colonies are thus obscured by the nonlymphoid colonies which develop. LPS-potentiated colonies probably differentiate more than do colonies potentiated in the other two ways, and the disperse nature of the colony cells minimizes the number of B cells that can be cultured. Finally, SRBC-containing cul-tures must be fixed with acetic acid to reveal B-cell colonies and this restricts further manipulations with the colony cells.

E. Incubation

Correct incubation conditions are crucial for optimal B-cell cloning. Proper humid-ification is essential to prevent drying of the cultures, and all surfaces of the incubator should be damp. A pan of water placed in the bottom of the incubator usually provides less humidification than pouring it directly on the chamber floor. It should be noted that CO_2 detectors on automatic incubators are very sensitive to changes in humidity. The pH of the cultures is governed by the CO_2 concentration, and since B cells form colonies in atmospheres of 5 to 10% CO_2 in air, we now use 7%. A small portable CO_2 detector (Fryryte, Bacharach Instrument Co., Pittsburgh, Pa.) is extremely help-ful for calibrating and monitoring incubator performance. We find that 6 days of incubation is optimal for colony formation and colonies degenerate after 7 days. Cul-tures should not be briefly removed, examined, and then returned to the incubator. This is detrimental for B-cell cultures, possibly due to their sensitivity to pH changes during the incubation period. Because of this, it is impractical to add things to the cultures after the third or fourth day of incubation, and examining them before scoring on the sixth day of culture is not recommended. Humid incubators provide ideal envi-ronments for mold growth, and care should be taken to avoid spilling medium on the trays. Between uses, trays should be washed or at least wiped off with 70% ethanol. When contamination becomes a problem, the incubator must be cleaned, and this is not a simple undertaking. For automatic units, the power must not be turned off unless the chamber is completely dry, so we shut off the gas supply and leave the unit on during cleaning. It is important not to use strong cleansers or disinfectants, as aerosols of these may remain for weeks and inhibit colony growth. We use dilute tissue culture detergent and follow this with numerous rinses with distilled H_2O. It is advisable to occasionally check replicate cultures placed in different locations within the incubator, or in different incubators, to reveal subtle gradients or incubator differences.

F. Scoring and Colony Morphology

Proliferating foci in semisolid cultures are three-dimensional and are conveniently enumerated with a stereoscopic dissecting microscope using slightly indirect, transmit-ted illumination at 40X magnification. There is an apparently continuous size distri-bution from very small aggregates to colonies of 500 or more cells. We arbitrarily consider aggregates of 20 or more cells to be colonies, but the cells which divide less than four times are responding B cells as well. It is necessary to continuously focus up and down with one hand while moving the dish with the other. When individual cul-tures contain more than 150 colonies, it is expedient to score only a proportion of the dish. For this purpose we use an inverted 60 × 15 mm tissue-culture dish with 2-mm grids (Lux®, Cat. No. 5216). An area corresponding to one third of the total plate is ruled off with a marking pen, and this serves as a platform for the 35-mm dish to be scored. If SRBC are used, these must by lysed by addition of less than 0.5 mℓ of 3% glacial acetic acid in H_2O. This should be carefully added drop-by-drop to avoid dis-rupting the gel. If it is impossible because of lack of time to score the colonies after 6 to 7 days of incubation, it is better to fix them all in this way and return them to the incubator for an additional day, than to continue incubation. Holding fixed cultures for prolonged periods makes them difficult to score, however, and we prefer to exam-ine LPS-potentiated cultures without fixing. When less than 10^6 lymphocytes are cul-tured, nonresponding cells lyse, leaving a background-free field on which to observe colonies. If, for any reason, more cells are added, or if the cell suspension is rich in monocyte-macrophages, a lawn of single cells will persist for the entire culture period. The gross appearance of colonies varies with the different potentiators. With SRBC, colonies are relatively tight with a majority of the cells actually touching. Their compactness makes it possible to score up to 500 colonies in a single culture. B-lymphocyte colonies in macrophage feeder-layer-potentiated cultures are very large and individual cells are usually slightly separated. With LPS-potentiated cultures the cells are very disperse and colonies are somewhat asymmetrical. B lymphocytes examined in this way generally look smaller and less refractile than cells in nonlymphoid colonies, and for most applications it is not necessary to identify the individual colonies as being lymphoid. However, when large numbers of fetal liver, adult bone marrow, or even spleen cells are cultured, there is sufficient endogenously produced CSA to result in some nonlymphoid colonies. This is particulary noticeable with tissues that are regenerating after irradiation. In these situations it is practical to set up replicate cultures containing anti-Ig antibodies.[11] This effectively prevents B-lymphocyte colony formation without inhibiting granulocyte-macrophage colonies. Alternatively, individual colonies can be removed and examined by immunofluorescence, or stained. We get poor cell recovery in suspensions of individual colonies, so generally immunofluorescene is done with pooled colony cells. Colonies can be transferred to ruled squares on microscope slides with disruption and 2.0% aceto-orcein (GIBCO®, Grand Island, N.Y.) used to reveal nuclear morphology. A much better classification can be achieved with a staining procedure intended for eosinophil colonies.[12]

G. Nonlymphoid Colonies

This B-lymphocyte cloning procedure is essentially an adaptation of techniques long used to clone granulocyte-macrophage progenitors,[13] and once the medium and equipment are available, by simply omitting 2ME and adding an appropriate source of CSA to the cultures, these can be studied as well. This has often provided an expedient control for toxicity or specificity of antibodies and other substances. The most readily obtained source of CSA is serum from mice injected 3 hr previously with 5 μg of LPS intravenously.[14] A wide variety of normal and neoplatic cells elaborate these factors, however, and for specific applications one might wish to review the considerable literature on this subject.[15]

H. Preparation of Agar-Derived Mitogens

On occasion we have found it interesting to study the effects of agar mitogens on B-cell proliferation and differentiation in conventional liquid cultures. Mitogens can be extracted from Bacto® agar with warm H_2O and then lyophilized with a typical yield of 80 mg/g of agar.[3]

III. RESULTS AND DISCUSSION

A. Subpopulations of B Cells Detected

The actual plating efficiency of this technique will not be known until the categories of responding B cells are fully defined. That is, some functionally restricted types of cells may not be detected, and their incidence in various populations has not been determined. With respect to B cells as a whole, and using any one potentiator alone, approximately 2 to 4% of the surface Ig positive (sIg⁺) cells divide to form colonies. This number exceeds 13% when all three potentiators are used in culture of lymph node cells.[8] In addition, there are many small B-cell aggregates present in these cultures which are difficult to enumerate. Homogeneous B-cell tumor lines clone under these conditions with up to 74% efficiency. We have tried adding lecithin, cholesterol, selenium, DEAE dextran, BAF, thymocytes, platelets, nucleotides, and conditioned medium from various tumor cell lines to the cultures, and varied concentrations of components of the medium, in an effort to improve cloning efficiency. None of these dramatically improved colony formation, and we consider serum selection and incubation conditions to be the most crucial variables.

A number of observations suggest that surface Ig negative (sIg⁻) precursors of B cells do not proliferate in semisolid agar cultures. Colony-forming cells emerge in fetal liver at the same time, 16.5 days, as sIg⁺ B cells.[7,16] Repeated injection of neonatal mice with purified anti-μ antibodies aborts B-cell development but spares cIg⁺, sIg⁻ "pre-B" cells.[17] The degree of suppression of sIg⁺ cells in various tissues of these mice coincides with reductions in numbers of clonable B cells. Over 95% of the sIg⁺ cells in suspensions of bone marrow, spleen, or lymph nodes can be removed by incubation on anti-Ig coated dishes, and colony-forming potential is reduced accordingly. Colony formation is also inhibited by the direct addition of anti-μ or anti-κ antibodies to the cultures. Finally, pre-B cells in marrow are thought to be actively dividing, whereas colony-forming cells in that tissue are largely out of cycle. These findings suggest that when pre-B cells are dispersed in semisolid cultures they fail to reach a functionally mature state during the initial culture period. On the other hand, if suspensions of sIg⁻ cells from fetal liver or bone marrow are cultured at relatively high cell density in liquid medium, functional sIg⁺ B cells spontaneously appear.[7,17] By using liquid cultures in tandem with the cloning technique, it should be possible to determine which kinds of cell-cell interactions govern the pre-B to functional B-cell transition. One could also examine the rate and mechanism of B-cell production in young, as compared to aged, mice.

The most immature B cells in fetal liver and spleen which form colonies are sIgM⁺ and bear the Lyb-2 alloantigen. Unlike clonable B cells found in all adult tissues, they resist killing with anti-Ia antisera plus complement and are not inhibited by anti-δ antibodies added directly to the cultures. These early B cells and a proportion of similar cells in neonatal spleen are also uniquely sensitive to preexposure to anti-Ig antibodies.[18] Essentially, all colony-forming B cells in adult tissues express Ia antigens, and they can be subdivided into three categories on the basis of IgD receptor expression and function. For example, approximatly 90% of the colony-forming cells in spleen must be sIgD⁺ because they are specifically depleted in dishes coated with hybridoma anti-δ antibody. If the anti-δ is added directly to the cultures, even in nanogram quantities, clonal proliferation is inhibited by about 60%. This suggests that spleen contains sIgD⁻ B cells, sIgD⁺ B cells whose function is insensitive to anti-δ, and a third category that receive a negative signal with respect to proliferation through surface IgD receptors.

Clonable cells are heterogeneous as B cells on the whole, with respect to complement receptor expression, buoyant density, size, and adherence.[19] Approximately 90% of splenic B cells adhere to nylon wool.[20] The non-adherent B cells do not bind during a second exposure to nylon, and these have three times the cloning potential of unfractionated B cells. The result is that column passage of spleen cells reduces numbers of colony-forming cells by only 60%. This illustrates heterogeneity of clonable cells with respect to adherence and should also be a caution to those who would employ this method of B-cell depletion.

When two potentiators are used together, the number of colonies obtained exceeds that which would result with either used alone. Often the number of proliferating foci in cultures containing SRBC and LPS approximates the sum obtained with each potentiator used separately.[3,8] This raises the possibility that the B cells detected in SRBC potentiated cultures may not be identical to those responding in LPS-containing cultures. Mindful of this possibility, most of our experiments are routinely performed in duplicate under the different conditions. To date it is not possible to conclude that completely different B cells are detected, but it is clear that the behavior of clones within SRBC- , as compared to LPS-containing cultures, is dissimilar. The relative cloning efficiency of B cells in newborn spleen, adult bone marrow, spleen, lymph nodes, and peripheral blood are roughly equivalent in LPS-containing cultures.[18] However, this is not true if SRBC are employed and then bone marrow B cells clone less well than do spleen cells.[21] Recently, we found that only LPS permits the detection of a very unusual category of B cells in the tissues of NZB mice.[22] These anti-μ resistant B cells were not observed with SRBC potentiated cultures. Also, SRBC cultures are more sensitive to inhibition with normal mouse serum than LPS-containing cultures.

The observations discussed thus far suggest that a wide variety of B-cell subpopulations, with the exception of pre-B cells, can be detected by this assay. However, another series of studies suggest that all B cells are not functional in this system. CBA/N strain mice have a partial immune deficiency which affects only some B cells and B-cell functions. For example, B cells from these mice are totally nonresponsive to certain nonmitogenic, T cell-independent antigens like haptenated Ficoll®, whereas substantial amounts of antibody are produced to antigens like SRBC. We have been unable to detect clonable B cells in any of the tissues of these mice at any stage of development.[7,10] B cells from CBA/N mice are responsive to mitogens, including the ones native to agar.[10] However, they neither proliferate or differentiate in low-cell density conditions such as pertain in semisolid cultures. This abnormality is controlled by an X-linked gene and whereas F$_1$ male CBA/N × CBA/H mice have no clonable cells, their female littermates have half the number of these found in homozygous normal CBA/H females.[23] Functional B cells are restored in lethally irradiated CBA/N mice given hemopoietic cells from normal CBA/H-T6T6 mice, and the donor chromosome marker is present in all of the newly-formed colony-forming cells.[7,23] It is also possible to graft CBA/N mice without prior irradiation, and this results in chimerism of B cells only.[24] The defect in these mice might selectively arrest the development of certain functionally specialized categories of B cells including those which are responsive in this system. In that case, it must be reasoned that the mutant gene product is important for an early event in B-lineage development.[25] Alternatively, even their residual B cells may be defective in some way. Presumably this question could be resolved by separating B cells from normal mice that have similar physical properties and markers to CBA/N cells, and then determining if these are clonable. Many of our studies of early events in B-cell differentiation have been facilitated by the use of CBA/N mice as recipients of various normal CBA/H-T6T6 precursor cells. Emergence of donor B cells can be unambiguously monitored with the cloning assay, and penetration of other hemopoietic compartments can be revealed by means of the chromosome marker.

B. Intrinsic Mitogens and the Importance of Endotoxin

That B-lymphocyte cloning was mitogen dependent followed from the observation that no colonies formed when agarose or methyl cellulose were used as a supporting matrix.[3] An aqueous extract of Bacto agar contained polysaccharide substances which were mitogenic for murine B cells in conventional liquid cultures, and this material allowed colony formation in agarose. From the limited studies that we have done on agar-derived mitogens, it appears that they correspond to the sulfated and nonsulfated polygalactans previously described in agar. [26] It is similar to dextran sulfate in that it stimulates division without much differentiation to antibody-secreting cells in liquid cultures, and proliferative responses to both mitogens differ from that of LPS in sensitivity to anti-μ antibodies.

Colony formation is enhanced by the deliberate addition of LPS, and numbers of cells which clone in SRBC-containing cultures are subnormal in C3H/HeJ[10] and C57BL/10CR strain mice. Both of these strains of mice are genetically unable to recognize the lipid A moiety of endotoxin, and this suggests that the presence of LPS in the culture system may be a requirement for optimal proliferation, even when SRBC are used. Alternatively, these mice may have a deficiency in numbers of these particular functional B cells. To determine which of these interpretations is correct, we added polymyxin B and anti-lipid A antiserum to the cultures. Both of these are known to efficiently complex with and inactivate LPS. When amounts of these inhibitors were added sufficient to bind 5 μg/mℓ of LPS, cloning of normal B cells in SRBC-containing cultures was not inhibited. From this result we tentatively conclude that the gene which controls LPS recognition in these mice influences, perhaps indirectly, development of functional B cells.

C. Regulation of the Response

An advantage of cloning procedures is that one can directly study the effects of humoral factors on individual cells. In this particular system, factors can be allowed to diffuse from a separate layer of cells or they may be added directly during plating. We have found a number of substances which affect B-cell activation and proliferation, and in some cases this can be used to reveal B-cell heterogeneity. The marked enhancing effect of diffusible substances from macrophages has been described above. In addition, macrophages elaborate prostaglandins and these similarly inhibit colonies developing in SRBC- or LPS-potentiated cultures.[8] Microgram quantities of divalent anti-μ or anti-$\varkappa$ antibodies inhibit clonal proliferation, and the Fc portion of the antibody molecules is not involved.[11] As discussed above, a proportion of B cells is sensitive to nanogram quantities of anti-δ antibodies, and antiserum to Ia antigens is also inhibitory. Deliberate binding of immune complexes to presumed Fc receptors does not affect the function of clonable cells. Normal mouse serum is inhibitory and our preliminary analysis suggests that more than one serum constituent is responsible. It is interesting that SRBC-potentiated cultures are more sensitive to inhibition by normal serum than LPS-containing cultures. Con-A-stimulated spleen-cell supernates also inhibit B-cell activation, presumably due to T-cell-derived factors similar to soluble immune response suppressor (SIRS).[27]

D. Limitations of the Method

Clonal proliferation in this system is mitogen-induced, and it is cumbersome to recover cells from the agar at the end of culture. In addition, very little differentiation of the responding cells to an Ig-secreting stage occurs, particulary if LPS is not used. For these reasons, the method is inappropriate for studies of specific humoral immune responses. Analyses of V-region gene expression can best be done with culture of splenic foci or liquid culture techniques employing filler cells.[28,29] Although a wide variety of B-cell categories are clonable, the studies with CBA/N mice suggest that one or more lineages of B cells may not be detectable. This selectivity could be advantageous or a limitation, depending on the application. It would be desirable to be able to serially propagate B-cell clones for extensive analysis, but subculturing has thus far not been successful. Perhaps a factor analogous to T-cell growth factor(s) will be found which will make this feasible.[30] The most notable limitation of this method is the fact that it only works for murine cells. We have been unable to clone B cells from rats, rabbits, guinea pigs, hamsters, chickens, or humans. It is probable that agar-associated mitogens do not efficiently stimulate the B cells of these species. Attempts by ourselves and others to grow human B-cell colonies with Staphylococcal mitogens have only resulted in marginal T-cell proliferation.[31]

E. Comparison With Other Cloning Techniques

This procedure is mechanistically similar to semisolid agar cloning techniques for progenitors of granulocytes, macrophages, megakaryocytes, eosinophils, and a type of immature precursor that forms mixed colonies composed of granulocytes, megakaryocytes, and erythroid cells.[13] Each of these are dependent on macromolecules, and it is believed that their analysis will reveal mechanisms whereby hemopoiesis is controlled. Several laboratories have successfully cloned T lymphocytes with appropriate mitogens, and it appears likely that this would be facilitated by a growth factor present in certain conditioned media.[32-34] Other limiting dilution assays partition B cells in irradiated spleens, or in an excess of filler cells, rather than the three-dimensional gel approach detailed here.[28,35,36] Perhaps the broadest spectrum of cell types can be detected with the splenic focus technique.[28,37] Here limiting numbers of B cells are injected into lethally irradiated, carrier-immunized mice, the spleens are removed and diced, and the fragments are cultured with antigen. The quality and quantity of antibody produced is usually determined by radioimmunoassay of the culture supernates. Approximately 80% of the B cells which settle in the spleen fragments produce antibody, and adaptations of the technique have revealed distinctions in immature, mature virgin, and memory B-cell populations. It would probably not be convenient to use this procedure to assess "burst" size or numbers of antibody-secreting cells per clone, and it is interesting that only T-dependent antigens are effective in this assay. Others use irradiated spleen cells and/or thymocytes as fillers for limiting dilution of B cells in liquid cultures.[35,36] LPS stimulation may be more efficient in such a system than in mitogen-stimulated bulk cultures or semisolid cultures, and the technique is more suitable for studying differentiation than for proliferative responses. About one out of every three LPS-stimulated B cells produce Ig-secreting cells which can then be conveniently enumerated with a reverse plaque assay.[36] Antigen-specific responses of clones in liquid cultures has provided evidence for an exceptional type of B-cell heterogeneity. It has been shown that the same hapten, presented on carriers which differ in mitogenicity and/or T-cell dependence, may stimulate different populations of B cells, even when relatively monoclonal responses are considered.[38-40] It should be noted that all of these procedures are unwieldy if the approximate frequency of responding cells is unknown. Proliferating foci in semisolid cultures can be accurately enumerated over at least a log range, and this is an advantage when comparing large numbers of cell suspension which contain unknown numbers of functional B cells. Other have held lymphocytes with mitogens in liquid culture for several days before plating them in semisolid cultures,[41] and we have confirmed that B lymphoblasts are capable of colony formation. However, the relationship between starting numbers of B cells and numbers of resulting colonies is complicated by this procedure, and we have not found it to be advantageous.

ACKNOWLEDGMENTS

Liberal use has been made of unpublished observations in this chapter. Most of these resulted from collaborative studies with Grace Lee, Christopher Paige, and Margrit Scheid. Our work is supported by grants AI-12741, CA-17404, CA-08748, and Research Career Development Award AI-00265 from the U.S. Public Health Service.

REFERENCES

1. Metcalf, D., Nossal, G. J. V., Warner, N. L., Miller, J. F. A. P., Mandel, T. E., Layton, J. E., and Gutman, G. A., Growth of B-lymphocyte colonies in vitro, *J. Exp. Med.*, 142, 1534, 1975.
2. Polet, H. and Spieker-Polet, H., Serum albumin is essential for in vitro growth of activated human lymphocytes, *J. Exp. Med.*, 142, 949, 1975.
3. Kincade, P. W., Ralph, P., and Moore, M. A. S., Growth of B-lymphocyte clones in semisolid culture is mitogen dependent, *J. Exp. Med.*, 143, 1265, 1976.
4. Metcalf, D., Role of mercaptoethanol and endotoxin in stimulating B lymphocyte colony formation in vitro, *J. Immunol.*, 116, 635, 1976.
5. Shortman, K., Separation methods for lymphocyte populations, *Contemp. Top. Mol. Immunol.*, 3, 161, 1964.
6. McCarthy, J. H., Differential effects of red cells on the formation of normal and neoplastic mouse B lymphocyte colonies in vitro, *Exp. Hematol.*, 6, 709, 1978.
7. Paige, C. J., Analysis of B cell precursors in fetal and adult mice, Ph.D. thesis, Cornell University,
8. Kurland, J. I., Kincade, P. W., and Moore, M. A. S., Regulation of B lymphocyte clonal proliferation by stimulatory and inhibitory macrophage-derived factors, *J. Exp. Med.*, 146, 1420, 1977.
9. Wood, D. D. and Gaul, S. L., Enhancement of the humoral response of T cell-depleted murine spleens by a factor derived from human monocytes in vitro, *J. Immunol.*, 113, 925, 1974.
10. Kincade, P. W., Defective colony formation by B-lymphocytes from CBA/N and C3H/HeJ mice, *J. Exp. Med.*, 145, 249, 1977.
11. Kincade, P. W. and Ralph, P., Regulation of clonal B lymphocyte proliferation by anti-immunoglobulin or anti-Ia antibodies, *Cold Spring Harbor Symp.*, 41, 245, 1976.
12. Nicola, N. A., Metcalf, D., Johnson, G. R., and Burgess, A. W., Preparation of colony stimulating factors from human placental conditioned medium, *Leuk. Res.*, 2, 313, 1978.
13. Metcalf, D., *Hemopoietic Colonies,* Springer-Verlag, New York, 1977.
14. Metcalf, D., Acute antigen-induced elevation of serum colony stimulating factor (CSF) levels, *Immunology*, 21, 427, 1971.
15. Burgess, A. W., Metcalf, D., and Russell, S., Regulation of Hematopoietic Differentiation and Proliferation by Colony-stimulating Factors, Vol. 5, *Cold Spring Harbor Conf. Cell Proliferation*, 1978, 339.
16. Johnson, G. R., Metcalf, D., and Wilson, J. W., Development of B-lymphocyte colony-forming cells in foetal mouse tissues, *Immunology*, 30, 907, 1976.
17. Burrows, P. D., Kearney, J. F., Lawton, A. R., and Cooper, M. D., Pre-B cells: Bone marrow persistence in anti-μ suppressed mice, conversion to B lymphocytes, and recovery following destruction by cyclophosphamide, *J. Immunol.*, 120, 1526, 1978.
18. Kincade, P. W., Piage, C. J., Parkhouse, R. M. E., and Lee, G., Characterization of murine colony-forming B cells. I. Distribution, resistance to anti-immunologlobulin antibodies, and expression of Ia antigens, *J. Immunol.*, 120, 1289, 1978.
19. Metcalf, D., Wilson, J. W., Shortman, K., Miller, J. F. A. P., and Stocker, J., The nature of the cells generating B-lymphocyte colonies in vitro, *J. Cell Physiol.*, 88, 107, 1976.
20. Julius, M. H., Simpson, E., and Herzenberg, L. A., A rapid method for the isolation of functional thymus-derived murine lympocytes, *Eur. J. Immunol.*, 3, 645, 1973.
21. Lala, P. K., Johnson, G. R., Battye, F. L., and Nossal, G. J. V., Maturation of B lymphocytes. I. Concurrent appearance of increasing Ig, Ia, and mitogen responsiveness, *J. Immunol.*, 122, 334, 1979.
22. Kincade, P. W., Lee, G., Fernandes, G. Moore, M. A. S., Williams, N., and Good, R. A., Abnormalities in clonable B lymphocytes and myeloid progenitors in autoimmune NZB mice, *Proc. Natl. Acad. Sci. U.S.A.*, 76, 3464, 1979.
23. Kincade, P. W., Moore, M. A. S., Lee, G., and Paige, C. J., Colony forming B cells in F₁ hybrid and transplanted CBA/N mice, *Cell. Immunol.*, 40, 294, 1978.
24. Paige, C. J., Kincade, P. W., Moore, M. A. S., and Lee, G., The fate of fetal and adult B-cell progenitors grafted into immunodeficient CBA/N mice, *J. Exp. Med.*, 150, 548, 1979.
25. Kincade, P. W. and Paige, C. J., B cell development in immunodeficient CBA/N mice, in *B lymphocytes in the immune response,* Cooper, M., Mosier, D., and Scher, I., Eds., Elsevier, Amsterdam, 1979, 349.
26. Izumi, K., Chemical heterogeneity of the agar from *Gracilaria verrucosa, J. Biochem.*, 72, 135, 1972.
27. Claesson, M. H., Soluble suppressor activity of concanavalin A activated spleen cells on B-lymphocyte colony formation in vitro, *Cell Immunol.*, 42, 1979, 344.
28. Sigal, N. H. and Klinman, N. R., The B-cell clonotype repertoire, *Adv. Immunol.*, 26, 255, 1978.

29. **Andersson, J., Coutinho, A., and Melchers, F.,** Frequencies of mitogen-reactive B cells in the mouse. II. Frequencies of B cells producing antibodies which lyse sheep or horse erythrocytes, and trinitrophenylated or nitroiodophenylated sheep erthrocytes, *J. Exp. Med.,* 145, 1520, 1977.

30. **Gillis, S., Ferm, M. M., Ou, W., and Smith, K. A.,** T-cell growth factor: parameters of production and a quantitative microassay from activity, *J. Immunol.,* 120, 2027, 1978.

31. **Shibasaki, M., Nemoto, H., Suzuki, S., and Kuroume, T.,** Induction of lymphocyte colony formation in vitro by protein A, *J. Immunol.,* 121, 2278, 1978.

32. **Sredni, B., Kalechman, Y., Michlin, H., and Rozenszain, L. A.,** Development of colonies in vitro of mitogen-stimulated mouse T lymphocytes, *Nature (London),* 259, 130, 1976.

33. **Claesson, M. H., Rodger, M. B., Johnson, G. R., Whittingham, S., and Metcalf, D.,** Colony formation by human T lymphocytes in agar medium, *Clin. Exp. Immunol.,* 28, 526, 1977.

34. **Jacobs, S. W. and Miller, R. G.,** Characterization of in vitro T-lymphocyte colonies from spleens of nude mice, *J. Immunol.,* 122, 582, 1979.

35. **Lefkovits, I.,** Induction of antibody-forming cell clones in microcultures, *Eur. J. Immunol.,* 2, 360, 1972.

36. **Andersson, J., Coutinho, A., Lernhardt, W., and Melchers, F.,** Clonal growth and maturation to immunoglobulin secretion "in vitro" of every growth-inducible B-lymphocyte, *Cell,* 10, 27, 1977.

27. **Teale, J. M., Howard, M. C., Falzon, E., and Nossal, G. J. V.,** B lymphocyte subpopulations separated by velocity sedimentation. I. Characterization of immune function in an in vitro splenic focus assay, *J. Immunol.,* 121, 2554, 1978.

38. **Quintans, J. and Cosenza, H.,** Antibody response to phosphorylcholine in vitro. II. Analysis of T-dependent of T-independent responses, *Eur. J. Immunol.,* 6, 399, 1976.

39. **Lewis, G. K. and Goodman, J. W.,** Carrier-directed anti-hapten responses by B-cell subsets, *J. Exp. Med.,* 146, 1, 1977.

40. **Tittle, T. V. and Rittenberg, M. B.,** Distinct subpopulations of IgG memory B cells respond to different molecular forms of the same hapten, *J. Immunol.,* 121, 936, 1978.

41. **Rozenszajn, L. A., Michlin, H., Kalechman, Y., and Sredni, B.,** Colony growth in vitro of mitogen-stimulated mouse B lymphocytes, *Immunology,* 32, 319, 1977.

Chapter 6

IN VITRO ANTIBODY RESPONSE IN AGING ANIMALS

A. A. Nordin and M. A. Buchholz

TABLE OF CONTENTS

I. INTRODUCTION

The technique of culturing dispersed lymphoid cell suspensions in tissue culture, as originally described by Mishell and Dutton,[1,2] has been used extensively in an attempt to clarify the cellular mechanism of antibody formation. This technique permits the examination of cells outside the complex in vivo situation and more importantly has allowed the investigator to manipulate cell populations by various biological and physical means prior to establishing the in vitro cultures. The separation and subsequent identification and classification of lymphocyte populations when combined with the in vitro culture system has provided a means of determining the cellular requirements essential for antibody synthesis.

The tissue culture system used for the in vitro immune response contains many variables which have resulted in both quantitative and qualitative differences. Several sources of the variability within the tissue culture system have been considered in a previous publication.[3] These problems most seriously affect attempts to determine the cellular mechanisms and interactions involved in the immune response. However, the in vitro system has proven to be invaluable in establishing the cellular requirements of the immune response.

It is now well documented in many experimental models that immune function declines with advancing age. The most recent studies in this field are directed towards determining the reasons for immunodeficiences among aging individuals. It seems appropriate, then, to apply the techniques of cell separation and in vitro culturing of lymphoid suspensions to determine what effects advancing age may exert on the cellular constituents of the humoral immune response. The technique of in vitro culturing of lymphoid cells is useful for studies in which cellular populations are changing with age in that suspected cellular deficiencies can be replaced by adding the proper cell populations derived from young syngeneic animals. On the other hand, if a suppressive population of cells is suspected of reducing the response of the old animals, this population can be added to young syngeneic cells to determine the efficiency of the suppressive cells. The in vitro culture system should represent one means of approach to identify deficiencies among the cellular constitutents of the immune systems as a result of age. As more information becomes available concerning the various cellular mechanisms, the in vitro technique may be quite useful in delineating the underlying mechanisms of immunosenescence.

In previous publications,[3,4] several sources of variability that influence the in vitro culture technique have been extensively considered. Since these apply irrespective of the age of mice donating the cells, these subjects will not be presented here. This article is meant to detail the tissue culture methodology used in our laboratory with several established methods of cell preparations. Representative results and the limitations of the techniques with respect to using aging mice in the in vitro system of the immune response are presented.

II. MATERIALS

A. Animals

The only experimental model that will be described involves C57BL/6 mice. The mice were all purchased from a single commercial source at 5 weeks of age and then maintained at the Gerontology Research Center, National Institute of Aging. The majority of studies used virgin female mice of at least 24 months of age. At sacrifice, all animals were examined for any gross pathology which may or may not eliminate a particular mouse from the study. The chapter by van Zwieten, et al.[5] has dealt with the possible effects of various pathological states on in vitro studies.

B. Medium

The tissue culture medium used was RPMI-1640 purchased from the Grand Island Biological Company. The same medium was also purchased as a powder and prepared and sterilized by filtration. This medium was supplemented with 20 %/v of fetal calf serum (FCS). It is essential to pretest FCS for their ability to support the in vitro immune response. This testing was done using young (3 to 4 month) C57BL/6 mice from the same commercial source that supplied the mice in the aging colony. The lots of FCS that were supportive of the in vitro cultures were further tested for endotoxin content by the Limulus assay [6] A FCS that is free of endotoxin activity and supports the in vitro immune response to yield plaque-forming cells (PFC) in numbers equivalent to the in vivo response is an ideal serum. The frequency of such lots is less than 30% of the tested samples from various commercial sources.

The addition of β-mercaptoethanol has been shown to be beneficial for culturing murine lymphoid cells.[7,8,9] This same beneficial effect is seen irrespective of the age of the mice and the optimal concentration is unchanged (5×10^{-5} M). Gentamycin at a concentration of 50mg/mℓ is added to the medium to yield a final concentration of 0.10 mg/mℓ. RPMI-1640 supplemented with 20% FCS and gentamycin was stable for at least one week at 4°C.

C. Antigens

The antigenic properties of sheep erythrocytes have been shown to vary greatly among different sheep and therefore several donors must be tested. Once an appropriate source of sheep erythrocytes has been established the same animal can be used over a period of at least four years. The blood is collected aseptically in Alsever's solution without preservatives and is stable for at least 2 months. An aliquot of the diluted blood is removed and washed three times with sterile Dulbecco's medium. After the final wash, 0.1 mℓ of packed erythrocytes are added to 5 mℓ of the appropriate tissue culture medium and 0.1 mℓ of this suspension is added to 10×10^6 spleen cells. In our hands this volume of diluted SRC suspension contains approximately 10^7 erythrocytes.

Dinitrophenyl-β-alanylglycylglycyl-Ficoll® (DAGG-Ficoll®) is known to be a T-helper cell independent antigen.[10] The preparation of this antigen as described by Inman[11] yielded a molar ratio of hapten:Ficoll® of 48:1. A stock solution was prepared from the lypholized DAGG-Ficoll® at a concentration of 1 mg/mℓ. For in vitro immunization the stock solution was diluted in tissue culture medium to a concentration of 1 μg/mℓ. The optimal antigenic dose for 10×10^6 spleen cells was found to be 10 ng.

D. Culture Vessels

The two types of culture vessels most commonly used are (1) tissue-culture plates which consists of six wells 35 mm in diameter, and (2) micro culture plates which consist of 96 flat-bottom wells, 6.4 mm in diameter. In the former, 10×10^6 spleen cells contained 1 mℓ of tissue culture medium yield optimal results, while in the latter, 1×10^6 spleen cells contained in 0.2 mℓ were optimal.

E. Conditions During Incubation

The cell cultures are incubated at 37°C in a humid atmosphere composed of 83% N_2, 7% O_2, and 10% CO_2. In order to maintain the gaseous environment the culture plates are placed in Lucite® chambers which can be flushed with the gas mixture and tightly sealed. Such chambers are commercially available or can be easily fabricated. The chamber is then placed on a rocking platform (Bellco Glass, Inc., Vineland, N.J.) in a 37°C incubator. In our hands, the cultures contained in 35-mm diameter wells responded considerably better when rocked but the response of the cultures contained in the micro culture plates were not affected by rocking.

III. PROCEDURES

A. Cell Preparations

1. Spleen Cell Suspensions

Mice were sacrificed by cervical dislocation and their spleens removed asceptically and placed into 60-mm petri dishes that contained 10 mℓ of Dulbecco's medium. A single cell suspension is prepared in Dulbecco's medium by gently pressing the spleens through a #200 stainless steel screen. The cell suspension is then placed into a 15-mℓ round-bottom polycarbonate tube and allowed to settle for 10 min. The cell suspension is then transferred into a polycarbonate centrifuge tube and centrifuged at 400 xg for 10 min. The supernatant fluid is removed and the cells are resuspended in tissue culture medium. A viable cell count is obtained using trypan blue exclusion.

For the removal of phagocytic cells from spleen cell suspensions, the cells are resuspended in the medium described by Mishell and Dutton[1,2] containing 0.1 mg/mℓ gentamycin in place of penicillin and streptomycin. For every 10^8 spleen cell to be treated, 25 mg of dry-heat-sterilized carbonyl-iron (GAF Corporation, 140 West 51st Street, N.Y., 10020) is resuspended in a small amount of the medium and transferred into a tissue culture flask. Since the final concentration of the spleen cells to be treated should be 5×10^6 per mℓ, additional medium is added and finally the proper number of spleen cells is introduced. The cell suspension is incubated at 37°C for 40 min in an atmosphere of 5% CO_2 in air. Cells that have ingested carbonyl-iron as well as the free carbonyl-iron were collected into one area at the bottom of the flask with the use of a strong magnet. The cell suspension is then poured off into another flask which contains the proper amount of carbonyl-iron suspended in 2 to 5 mℓ of the medium. The incubation and removal of the carbonyl-iron with the magnet is repeated. The cell suspension is then poured off into a polycarbonate centrifuge tube, and the cells sedimented at 400 xg for 10 min. The cells are then resuspended in tissue culture medium and the last traces of carbonyl-iron are removed by passing the cell suspension through a Lymphocyte Separator (Technicon Instruments Corporation, Tarrytown, N.Y., 10591). Viable cells are counted using trypan blue dye, and the cell density adjusted to the desired concentration. Cell recovery following carbonyl-iron treatment is 70 to 75% of the original cell number.

2. Peritoneal Cells

Prior to removing the spleen the peritoneal cavity is flushed with 3 mℓ of 0.34 *M* sucrose. The washings are collected in silicone-coated conical glass test tubes kept in a melting ice bath. Cells are washed once with cold Dulbecco's phosphate buffered saline without Ca^{++} and Mg^{++} and then resuspended in tissue culture medium. Viable cell counts are done using trypan blue dye and the cell density is adjusted to the desired concentration.

3. Thymus-Derived Cells

The isolation of T lymphocytes from mouse spleen is done using nylon wool columns as described by Julius et al.[12] with minor modifications. Nylon wool from Leuko-Pak (Fenwall Lab., Deerfield, Ill.) is boiled six times in 2 to 3ℓ of distilled water and then dried overnight at 37°C. Approximately 0.6 g of nylon wool is completely pulled apart and put into a 10-mℓ plastic syringe with the aid of a Pasteur pipette. The syringe containing the nylon wool is wrapped in aluminum foil and sterilized by autoclaving at 15 lb pressure for 15 min. The sterilized column is placed at 37°C and rinsed slowly with prewarmed Dulbecco's phosphate buffered saline containing 5% heat-inactivated fetal calf serum and incubated at 37°C for at least 1 hr prior to the addition of the spleen cells. The spleen cells are washed in Dulbecco's phosphate buffered saline with 5% heat-inactivated FCS and adjusted to a density of 50×10^6 cells per mℓ. Before the cells are applied, the column is flushed again with 30 mℓ of the medium. A total of 1×10^8 spleen cells are introduced onto the column and washed into the nylon wool with approximately 1 mℓ of the medium. The column is sealed to prevent evaporation and incubated for 45 min at 37°C. The cells are eluted with 10 mℓ of the warmed medium and collected in a polycarbonate centrifuge tube. The cells are collected by centrifugation at 400 xg for 10 min and resuspended in the tissue culture medium. A viable count is performed using trypan blue dye. The recovery is 20 to 25% of the total cells applied to the column and in our hands 5 to 8% of these cells show membrane immunoglobulin by fluorescent microscopy.

B. Tissue Culture Technique

The in vitro culture technique was the same as that described by Mishell and Dutton,[1,2] with the modifications described by Schreier and Nordin.[3] With this technique, the spleen cell concentration is 10×10^6 cells per mℓ, and the total volume in each culture is 1 mℓ. Antigen and/or mercaptoethanol is added to each individual culture. Old mice show individual patterns of immuno-deficiency, which demand that each animal be assayed separately, and the large number of spleen cells required in this tissue culture system often limits the experimental design. The micro culture system, as described by Pike,[12] is more suited for studies of the in vitro response of aging animals, mainly because this system requires not more than 10^6 cells per culture. For the micro culture system the cells to be placed in culture are first prepared in 12×75 mm sterile plastic tubes. The initial concentration of spleen cells, carbonyl-iron-treated spleen cells, peritoneal cells, and splenic T lymphocytes was adjusted to the required density so that when these cell preparations were combined in the 12×75 mm tubes, the final concentration contained in 0.2 mℓ was 10^6, 10^5, and $2.5 - 1.0 \times 10^5$, respectively. A total volume of 1.2 mℓ of the final cell mixtures is contained in each culture tube, so that five individual cultures can be easily prepared from each tube. To the appropriate tubes, 10 $\mu\ell$ of DAGG-Ficoll® at 1.0 μg/mℓ or 10 $\mu\ell$ of a suspension of SRC at 10^8 cells per mℓ are added, along with 12 $\mu\ell$ of a 5×10^{-3} M solution of mercaptoethanol. The cell mixtures, with or without antigen and mercaptoethanol are thoroughly mixed by vortex action, and five individual 0.2-mℓ cultures are pipetted into a Costar® 96-well, flat-bottom, tissue-culture plate.

The preparation of splenic adherent cells using the 35-mm tissue-culture plate has been previously described.[3] In the micro culture system, the spleen cells from which the adherent population is to be prepared are adjusted to a concentration of 2×10^6 cells per mℓ in the tissue culture medium described by Mishell and Dutton.[1,2] To the appropriate number of wells, 0.2 mℓ of this cell suspension is added, and the tissue culture plates are incubated for 1 hr at 37°C in the previously described gaseous environment. Nonadherent cells are removed and each well is washed three times with 0.2 mℓ of Dulbecco's medium. At each washing the wells are gently flushed with 0.2 mℓ of Dulbecco's medium, with a sterile Pasteur pipette to remove the loosely attached cells. After the final wash 0.2 mℓ of the tissue culture medium is added to each well and the plates are placed back at 37°C in the gaseous environment until needed. When the appropriate cell mixtures are to be cocultivated with the splenic adherent cells, the 0.2 mℓ of medium is removed and replaced with the appropriate cell suspension.

C. Assay for Antibody-Producing Cells

The assay procedures for detecting antibody-producing cells do not require the use of sterile technique. Culture fluid and cells from each individual well is removed using a Pasteur pipette. Each well is then washed with minimal essential media (MEM) containing 25 mM HEPES, the well is flushed and the wash fluid is added to the appropriate tube. For each 35-mm well, 1 mℓ of MEM with 25mM HEPES is added and 0.2 mℓ is added to each well in the micro culture plates. The tubes are centrifuged at 350 xg at room temperature, the supernate removed, and the cells resuspended in the desired volume of MEM with 25 mM HEPES. The amount of medium added to each tube is dependent on the number of PFC contained in the culture. Though this can be judged only after some experience with the in vitro culture system, the cells recovered from the 35mm tissue culture plates are usually suspended in 4 to 10 mℓ of medium while the cells recovered from the micro cultures are resuspended in 1 to 2 mℓ of medium.

The medium used in the plaque assay is a semisolid agar composed of 0.5% agarose (Microbiological Associates, Bethesda, Md.) in MEM with 25 mM HEPES. This solution is prepared by mixing together equal volumes of 1% agarose in water and 2x concentrated and warmed MEM. With a prewarmed pipette, 0.4 mℓ of this mixture is pipetted into 12 × 75 mm prewashed, disposable glass test tubes that are placed in a 48°C water bath. Microscope slides (2 × 3) are prepared in advance of the assay by adding several drops of a mixture containing 0.5% agarose in 0.3% NaCl to slides that have been previously placed on a slide warming table. The agarose is spread over the slide with the aid of a glass rod and the excess then removed from the slide. The thin film of agarose is allowed to dry on the slide and has been found necessary to aid in the adherence of the plating medium. SRC or hapten-conjugated SRC are washed three times and adjusted to a 15% (SRC) or a 20% (hapten-SRC) suspension. Fifty microliters of the SRC suspension is pipetted into the semisolid agarose. To this mixture is added the proper volume of the in vitro cultured cell suspension. Any volume of cultured cells up to 200 $\mu\ell$ can be safely added without disturbing the gelling properties of the agarose solution. The usual volume of cells plated in our laboratory is 100 $\mu\ell$. After the addition of the cells, the tube is removed from the water bath and mixed thoroughly, and the contents poured onto prewarmed, agarose-coated slides. The agarose mixture containing the cells is spread evenly over the slide with the aid of a glass rod. The slide is then placed on a level surface and the agarose allowed to solidify. The slides are then placed face down into a Lucite® tray (See Chapter 7) specifically designed for the assay, and MEM containing 25mM HEPES is introduced under the slides. Each of these trays contains eight slides and requires approximately 25 mℓ of medium. The trays are then placed into a 37°C incubator with 5% CO_2 for 1 hr. After the incubation, the slides are removed and placed into Wheaton® staining dishes (Thomas Co., Philadelphia, Pa.) designed to hold 2 × 3 slides, and that contain 0.85% NaCl. The medium is emptied from the trays, and the trays washed with distilled water and dried. The slides are then removed from the 0.85% NaCl and placed back into the trays. MEM with 25mM HEPES and guinea pig complement at a dilution of 1/30 to 1/50 is added, and the trays placed back into the incubator for 45 to 60 min. The slides are again removed from the tray and placed into dishes as described above containing 0.85% NaCl. This technique will detect direct or IgM PFC. If the indirect or IgG PFC are to be detected,[16,17] a similar procedure is done, except that after the first one hr incubation period the slides are incubated with the proper dilution of antisera contained in the MEM medium. The slides are incubated with the enhancing antisera for approximately 45 min before they are washed and exposed to the guinea pig complement. After the plaques have been developed and the slides have been washed in 0.85% NaC1, they are fixed in acetone for 3 min and in 95% ethanol for 5 min. The agarose plating medium is then dried with forced hot air, and the slides can be stored indefinitely in this state. The hemolytic plaques are counted using a stereo microscope, and the results are usually recorded as the number of PFC per culture. Plaque counting using the stereo microscope system is time consuming and can be replaced by using the automatic counting devices that are now commercially available (Artek Systems Corp., Farmingdale, N.Y.).

The Cunningham chamber technique[18] for detecting PFC shows the same sensitivity as the previously described slide technique, but has been more useful when hapten inhibition of plaques is examined. However, when hapten-conjugated erythrocytes were used in this assay, it was necessary in our laboratory to reduce the amount of hapten conjugated to the SRC. With the reagents we used and the technique of conjugation described by Inman,[19] the hapten-conjugated SRC consistently lysed during the incubation. To prevent this lysis, the amount of hapten was reduced to one fourth of that used in conjugating the red cells for the slide assay. However, the number of PFC detected using the two techniques with the different preparations of conjugated SRC was not significantly different.

IV. SUMMARY AND FURTHER CONSIDERATIONS

The importance of FCS in the tissue culture medium has been well recognized in the in vitro technique of the immune response. The reasons for variation among lots of FCS has yet to be established, and a particular lot of FCS supportive of one strain of mice may be nonsupportive for another strain. However, our experience has shown that the age of the mice is not a critical element with respect to the FCS. Although the in vitro immune response of aging mice is consistently low, FCS lots that are supportive in the young control cultures give the maximal response in cultures of spleen cells of aging mice. Likewise, partially or nonsupportive FSC lots are equally noneffective when old mice are used as the source of spleen cells. Such deficient lots of FCS have been shown to be improved by the addition of ME. The optimal concentration of ME is 5×10^{-5} M, irrespective of whether young or old mice are used as a source of spleen cells. FCS that is fully supportive without the addition of ME in cultures of young spleen cells does not improve the response of old spleen cells if ME is added. Iscove and Melchers[20] described a medium in which albumin, transferin, and lipids completely replaced the serum requirement for LPS stimulation of murine B lymphocytes. Schreier,[21] using this same medium, has recently described and in vitro helper cell assay. The development of such a fully supportive serum-free medium is of significant advantage for the in vitro technique.

The number of PFC generated in the in vitro immune response is dependent on the concentration of antigen added. The optimal concentrations of SRC and DAGG-Ficoll® do not change as a result of the age of the mice. In addition, spleen cell cultures to which no antigen was added did not show different background levels of PFC with respect to the age of the mice.

The observation that aging mice show individual patterns of immuno-dificiencies adds a significant limitation to the studies of the in vitro immune response. Examples of the wide variations in the number of PFC generated in the in vitro immune response to SRC or DAGG-Ficoll® are shown in Table 1. The mice were all 24-month-old C57BL/6 females housed under identical conditions. The spleen cells were cultured under identical conditions and cultures of young spleen cells were included as a control of the tissue culture conditions. It should also be pointed out that the kinetics of the in vitro response do not change, except for the magnitude of the response, as a function

Table 1

THE IN VITRO PRIMARY
IMMUNE RESPONSE OF 10
C57BL/6 FEMALE MICE AT 24
MONTHS OF AGE TO DAGG-
FICOLL® AND SRC

| Mouse | PFC/Culture[a,b] | |
	DAGG-Ficoll®	SRC
1	231	3
2	90	20
3	113	8
4	146	0
5	466	12
6	484	55
7	370	111
8	840	156
9	125	0
10	28	0
Young control	2784	3738

a) 1×10^6 spleen cells were cultured in each
of five wells in a Costar® microplate.
b) The number of PFC is the average of the
five cultures.

of age. The peak response to SRC is between 4 to 5 days, and for DAGG-Ficoll® the peak response is consistently seen on day 4. The response to various mitogens (Adler, W. H., Chapter 12, this volume), and the in vitro generation of cytotoxic killer cells, also show large variations in results among aging mice and without a change in kinetics when compared to young mice.

Because of the various patterns of immune reactivity observed among old mice, it is not possible to pool spleen cells for in vitro studies. Not only is it impossible to repeat data when using pools of cells, but in old mice the results obtained from a pool of spleen cells are consistently significantly lower than the calculated mean.

The number of cells recovered from the spleens of aging mice is quite variable and is generally lower than the number recovered from young mice. In mice 24 months and older, the recovery of spleen cells often limits the number of parameters to be assayed. Because of this problem, we have adopted the micro culture technique for our investigations. The cell survival in the microculture technique was examined using spleen cells from 6-, 12-, 18-, and 24-month-old mice. The spleen cells were cultured in the presence of ME and were stimulated with DAGG-Ficoll®. The number of cells recovered 4 days after the initiation of the cultures was the same for all age groups while the number of PFC declined steadily. This decline could be due to deficiencies in any of the three cell types known to participate in the immune response, a combination of deficiencies involving more than one cell type, or to a high level of suppressor cells. In our hands, the addition of PC from young mice to cultures of old mice spleen cells slightly improves the in vitro immune responses. The addition of splenic T cells eluted from nylon wool columns does not improve the response of old mice spleen cells unless PC from young mice are also added to the cultures. When both PC and T cells from young animals were co-cultivated with spleen cells from old mice approximately 30% of the old mice examined yield PFC levels that could be considered equiv-

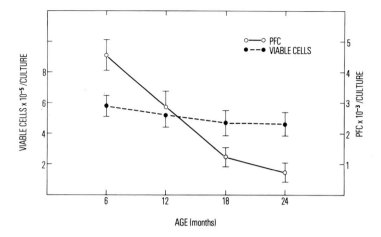

FIGURE 1. The effect of age on the number of PFC (O——O) and number of viable cells (●- - - ●) per 1 × 10⁶ spleen cells cultured for 4 days. Each point represents the mean of eight to ten individually assayed mice.

alent to the response of young animals. The remaining old mice could have a B-cell deficiency and/or a high level of suppressor cells. There is evidence for both viewpoints, and there is increasing evidence to suggest that the immunodeficiencies of aging mice are not a singular, uniform cellular change, but rather combinations and permeations of cellular changes involving all cell types participating in the immune response. The in vitro culture technique in combination with methods of cellular separation and identification should add significant contributions to the underlying causes of immunosenescents.

REFERENCES

1. **Mishell, R. I. and Dutton, R. W.,** Immunization of Normal Mouse Spleen Cell Suspensions In Vitro, *Science,* 153, 1004, 1966.
2. **Mishell, R. I. and Dutton, R. W.,** Immunization of Dissociated Spleen Cell Cultures from Normal Mice, *J. Exp. Med.,* 125, 423, 1967.
3. **Schreier, M. H. and Nordin, A. A.,** An Evaluation of the Immune Response In Vitro, in *B and T Cells in Immune Recognition,* Loor, F. and Roelants, G. E., Eds., John Wiley & Sons, New York, 1977, 127.
4. **Schreier, M. H.,** In Vitro Immunization of Dissociated Murine Spleen Cells, in *Immunological Methods,* Lefkovits, I. and Pernes, B., Eds., Academic Press, New York, 1978, 327.
5. **van Zwieten, N. J., Zurchur, C., Solleveld, H. A., and Hollander, C. F.,** Pathology, in *Immunological Techniques Applied to Aging Research,* Adler, W. H. and Nordin, A. A., Eds., CRC Press, Boca Raton, Fla., 1980, chap 1.
6. **Leven, J. Jomasulo, P. A. and Oser, R. S.,** Detection of endotoxin in human blood and demonstration of an inhibitor, *J. Lab. Clin. Med.,* 75, 903, 1970.
7. **Click, R. E., Benck, L., and Alter, B. J.,** Enhancement of antibody synthesis in vitro by mercaptoethanol, *Cell. Immunol.,* 3, 156, 1972.
8. **Broome, J. D. and Jeng, M. W.,** Promotion of replication in lymphoid cells by specific thiols and disulphides in vitro. Effects on mouse lymphoma cells in comparison with splenic lymphocytes, *J. Exp. Med.,* 138, 574, 1973.

9. **Bevan, M. J., Epstein, R., and Cohen, N.,** The effect of 2-mercaptoethanol on murine mixed lymphocyte cultures, *J. Exp. Med.,* 139, 1025, 1974.

10. **Mosier, D. E., Johnson, D. M., Paul, W. E., and McMaster, P. R. B.,** Cellular requirements for the primary in vitro antibody response to DNP-Ficoll, *J. Exp. Med.,* 139, 1354, 1974.

11. **Inman, J. K.,** Thymus-independent Antigens: The preparation of covalent, hapten-Ficoll conjugates, *J. Immunol.,* 114, 704, 1975.

12. **Julius, M., Simpson, E., and Herzenberg, L. A.,** A rapid method for the isolation of functional thymus-derived murine lymphocytes, *Eur. J. Immunol.,* 3, 645, 1973.

13. **Pike, B. L.,** A microculture method for the generation of primary immune responses in vitro, *J. Immunol. Meth.,* 9, 85, 1975.

14. **Jerne, N. K. and Nordin, A. A.,** Plaque formation in agar by single antibody-producing cells, *Science,* 140, 405, 1963.

15. **Jerne, N. K., Nordin, A. A., and Henry, C.,** The agar plaque technique for recognizing antibody-producing cells, in *Cell-Bound Antibodies,* Amos, B. and Koprowski, H., Eds., Wistar Institute Press, Philadelphia, 1963, 109.

16. **Sterzl, J. and Riha, I.,** A localized hemolysis in gel method for the detection of cells producing 7S antibody, *Nature (London),* 208, 858, 1965.

17. **Dresser, D. W. and Wortis, H. H.,** Use of an antiglobulin serum to detect cells producing antibody with low hemolytic efficiency, *Nature (London),* 208, 859, 1967.

18. **Cunningham, A. J. and Svenberg, A.,** Further improvements in the plaque technique for detecting single antibody-forming cells, *Immunology,* 14, 599, 1968.

19. **Inman, J. K., Merchant, B., Claflin, L., and Tate, S. E.,** Coupling of large haptens to proteins in cell surfaces: preparation of stable, optimally sensitized erythrocytes for hapten-specific, hemolytic plaque assays, *Immunochemistry,* 10, 165, 1973.

20. **Iscove, N. N. and Melchers, F.,** Complete replacement of serum by albumin, transferren, and soybean lipid in cultures of lipopolysaccharide-reactive B lymphocytes, *J. Exp Med.,* 147, 923, 1978.

21. **Schreier, M.,** B-cell precursors specific to sheep erythrocytes. Estimation of frequency in a specific helper assay, *J. Exp. Med.,* 148, 1612, 1978.

Chapter 7

ENUMERATION OF INDIVIDUAL ANTIBODY SYNTHESIZING CELLS IN VITRO

J.E. Nagel and F. J. Chrest

TABLE OF CONTENTS

I. INTRODUCTION

In 1963 Jerne and Nordin[1] described a technique to quantitate individual antibody producing cells in vitro. Since that time their technique, and modifications of it, has become one of the standard methods for analysis and study of the mechanisms of activation, specificity, and enumeration of not only what are now known as B lymphocytes, but also for other cell populations and products which interact with antibody synthesizing cells.

The original "Jerne-Nordin" plaque assay in agar is also frequently referred to as the "direct plaque assay" technique since the antibody detected by it is specifically directed against the surface determinants of sheep erythrocyte (SRBC) indicator cells resulting in their lysis when complement is added. Complex antigens, haptens, and peptide fragments may be coupled or conjugated to the surface of the indicator cells thus increasing the variety and sensitivity (in the murine system) but not class of specific antibody that may be detected.[2-4] Because of the greater affinity, molecule for molecule, of 19S or IgM antibodies to bind complement, virtually all antibody detected in the "direct" plaque assay is of the IgM class. Popular modifications of this assay method are the "Cunningham" technique in which the lymphoid cells and indicator erythrocytes are incubated in microchambers using liquid media, and the ultra-thin layer gel technique.[5,6]

The limitation of the direct plaque assay, namely that it detects only IgM class antibodies was overcome by the development of several "indirect" techniques[7,8] which permit the enumeration of cells producing other immunoglobulin classes. In 1976 Gronowicz, Coutinho, and Melchers, incorporating the observation that protein A, a cell wall component of *Staphylococcus aureus,* has the ability to covalently bind the Fc portion of IgG,* described yet another modification of the hemolytic plaque assay which permits the quantitation by immunoglobulin class (or subclass) of any immunoprotein molecule for which complement binding antibodies are available irrespective of the antigen against which they are directed.[10] The basic principles underlying this assay are shown in Figure 1. Protein A is coupled, using chromic chloride, to SRBC and the resulting protein A/SRBC incorporated into an indicator layer. The antibody to be detected is then "developed" by treatment of this indicator cell matrix with either a poly or monospecific rabbit antisera containing the IgG class of antibody. This rabbit IgG "linking antibody" attaches to the protein A on the SRBC via the Fc portion of the molecule and with the antibody secreted from the lymphocyte via its antigen binding area. The resulting antigen-antibody reaction between the secreted immunoglobulin (Ig) and the protein A/SRBC coupled Ig then allows localized complement lysis of the sheep erythrocytes in the indicator layer leading to the appearance of plaques.

In the following discussion the details of a slide modification of the protein A hemolytic plaque technique will be presented. The technique is useful for enumerating naturally occurring and polyclonal activator (PCA) stimulated immunoglobulin-synthesizing cells isolated from the peripheral blood (PB) of humans. In addition to the description of general methods, specific problems encountered with the use of this assay in studies of human aging will be discussed.

II. MATERIALS AND METHODS UTILIZED FOR THE PLAQUE ASSAY

A. Cell Separation
Mononuclear cells are isolated by the density centrifugation method of Böyum.[11]

---

*   Recently types and subclasses of immunogloublin other than IgG have been shown to interact with protein A.[9]

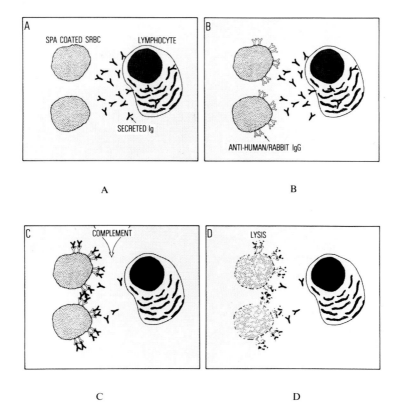

A   B

C   D

FIGURE 1. Mechanism of staphylococcal protein A (SPA)-coupled SRBC plaque assay for human lymphocytes. (A) Immunoglobulin is secreted from a lymphocyte incorporated in an agarose/SRBC indicator layer. (B) Rabbit IgG "linking antibody", specific for the class or subclass of human immunoglobulin to be detected, is added. The Fc terminal end of the rabbit antibody is bound to the SRBC by SPA. (C) The human immunoglobulin specifically binds to antigen receptor of the rabbit IgG. The addition of complement results in (D), regional lysis of the SRBC indicator layer, producing plaques.

The blood specimen is first anticoagulated either with heparin (10 U/mℓ) or defibrinated with 3- to 4-mm glass beads under sterile conditions. The anticoagulated blood is diluted 1:4 with RPMI-1640 and 5 to 6 mℓ are gently layered, to preserve the interface, on 5 mℓ of sterile Ficoll®/sodium diatrizoate (S.G. 1.078)* in sterile 17 × 100 mm round-bottom tubes (Falcon Plastics #2057, Oxnard, Calif.). The tubes are centrifuged at 400 × g for 40 min at 18 to 22°C and the centrifuge allowed to decelerate without use of the brake. The mononuclear cells are harvested from the interface with a sterile pasteur pipette and washed twice with RPMI. They are then counted in a hemocytometer, with a morphological differentiation of mononuclear and granulocytic cells. The usual cell yield from normal adults is 1 to 2 × 10⁶ mononuclear cells per mℓ of whole blood with approximately 95% viability by trypan blue dye exclusion and less that 10% granulocyte contamination.

---

*   The Ficoll® (Pharmacia Fine Chemicals, Piscataway, N.J.) and sodium diatrizoate, (Hypaque®, Winthrop Laboratories, N.Y., N.Y.) separation media for human cells may be purchased as a sterile and ready to use solution under several brand names (LSM®, Litton Bionetics; Lymphoprep, Nyegaard, Oslo; Ficoll-Paque®, Pharmacia) or prepared by mixing approximately 24 parts 9% Ficoll® in distilled water with 10 parts 33.9% sodium diatrizoate in distilled water, adjusting the specific gravity to 1.078 and sterilizing by 0.45μm filtration. Note: Ficoll® lowers the specific gravity, Hypaque® raises it.

B. Culture Conditions

The washed mononuclear cells are adjusted to a concentration of $2.5 \times 10^5/ml$ in RPMI-1640 supplemented with 10% fetal calf serum (North American Biologicals, Miami, Fla.), 2 mM L-glutamine, penicillin (50 U/ml), streptomycin (50 μg/ml), and gentamycin (50 μg/ml) (Schering Corporation, Kenilworth, N.J.). Some investigators routinely use human sera to supplement the culture media, however, we have found that AB sera, despite prior adsorption (2×) with SRBC, still contain enough antibody to later cause lysis of the SRBC in the plaque "lawn". In addition, some lots have an inhibitory effect on plaque production. Duplicate 10-ml cell suspensions (2.5×10^5 lymphocytes per ml) are prepared in 17×100 polystyrene tubes. The polyclonal B-cell activator, pokeweed lectin (Sigma Chemical, St. Louis, Mo.) is added to one of the cell preparations, and both tubes are incubated at 37°C 100% humidity in 5% CO_2, 95% air atmosphere. The concentration of pokeweed for maximal plaque formation is approximately 1 log or less than the concentration for optimal thymidine incorporation at the same incubation period. The PFC-stimulating ability of pokeweed preparations obtained from different manufacturers may differ and each lot must be routinely tested. The non-stimulated culture serves as a control for determination of spontaneously occurring PFCs.

C. Preparation of Cells for Plaque Assay

Ater 6 days in culture, the cells are resuspended, and their number and viability assessed with fluorescent microscopy using ethidium bromide (EB) and fluorescein diacetate (FDA) (Sigma Chemical)*. This is a combination of the methods orignally described by Rotman and Papermaster[12] for FDA, and Edidin[13] for EB.

One ml of the cultured cell suspension is removed, and 1 ml of the EB solution and 1 ml of the FDA working solution are added, the mixture vortexed and counted on a hemocytometer using a fluorescence microscope. The order of addition of the cells and stain does not appear critical. The counting should, however, be performed within 10 to 15 min of staining since background fluorescence increases, making accurate counting difficult. Viable cells, which are able to hydrolyze the nonfluorescent FDA, stain a brilliant green, and dead cells bright red with EB. RBC's do not stain. Viable cells comprise approximately 70 to 90% of the day-6 culture. Two × 10^5 viable cells per slide and three slides per culture are usually prepared, therefore, 6×10^5 viable cells are removed from each culture tube, washed twice with MEM** without serum supplementation, and resuspended in MEM to a final volume of 0.3 ml.

D. Preparation of Protein A Labeled SRBC

Sheep red blood cells (SRBC) (Colorado Serum Co., Denver, Colo.) in Alsever's solution are washed three to four times with 0.85% saline. After the final wash, the supernatant and some SRBC are removed by suction to adjust the volume of packed SRBCs to 1 ml. A staphylococcal protein A (SPA) solution (Pharmacia Fine Chemicals) is prepared by mixing 0.5 mg of protein A with 1 ml of 0.85% saline. Chromic chloride ($CrCl_3 \cdot 6H_2O$) 6 mg/100 ml is also prepared in 0.85% saline. To the 1 ml of packed SRBC, 0.5 ml of the protein A solution is added. After thorough mixing of

---

*   The ethidium bromide (EB) solution is prepared in a concentration of 2 mg/100ml in RPMI-1640. Fluorescein diacetate (FDA) 5 mg/ml in acetone is prepared as a stock solution. The FDA working solution, which is prepared daily, contains 50 μl of the stock solution in 10 ml of RPMI-1640. The stock reagents should be kept cold and protected from lights when not is use.

** Hanks' base Eagle MEM without glutamine or antibotics containing 15 ml of 7.5% $NaHCO_3$ and 20 ml of 1 M (pH 7.2) HEPES per l MEM with Earle's salts may cause precipitation of the phosphates in the agarose and therefore should not be used.

the SRBC and SPA, 5 ml of the chromic chloride solution is added dropwise with constant vortexing during addition. The CrCl₃/SPA/SRBC mixture is then incubated at room temperature for 30 min, followed by washing with 0.85% saline and then with two additional washes using phosphate buffered saline (PBS) pH 7.2. After the last wash, the SRBC's are resuspended to 30% v/v with PBS. Because of the time involved, the protein A-coupled SRBC are usually prepared the day prior to the actual plating of the cultures. The SPA coated SRBC are usable for 3 to 4 days if diluted before storage at 4°C. The cells should be washed several times with PBS and resuspended to 30% v/v before each subsequent use.

E. Antisera Production

Rabbit antihuman immunoglobulin antisera is prepared by injecting 1.5 mg of Cohn fraction II human gamma globulin (Sigma) emulsified in complete Freund's adjuvant into New Zealand white rabbits. After 2 weeks a booster injection of 1.5 mg of Cohn fraction II in incomplete Freund's adjuvant is given. One week following the second injection, each rabbit is test bled, the serum heat inactivated, and the antibody level determined by the protein A hemolytic plaque assay using an individual known to produce plaques in response to PWM, and several dilutions of the crude antisera. Usually the polyvalent antisera produced by this method can be diluted between 1:50 and 1:200 for use. Because of the differences in antibody levels between rabbits it is advisable not to pool antisera.

Commerically obtained poly- and monospecific rabbit antihuman immunoglobulin (DAKO, Copenhagen, Denmark) can be diluted approximately 1:400 to 1:600 for use. Antisera prepared in other animals such as goat, presumably because of a lower binding efficiency with the protein A coupled SRBC°, are generally not able to be used in this assay system.

F. PFC Determination

There are many modifications of the techniques for quantitating immunoprotein synthesizing cells in agar gels. The method presented in detail below has been in use in our laboratory for over 3 years.

Agarose is now used as the supporting media for plaque assays rather than an unrefined agar (Difco®, Noble, Bacto®, Ionogar). This alleviates the need to add DEAE-dextran and gives superior results. Glass slides (2 by 3 in.) are precoated with a 0.5% agarose (Seakem® Agarose, Marine Colloids, Rockland, Maine) in a 0.3% saline solution. This is accomplished by Pasteur pipetting a few drops of the melted agarose coating solution onto a prewarmed (40 to 45°C) slide, and spreading it evenly over the entire slide with a clean glass rod. The slide is then placed back on the slide warmer and allowed to dry. The coating film should be almost invisible with no bubbles or salt crystals, since they will cause local defects or lysis of the SRBC. It is advisable to store the coated dry slides in a rack with the coated sides all facing the same direction, so that the coated side can be readily identified. The slides may be coated ahead of time and will keep in a dry environment. Because the slides are ultimately dehydrated and fixed in ethanol and acetone, they must be identified using a diamond or carbide pencil.

At the time of assay, a 1% agarose solution in distilled water is melted and mixed with an equal volume of warmed 2× MEM*. It is convenient to melt the agarose in a beaker placed in an electric pressure cooker (250° for 10 to 15 min). The warm MEM-

---

* Hank's base Eagles MEM (10×) is diluted 1:5 to give 2×, then 3.5 ml of 7.5% NaHCO₃ and 2 ml of 1 M HEPES, pH 7.2 is added per 100 ml.

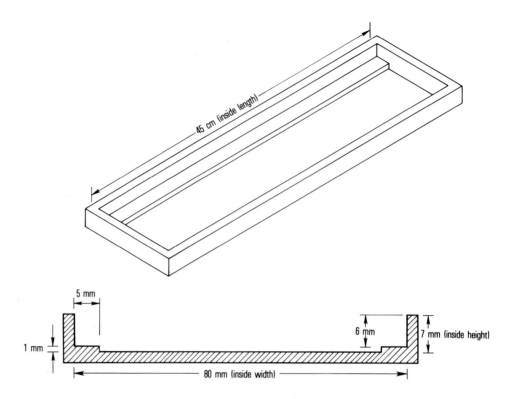

FIGURE 2.   General dimensions of a slide tray used in the slide modification of the plaque assay. Approximately 30 m*l* are required to fill the tray to a depth of 1 mm.

agarose solution (0.4 m*l*) is pipetted (Cornwall repeating syringe, Becton Dickinson, Rutherford, N.J.) into individual warmed (49°C waterbath) 12 × 75 mm glass tubes. Because of the pH change that occurs in the agarose-media mixture while standing, it is best to only fill a maximum of 50 to 60 tubes at one time immediately prior to the addition of the cells.

To prepare the slides for the PFC assay an agarose containing tube is removed from the waterbath and 20 μ*l* of SPA coupled SRBC are added. This is immediately followed by the addition of 100 μ*l* (2 × 10^5 lymphocytes per 0.1 m*l*) of cells from the resuspended cultures. These additions are most easily accomplished by using a semiautomatic pipette (Eppendorf, Oxford®, Finn, etc.). The tube is then gently mixed and the contents poured onto the agarose coated surface of a prewarmed slide (45 to 48°C slide warmer). The mixture is spread evenly with a clean 6-in-glass rod by drawing it over the slide except for approximately 5 mm at each narrow end. The slide is gently rotated to distribute the agarose-cell mixture to an even thickness. Then the agarose is allowed to solidify by placing the slide on a level bench top. While one slide is solidifying several others can be prepared. The agarose should form a firm gel, but should not be allowed to dry out. Once firm, the slides are inverted in a tray (Figure 2) which allows them to be suspended on the uncoated, narrow slide ends. The tray is filled with MEM avoiding the formation of air bubbles under the slides. An eight-slide tray requires approximately 30 m*l* of media to fill it. It is possible to add SRBC to 2 to 3 agarose-containing tubes at one time but one must watch that these cells do not agglutinate in the heated agarose prior to plating.

After several trays are filled with slides and media, they are placed for 60 min in a 37°C incubator in a humidified 5% CO_2 atmosphere. After this initial incubation, the slides are removed from the trays, placed in glass slide racks, and rinsed for 1 to 2 min by immersion in 0.85% saline. After washing, the slides are again placed face down in the trays and rabbit antihuman immunoglobulin added. The antibody concentration of each antisera lot differs and the optimal dilution must be determined experimentally. The range of dilutions can be 1:100 for a crude antisera and between 1:400 and 1:1000 for a more refined Ig fraction. The antisera is kept frozen in small aliquots and diluted immediately prior to use. The slides are incubated with the antisera for 30 min at 37°C in the CO_2 incubator. It is possible to combine the cells and antisera during the first incubation which will save time, however, if difficulties arise it is impossible to pinpoint the source of trouble.

After the antisera incubation, the slides are again washed with 0.85% saline and then incubated with guinea pig complement (GIBCO®, Grand Island, N.Y.) diluted in MEM. The best dilution of complement must be determined experimentally, and may vary between 1:50 and 1:200. The length of the complement incubation step also varies, for unlike direct SRBC plaquing techniques, the entire protein A/SRBC "lawn" will lyse if complement is left on for too long a time. It is advisable to incubate the slides for 30 min and then visually check them. Lysis is most apparent at the edges of the slide, but occurs over the entire surface. Most slides will totally lyse in 90 min when incubated in a 1:50 complement dilution.

After complement incubation, the slides are placed in slide racks, washed in 0.85% saline, and then dehydrated in acetone for 3 min, fixed in ethanol for 3 min, and blown dry with heated air. An inexpensive hair dryer works well. High-temperature heat guns (like the ones used for drying TLC plates) should be used with caution because excessive heat can melt the agarose on the slides. The acetone and alcohol can be reused one time, but after that it is too saturated with water to function as a dehydrating agent. Insufficient dehydration will be seen as white areas on dried slides. The PFC's can be counted rapidly on nonfixed slides, using a television-based, semiautomated plaque counter. If this equipment is not available, it is best to fix the slides prior to counting the plaques because of the difference in the time necessary for each procedure.

G. Plaque Counting

The final analysis of this procedure is the enumeration of the plaques which have formed in the SRBC/agarose suspension on a slide. Until recently, this has been accomplished by visualization and counting the number of lytic areas on a slide while observing it with a binocular sterozoom microscope with indirect lighting. It is essential that each lytic area be observed for the presence of a mononuclear cell (or cells) since aggregated SRBC, bubbles, and salt crystals in the agarose under-layer will also produce areas of "lysis" and pseudoplaques.[14] Some investigators stain the slides with Wrights's or Giemsa stain prior to counting the plaques to aid the detection of mononuclear cells.

Katz et al.[15] have recently described experiments using a semiautomated plaque counter (Fisher Count-All, Fisher Scientific; Artek Systems, Farmingdale, N.Y.) based on a high-resolution television camera with an electronic processing unit. Recent improvements in the resolving ability of these and similar devices make them a necessity for plaque enumeration in any laboratory routinely performing large numbers of assays. The time differential between manual and automated counting can obviate the need for additional technical staff.

III. DISCUSSION

There have been several extensive reviews of the various plaque assay techniques up

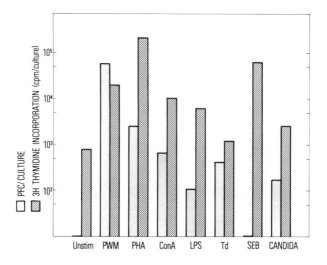

FIGURE 3.   Comparison of the relative efficiency of polyclonal
activators and antigens to stimulate SPA/SRBC hemolytic plaques
and 3H-thymidine incorporation.

to the introduction of the protein A coupled-assay system. Since these reviews are quite
good and deal extensively with both technical and theoretical considerations, only
points deserving special emphasis will now be considered.[16,17]

The PFC assay system amplifies a multimolecular submicroscopic event allowing it
to be quantitated visually. This in vitro induction of immunoglobulin synthesis requires
the presence of both viable T and B lymphocytes, however, other cell populations are
apparently nonessential.[18,19] Adherent cells, macrophages, or compounds substituting
for them may, under specific conditions, augment the number of antibody-producing
cells.[20]

Recently extensive use has been made of pokeweed lectin as an activator of PFC's
in humans. Lymphocyte cultures stimulated with PWM yield approximately 150 to
200% of the original number of viable cells present by day 6 when the culture is analyzed. This number of viable cells does not appear to change as a function of age in
humans, but remains, as in the murine system, relatively stable throughout life. Other
lymphocyte activators such as phytohemagglutinin, soluble protein A, and concanavalin A also produce large numbers of viable cells after several days in culture, however, because of the particular cell subsets which have been stimulated, these cultures
contain relatively few immunoprotein-synthesizing lymphocytes and produce meager
numbers of plaques. Antigen-stimulated cultures also produce few plaques (Figure 3).
This point seems especially pertinent to investigations of the effect of aging, since most
studies indicate that the major age-associated decline in lymphocyte function involves
only T- and not B-cell performance. Plaque enumeration measures not only B lymphocyte function, but also indirectly evaluates the interaction of T and B cells leading to
immunoglobulin synthesis. Because our understanding of this T- to B-cell interaction,
especially as a function of age, in only beginning to be investigated in humans, care
should be exercised in interpreting decreases in the numbers of PFC's as representing
decreases in the functional capacities of only B cells. Despite the widespread use of
pokeweed lectin as a polyclonal activator of human cells, little consideration also appears to have been made of the fact that pokeweed is a heterologous compound which,
by even simple electrophoretic techniques, is composed of at least five separate frac-

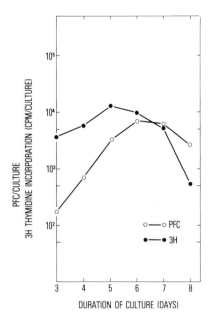

FIGURE 4. Comparison of numbers of
plaques and 3H-thymidine incorporation
as a function of time in culture of human
lymphocytes activated with optimal doses
of pokeweed lectin.

tions, some of which we have found to have more plaque-stimulating ability than others. It is also well recognized that PWM is a mitogen for human B lymphocytes and also some T cells as well.[21] As shown in Figure 4, the number of antibody-producing cells detected after stimulation of cultures with PWM may vary considerably, but the optimal culture time for maximal DNA synthesis, as assessed by tritiated thymidine uptake, is clearly different than that for maximal immunoglobulin secretion.

Exactly how the results of a SPA/SRBC PFC assay will correlate with other evaluations of B-cell numbers and functions is under investigation. Preliminary results comparing B-cell numbers, detected by cytoplasmic and surface immunofluorescence, with numbers of antibody-secreting cells by PFC assay, have not produced a discernable correlation between the two assays. It should be kept in mind, however, that the plaque assay is a functional test requiring individual cells to perform at high levels of competence to produce sufficient immunoglobulin to yield a hemolytic plaque. Immunofluorescence studies do not have such stringent temporal and functional requirements. Reports of the switching of individual B-cell clones from IgM to IgG production during maturation may also influence attempts to correlate these two assays.[22] Other studies of surface and cytoplasmic immunoglobulin on human B lymphocytes after PWM activation have also shown different patterns of maturation, depending upon the particular class of immunoglobulin ultimately synthesized.[23] Whatever class of immunoprotein is ultimately secreted after cellular activation by PWM is presently thought to be the product of only a partially differentiated lymphoblast, rather than a mature plasma cell.[24]

The growth medium for the culture of lymphocytes in the protein A/SRBC plaque assay is supplemented with fetal calf rather than human sera. When using cells cultured in human sera for plaquing, we have routinely experienced lysis of the SRBC's when the slides were incubated with complement. Adsorption of the human sera with SRBC did not eliminate this problem, since it appeared to be mediated via the coupling of immunoprotein in the human serum-supplemented growth media to the protein A rather than by the presence of specific anti-SRBC antibodies. Washing of the cell cultures several times prior to plaquing also did not totally eliminate the lysis. Since Anderson et al.[25] have found that the synthesis and secretion of IgG by murine B lymphocytes is dependent upon several factors, including the particular lot and concentration of FCS in the media, differences in serum supplementation should be carefully evaluated as a source of potential variability in the PFC assay. In an attempt to solve this problem, Iscove et al. have recently begun to successfully experiment in the murine system with a partially or totally synthetic mixture which is able to replace fetal calf sera.[26,27] Perhaps the development of a similar serum replacement for use with human cells will eliminate this area of uncertainty.

The number of cells producing immunoprotein in a PFC assay is generally expressed either as plaques per culture or as plaques per number of cells (usually 10^6). To use either of these methods with no knowledge of cell density and the number of viable cells plated per slide, may introduce uncertainty, if not error, into the subsequent interpretation of the results. Small differences in the absolute numbers of plaques may be greatly amplified and appear statistically significant. To complicate matters further the unstimulated cultures used to determine "background" plaques contain fewer cells, but are about 90% viable while the PWM-activated cultures have about 1.5 to 2 times the number of cells but a viability of only about 75%. It can readily be seen that to express results as PFC's per 10^6 cells creates a problem in how one should relate this number to the original cell density. We have therefore chosen to assess the viability of each culture and plaque 2×10^5 viable cells (disregarding the total number of cells) per slide, and then calculate the results on the basis of volume which allows us to sidestep this issue by expressing results as plaques per culture.

IV. SUMMARY

In this chapter a slide modification of the protein A-coupled, hemolytic-plaque technique has been described. The relative simplicity of this technique, coupled with its ability to assay cells secreting all classes of immunoglobulin, makes it especially useful to study human cells. The isolation, enumeration, and function of human B and T lymphocytes and their relationship to various infectious, autoimmune, and lymphoproliferative processes is at present an area of intense interest in both laboratory and clinical medicine. This and other plaque techniques, coupled with polyclonal B-cell activation, are already being used to study these diseases, as well as, immunodeficiencies, helper-suppressor factors and cells, drug and hormone activities, and antibody synthesis in humans.[28-33]

As the plaque assay represents the only method that *functionally* assesses the activation, cell-cell interaction, proliferation, and biosynthetic capacities of individual B cells, it seems destined to play an increasingly important role in the dissection and analysis of the human immune response.

REFERENCES

1. **Jerne, N. K. and Nordin, A. A.,** Plaque formation in agar by single antibody-producing cells, *Science,* 140, 405, 1963.
2. **Segre, D. and Segre, M.,** Hemolytic plaque formation by mouse spleen cells producing antibodies to ovalbumin, *Immunochemistry,* 5, 206, 1968.
3. **Layson, M. N. and Sehon, A. H.,** Detection of cells producing antibodies against the dinitrophenyl group, *Can. J. Biochem.,* 45, 1773, 1967.
4. **Golub, E. S., Mishell, R. I., Weigle, W. O., and Dutton, R. W.** A modification of the hemolytic plaque assay for use with protein antigens, *J. Immunol.,* 100, 133, 1968.
5. **Cunningham, A. J., and Szenberg, A.,** Further improvements in the plaque technique for detecting single antibody-forming cells, *Immunology,* 14, 599, 1968.
6. **Fauci, A. A. and Pratt, K. R.,** Activation of human B lymphocytes I. Direct plaque-forming cell assay for the measurement of polyclonal activation and antigenic stimulation of human B lymphocytes, *J. Exp. Med.,* 144, 674, 1976.
7. **Dresser, D. W. and Wortis, H. H.,** Use of an antiglobulin serum to detect cells producing antibody with low hemolytic efficiency, *Nature (London),* 208, 859, 1965.
8. **Sterzl, J. and Riha, I.,** Detection of cells producing 7S antibodies by the plaque technique, *Nature (London),* 208, 858, 1965.
9. **Harboe, M. and Følling, I.,** Recognition of two distinct groups of human IgM and IgA based on different binding to staphylococci, *Scand. J. Immunol.,* 3, 471, 1974.
10. **Gronowicz, E., Coutinho, A., and Melchers, F.,** A plaque assay for all cells secreting Ig of a given type or class, *Eur. J. Immunol.* 6, 588, 1976.
11. **Böyum, A.,** Isolation of mononuclear cells and granulocytes from human blood, *Scand. J. Clin. Lab. Invest.,* 21 (Supp. 97), 51, 1968.
12. **Rotman, B. and Papermaster, B. W.,** Membrane properties of living mammalian cells as studied by enzymatic hydrolysis of fluorogenic esters, *Proc. Nat. Acad. Sci. U.S.A.,* 55, 134, 1966.
13. **Edidin, M.,** A rapid quantitative fluorescence assay for cell damage by cytotoxic antibodies, *J. Immunol.,* 104, 1303, 1970.
14. **Muchmore, A. V., Koski, I., Dooley, N., and Blaese, R. M.,** Artifactual plaque formation *in vitro* and *in vivo* due to passive transfer of specific antibody, *J. Immunol.,* 116, 1016, 1976.
15. **Katz, D. H., Faulkner, M., Katz, L. R., Lindh, E., Leonhardt, C. C., Herr, K., and Tung, A. S.,** A rapid, semiautomated counting procedure for enumeration of antibody-forming cells in gel and nucleated cells in suspension, *J. Immunol. Methods,* 17, 285, 1977.
16. **Jerne, N. K., Henry, C., Nordin, A. A., Fuji, H., Koros, A. M. C., and Lefkovits, I.,** Plaque forming cells: methodology and theory, *Transplant Rev.,* 18, 130, 1974.
17. **Jerne, N. K., Henry, C., Nordin, A. A., Fuji, H., Koros, A. M. C., and Lefkovits, I.,** Plaque techniques for recognizing individual antibody-forming cells, in *Methods in Immunology and Immunochemistry,* Vol. 5, Williams, C. A. and Chase, M. W., Eds., Academic Press, New York, 1976, 335.
18. **MacDermott, R. P., Nash, G. S., Bertovich, M. J., Merkel, N. S., and Weinrieb, I. J.,** Human B-cell mitogenic responsiveness to lectins: the requirement for T-cells, *Cell. Immunol.,* 38, 198, 1978.
19. **Gmelig-Meyling, F., UytdeHaag, A. G. C. M., and Ballieux, R. E.,** Human B-cell activation in vitro; T-cell dependent pokeweed mitogen induced differentiation of blood B-lymphocytes, *Cell. Immunol.,* 33, 156, 1977.
20. **Nordin, A. A.,** The *in vitro* immune response to a T dependent antigen I. The effect of macrophages and 2-mercaptoethanol, *Eur. J. Immunol.,* 8, 776, 1978.
21. **Greaves, M., Janossy, G., and Doenhoff, M.,** Selective triggering of human T and B lymphocytes *in vitro* by polyclonal mitogens, *J. Exp. Med.,* 140, 1, 1974
22. **Andersson, J., Coutinho, A., and Melchers, F.,** The switch from IgM to IgG secretion in single mitogen-stimulated B-cell clones, *J. Exp. Med.,* 147, 1744, 1978.
23. **Morell, A., Skvaril, F., and Barandun, S.,** Terminal differentiation of PWM-stimulated human B lymphocytes, *Cell. Immunol.,* 42, 384, 1979.
24. **George, E. R. and Cohen, H. J.,** Kinetics of immunoglobulin synthesis and secretion by resting and pokeweed mitogen-transformed human lymphocytes, *Clin. Immunol. Immunopathol.,* 12, 94, 1979.
25. **Andersson, J., Coutinho, A., and Melchers, F.,** Stimulation of murine B lymphocytes to IgG synthesis and secretion by the mitogens lipopolysaccharide and lipoprotein and its inhibition by anti-immunoglobulin antibodies, *Eur. J. Immunol.,* 8, 336, 1978.
26. **Guilbert, L. J. and Iscove, N. N.,** Partial replacement of serum by selenite, transferrin, albumin and lecithin in haemopoietic cell cultures, *Nature (London),* 263, 594, 1976.

27. **Iscove, N. N. and Melchers, F.,** Complete replacement of serum by albumin, transferrin, and soybean lipid in cultures of lipoplysaccharide- reactive B lymphocytes, *J. Exp. Med.,* 147, 923, 1978.

28. **Dosch, H-M., Percy, M. E. and Gelfand, E. W.,** Functional differentiation of B lymphocytes in congenital agammaglobulinemia I. Generation of hemolytic plaque-forming cells, *J. Immunol.,* 119, 1959, 1977.

29. **Herrod, H. G. and Buckley, R. H.,** Use of a human plaque forming cell assay to study peripheral blood bursa-equivalent cell activation and excessive suppressor cell activity in human humoral immunodeficiency, *J. Clin. Invest.,* 63, 868, 1979.

30. **Nespoli, L., Vitiello, A., Maccario, R., Lanzavecchia, A., and Ugazio, A. G.,** Polyclonal activation of human B lymphocytes *in vitro* by pokeweed mitogen: A simple technique for the simultaneous assessment of cell proliferation, generation of plasma cells, plaque-forming cells and immunoglogulin production, *Scand. J. Immunol.,* 8, 489, 1978.

31. **Melmon, K. L., Bourne, H. R., Weinstein, Y., Shearer, G. M., Kram, J., and Bauminger, S.,** Hemolytic plaque formation by leukocytes *in vitro* : Control by vasoactive hormones, *J. Clin. Invest.,* 53, 13, 1974.

32. **Chiorazzi, N., Fu, S. M., and Kunkel, H. G.,** Induction of polyclonal antibody synthesis by human allogenic and autologous helper factors, *J. Exp. Med.,* 148, 1543, 1979.

33. **Heijnen, C. J., UytdeHaag, F., Gmelig-Meyling, F. H. J., and Ballieux, R. E.,** Localization of human antigen-specific helper and suppressor function in distinct T-cell subpopulations, *Cell. Immunol.,* 43, 282, 1979.

Chapter 8

IMMUNOGLOBULIN LEVELS AND ABNORMALITIES IN AGING
HUMANS AND MICE

Jiri Radl

TABLE OF CONTENTS

I. INTRODUCTION

The immunoglobulin levels in serum reflect directly the activity of the B-immune system and indirectly that of the T-immune system. In cooperation with T-helper cells, under the control of T-suppressor cells, and to a lesser extent also independently, thousands of various B-cell clones are continuously active in response to many diverse stimuli to which every individual is exposed at any time. While each individual B-cell clone will produce at a given time only one homogeneous population of immunoglobulins (Ig),i.e., antibodies, the sum of the products of the innumerable various clones pooled in the blood forms a heterogeneous (polyclonal) Ig spectrum under normal conditions. The levels of Ig divided according to the structure of the constant part of their heavy chains into different classes and subclasses vary widely among individuals, but they are relatively stable within the normal individual and their variation is small, even for a longer period of time. In disease, the level and the heterogeneity of Ig may change; their assessment may substantially contribute to the making of a correct diagnosis. For example, increased levels of serum Ig are found in various infections, autoimmune, and liver diseases. Lower than normal values are detected in different groups of immunodeficiency diseases. A finding of a high and still progressively increasing homogeneous Ig component (paraprotein) is a very valuable diagnostic sign of a B-cell malignancy such as myeloma and Waldenström's macroglobulinemia.

During aging, the serum Ig show some particular phenomena which mirror changes occurring in the immune system. These include quantitative changes, restriction of the heterogeneity of Ig, and the appearance of transient and persistent homogeneous immunoglobulins (H-Ig). Recent studies which have increased our understanding of these changes are the subject of this review.

II. METHODS FOR DETERMINATION OF IMMUNOGLOBULINS IN SERUM

A. Quantitative Techniques

In the majority of our studies, the single radial immunodiffusion technique of Mancini et al.[1] employing a modification described by Voormolen - Kalova et al.[2] was used. In some experiments where only a limited amount of serum from individual mice was available, a microfluorometric assay[3] was applied. Quantitation of human subclasses was performed by a radioimmunoassay.[4] These techniques, described in detail in the publications quoted above, give reliable results in the hands of skilled investigators and they present no special problems (except for inaccuracy in the determination of IgM in humans by the Mancini technique[5]), provided that the antisera and the standard preparations are properly defined and of good quality. The preparation and the quality control of specific antisera will be dealt with in a separate section of this chapter. The problems concerning a proper reference standard for Ig quantitation relate to the antigenic heterogeneity and the molecular forms of the Ig in the serum under investigation, and in the standard preparation. The molecular composition of a given Ig class in the reference preparation should be as closely comparable to that of the test samples as is possible. Therefore, pooled normal serum containing heterogeneous Ig is to be preferred as a standard over preparations of a single or multiple isolated paraproteins. Nevertheless, when testing sera with an abnormal Ig composition (e.g., Ig of restricted heterogeneity, H-Ig, or with a change in proportion between monomeric and polymeric forms), the determination will necessarily be less accurate. With respect to the testing of human material, the comparability of results among different laboratories has been greatly improved by the introduction of the international WHO Ig reference preparations.[6] The values for human Ig are now usually measured by using an internal standard (pooled normal human serum) in which the Ig levels are calibrated against the WHO reference serum.

No standards of a comparable nature are presently available for the determinations of Ig in murine sera. Preparations consisting of a mixture of paraproteins, one for each class or subclass, are commercially available. However, their use can be a source of great errors, especially if the antiserum used in the investigation has been prepared by immunization with the same paraprotein as present in the standard preparation. Such an antiserum also usually contains antibodies against idiotypic determinants of the paraprotein and thus erroneously leads to higher values in determinations for the corresponding Ig class or subclass. Therefore, Ig levels in sera of mice are preferably expressed as a percentage of an internal standard consisting of a large pool of sera from young adult normal mice of the strain under investigation. In follow-up studies, the values are easily comparable with those obtained in other laboratories. For comparison of results of cross-sectional studies, exchange of the relevant standards among different laboratories is necessary.

The concentration of H-Ig, paraproteins, was calculated from values obtained by photometric scanning of the electrophoretic pattern on agar plates or acetate cellulose strips by densitometry and by determination of the total serum protein concentration by the biuret method. In the case of a paraprotein with an α- or β-electrophoretic mobility or of a low-level paraprotein in a serum containing a high background of other heterogeneous Ig, the scanning procedure can be performed on the immunofixation plates[7] and the results compared with a known standard of the Ig class under investigation. The two latter techniques do not yield very accurate results, but are satisfactory, particularly since better techniques are not presently available or are too laborious and too costly.

B. Qualitative and Semiquantitative Techniques
1. Assessment of Homogeneous Immunoglobulins

A number of criteria should be fulfilled for an exact demonstration of a paraproteinemia. Theoretically, the Ig under examination must be shown to be homogeneous in both its constant (it belongs only to one class, subclass, light chain type, and allotype) and its variable part (it possesses unique idiotypic determinant and combines with only one antigen.) An isolated paraprotein gives only a few bands when tested by the isoelectric focusing technique. In practice, however, not all test systems and antisera are always available. Therefore, a combination of a sensitive electrophoretic technique (for demonstration of a homogeneous (M-) component in the β to γ region) and immunoelectrophoresis with specific antisera to Ig classes, subclasses, and light chain types (for specification and typing of H-Ig) is usually a common procedure for the detection of most of the paraproteins. It is proper to stress here that the technique of agar electrophoresis according to Wieme[8] proved to be superior for detection of homogeneous Ig components at low concentrations (Figure 1). As compared to a number of commercial electrophoretic techniques using acetate cellulose as a carrier, it is four to ten times more sensitive, and H-Ig in a concentration as low as 0.5 mg/ml can be detected. As far as the immunoelectrophoretic technique is concerned, most of the commercially available equipment and instructions give satisfactory results. However, two recommendations can be made to improve the quality of the Ig precipitin pattern, which is of special importance for a proper evaluation of sera containing H-Ig at a low concentration. When using agar with a high electroendosmosis, all immunoglobulins are "drifted" by it cathodally, and they form long assymetric (heterogeneous) precipitin lines which are not influenced and deviated by the starting well (Figure 2).

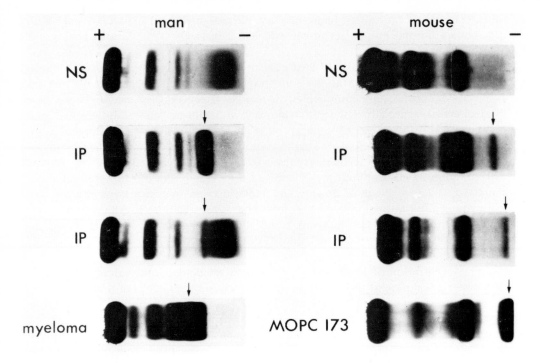

FIGURE 1.   Comparison of the agar electrophoretic pattern of human and mouse sera from normal individuals (NS), from individuals with an idiopathic paraproteinemia (IP), and from individuals suffering from
a malignant paraproteinemia (myeloma in man; plasma cell tumor in the BALB/c mouse). The paraproteins
are indicated by arrows. (From Van Camp B. and Radl, J., *Ned. T. Geront.* 9, 236, 1978. With permission.)

In this arrangement, even a low-level paraprotein may be revealed by a symmetric
(homogeneous) deviation of the precipitin line, regardless of the electrophoretic mobility of the paraprotein. Immunoelectrophoresis performed on microscopic slides is
inferior to that using larger plates where multiple samples can be investigated at the
same time. The latter arrangement allows the inclusion of a reference serum (against
which each test sample should be compared), and the antisera can diffuse and precipitate the proteins under investigation from two troughs which are parallel to the line
of electrophoretic migration. The one trough arrangement gives a less regular precipitin pattern and small abnormalities (especially of IgM) could be easily missed.

In doubtful cases where agar electrophoresis and immunoelectrophoresis failed to
prove unambiguously the homogeneity of a given Ig, additional techniques were used.
Immunofixation[7] performed on Wieme's agar electrophoretic plates[8] (Figure 3) is very
useful in situations where the homogeneous Ig components are overlapped by nonim-
munoglobulin protein components, that is, paraproteins migrating in the alpha, beta$_1$,
and beta$_2$ electrophoretic regions. The method of immunoselection[9,10] (Figure 4)
proved to be very helpful, especially in testing multiple paraproteins at a low concentration, imbalance in Ig subpopulations, and heavy chain disease proteins. In special
investigations, a reliable marker for the homogeneity of the variable part of the Ig
molecule is necessary. For this purpose, antisera to the idiotypic determinants of the
H-Ig can be raised in a relatively short period of time by a simple procedure, without
the necessity to isolate the relevant H-Ig.[11] Finally, the technique of isoelectric focusing
offers further possibilities, mainly if H-Ig of a known antibody specificity are investigated.[12]

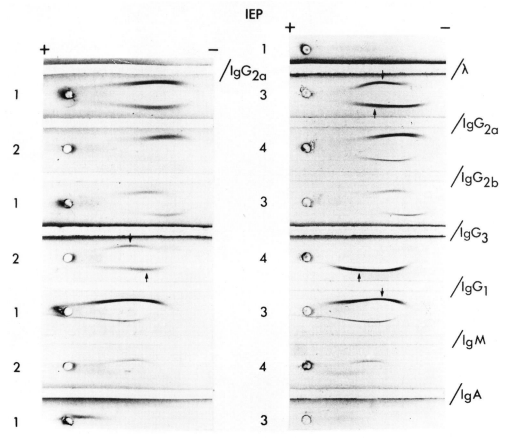

IEP

FIGURE 2. Demonstration of immunoglobulins of restricted heterogeneity in the sera of aging (over 1 year of age) thymusless nude mice on the BALB/c background (2,3,4) by means of immunoelectrophoresis. A serum from a normal one year old BALB/c mouse (1) is shown as a control. Note the symmetric deviations of the precipitin lines (arrows) indicating the presence of H-Ig of the IgG2a (3), IgG3 (2) and IgG1 (2,3,4) subclasses (in the serum of mouse 3, the IgG1 H-Ig is of the λ light chain type), the shortening of the IgG2a (2,3,4), IgG2b (3), and IgM (2,4) lines and the absence of the IgG2b (2), IgG3 (4) and IgA (2,3) precipitin lines.

Each of these techniques is used mainly for a qualitative assessment of Ig, that is, of their heterogeneity or homogeneity. However, they also offer to an experienced investigator some semiquantitative information, when performed under standard conditions and proper reference samples are included.

2. Assessment of Ig of Restricted Heterogeneity

The term immunoglobulins or antibodies of restricted heterogeneity is usually used in the literature for a specific immune response where only a very few clones are found to respond to an antigenic stimulation. We are using it here in a more broad sense and describe by it a general Ig pattern where the normally largely heterogeneous spectrum is reduced. This phenomenon can perhaps also be described as (multiple) partial or selective Ig deficiencies which, however, are often accompanied by the (usually transient) appearance of several small mono- or oligoclonal Ig components. The most representative examples of such Ig spectra can be seen in sera of immunodeficient children[13] or lethally irradiated laboratory animals[14] during the early reconstitution period after successful bone marrow transplantation (Figure 3). While the gamma globulin

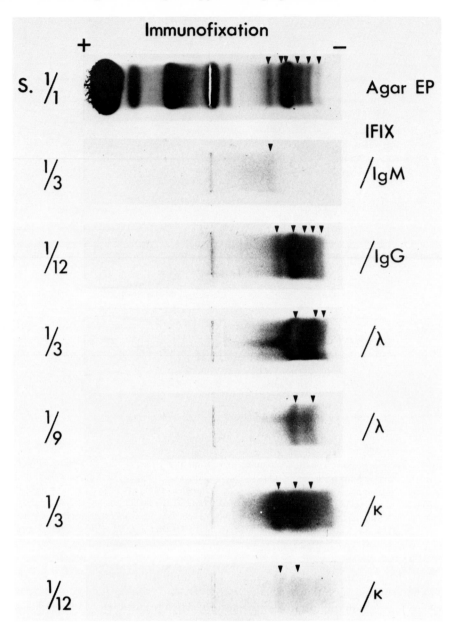

FIGURE 3.   Classification and light chain typing of multiple homogeneous immunoglobulin components by immunofixation. The serum of a boy treated by bone marrow transplantation for aplastic anemia was shown 2 months after transplantation to contain 1 IgM-ϰ,2 IgG-ϰ and 3 IgG-λ homogeneous Ig components. Note that the homogeneous bands detected by Wieme's agar electrophoresis (Agar-EP) can selectively be distinguished by specific antisera in properly diluted serum samples (dilution indicated on the left site) on the same plate by immunofixation (IFIX). The monospecific antisera used for the immunoprecipitation (fixation) are indicated on the right site of the plate. (From the material of the Children's Department of the University Hospital, Leiden, The Netherlands).

region on the agar electrophoretic plate may resemble a "washboard", the immuno-electrophoresis with specific sera to individual classes and subclasses may reveal a reduction in some, and a rather homogeneous increase in other Ig populations (Figure 2). In these cases, an imbalance of the kappa:lambda light-chain ratio within individual

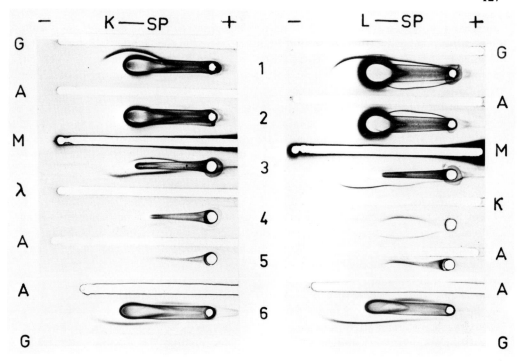

FIGURE 4. Analysis of immunoglobulin classes according to their light chain types by immunoselection. The samples investigated were: normal human serum (6), the serum (1,2), the serum euglobulin fraction (3), and the tears (4) of a boy suffering from severe combined immunodeficiency, 3 months after transplantation of bone marrow cells and foetal thymus. At that time, there were IgG-λ and IgA-$\varkappa$ paraproteins, normal IgG-$\varkappa$, no detectable IgA-λ, high IgM-λ and low IgM-$\varkappa$ in the serum. The tears of normal children (5) contain IgA of both light chain types, whereas only IgA-$\varkappa$ was detectable in this boy's tears. The troughs contained specific anti-IgG (G), anti-IgA (A), anti-IgM (M) and anti-$\varkappa$ ($\varkappa$) or anti-λ (λ) sera. Plate K-SP contained anti-$\varkappa$ light chain antiserum incorporated into the agar and accordingly all immunoglobulins with the $\varkappa$ light chain type were selected in the central precipitate; L-SP contained anti-λ serum (From Radl, J., *Immunology*, 19, 137, 1970. With permission.)

classes, as tested by immunoelectrophoresis, double-line immunodiffusion technique according to Skvaril and Barandun[15] and, in more detail, by immunoselection,[9] may also be a frequent finding. Useful information on the heterogeneity of specific antibodies can be obtained by investigation of the heterogeneity of their avidity.[16]

C. Antisera

The reliability of all the techniques used depends primarily on the quality of the antisera. Therefore, a separate section is devoted to their preparation and quality testing. It is necessary to stress that different techniques require antisera with different properties, titer, and grade of purity. For example, immunoprecipitation techniques such as radial immunodiffusion, immunoelectrophoresis, immunofixation, and immunoselection require precipitating antibodies only, the latter two of a very high titer. In radioimmunoassay and immunofluorescence, nonprecipitating antibodies are also active. Because of their high sensitivity, antisera for use in these methods must meet very strict requirements. Most routine, as well as research, laboratories depend wholly or largely on antisera of commercial origin. Such antisera sometimes lack proper specification (nature of the immunogen, antibody titer, method of absorption, other characteristics). In addition, subsequent batches of an antiserum may vary considerably. For these reasons, a sufficiently large stock of an appropriate and thoroughly tested antiserum should be available before starting any research project or study. It is quite imperative that each antiserum should finally be tested in the technique for which it is ultimately destined. Consequently, antisera prepared for, and tested exclusively in, immunodiffusion techniques should not be applied, as such, in immonofluorescence techniques.

Except for those to subclasses of human IgG and IgA (Nordic Immunological Laboratories, Tilburg, The Netherlands, or a gift from Dr. F. Skvaril, University of Bern, Switzerland) and to $\varkappa/\lambda$ light chains for the double-line technique (Dr. F. Skvaril) all antisera used in our studies were prepared in our laboratories. The following methods were used for their preparation.

1. Immunogens

For preparation of class-specific antisera to human Ig, mostly heterogeneous Ig of individual classes were isolated from pooled normal serum. A pool of five purified IgD paraproteins was available for immunization to the IgD class. Fab and Fc fragments of heterogeneous IgG were obtained by papain splitting and used for the preparation of anti Fab and anti IgG class-specific serum, respectively. Antisera to $\varkappa$ and λ light chains were raised against a pool of five different purified Bence Jones proteins of the corresponding type. Some antisera were prepared by immunization with individual paraproteins in an attempt to obtain antibodies recognizing particular subspecificities (subclass, idiotypic, and conformational determinants). They could also be used as class-specific antisera after proper absorption and/or pooling with other antisera of the appropriate specificity, provided that the quality tests did not show restrictions in their specificity to the relevant Ig class.

For the mouse Ig system, the following purified Ig preparations were used for immunization: heterogeneous IgG, Fab and Fc fragments of heterogeneous IgG, heterogeneous IgM cryoglobulin, isolated paraproteins (MOPC-315, IgAλ; TEPC-15, IgA$\varkappa$; MOPC-104E, IgMλ; MOPC-21, IgG1$\varkappa$; MOPC-195, IgG2b$\varkappa$; MOPC-173, IgG2a$\varkappa$; RPC-5, IgG2a$\varkappa$; HOPC-1, IgG2aλ; 10 different C57BL IgG2a$\varkappa$ paraproteins; J606, IgG3$\varkappa$; FLOPC-21, IgG3$\varkappa$; and isolated Bence Jones proteins (RPC-20, λ; MOPC-63, $\varkappa$; MOPC-41, $\varkappa$). For the isolation and purification of these Ig, conventional methods, as described earlier,[17] were used. All preparations were tested for their purity at 1% concentration by Ouchterlony analysis and by immunoelectrophoresis against a complete set of monospecific and polyspecific antisera; they gave a precipitin line only with the corresponding specific antiserum.

2. Immunization Procedure

Goats, sheep, rabbits, and guinea pigs belong to the animal species most frequently used for antisera production. All of these animals yield precipitating antibodies of the "rabbit type". In response to some antigens (e.g., free light chains of the λ type), goats and sheep may produce precipitating antibodies to one antigenic determinant and non-precipitating antibodies to another (i.e., "hidden" versus "surface" determinants of the λ light chains). The choice of the animal species is determined more by the housing facilities, the time factors, and the demands for the quantity of antiserum than by any "special superiority of properties" of antisera from any of the animals. The guinea pig yields the smallest volume of antiserum (15 to 25 mℓ), but it is the animal of choice when the antiserum is required in a short time period, as can be the case, e.g., in follow-up studies on H-Ig with the anti-idiotypic sera.[18] In this animal, only one injection of antigen in PBS, mixed with complete Freund's adjuvant, is administered in an amount of 0.1 mℓ into each foot pad.[11] Four weeks later, 6 to 8 mℓ of blood are drawn from the animal by heart puncture and this is repeated 1 week later. Six weeks after immunization, the animal is killed and completely exsanguinated.

Immunization of rabbits, goats, and sheep requires a series of injections. In principle, the same amount of antigen is given with each immunization, regardless of the species used. The dosage is dependent on the immunogenicity of the antigen, but, for most of the antisera, the following immunization scheme was used: the first injection consisted of 1 mg of antigen in 0.5 mℓ PBS mixed with 0.5 mℓ of Freund's complete adjuvant. The suspension was injected intradermally at multiple sites along the backbone of the animal. The rabbits also received a part of the suspension into foot pads. The same amount of antigen in complete Freund's, and after the third injection in incomplete Freund's adjuvant, was administered intradermally and subcutaneously every 14 days until a high antibody titer was obtained. Blood was withdrawn from the rabbits from the ear vein (about 30 mℓ) and from the goats and sheep from the jugular vein (about 120 mℓ) every two weeks. The separated sera were tested and pooled according to their quality. After top levels of antibodies were reached, the animals maintained the production of comparable lots of antiserum for months, even without further boosting.

Certain antigens (small molecules and split products), when presented as described above, do not give optimal results. Here, another immunization technique proved to be highly efficient.[18] After three initial injections of the antigen with complete Freund's adjuvant, the animals were allowed to rest for a period of 6 weeks. Afterwards, they received a series (twice a week) of intraveneous injections with increasing amounts of alum-precipitated antigen. One week after a total of six injections, the antibody titer reached its highest level and declined slowly afterwards. This technique was the only one of several tried which yielded antisera of a very high titer of antibodies to the surface determinants of Ig light chains which were needed for the method of immunoselection.[9]

3. Absorption of Antisera

Most of the antisera obtained by immunization, even with highly purified antigens, still have to be absorbed in order to make them specific. Antisera to complete Ig molecules contain antibodies not only to class (subclass)-specific determinants but also to determinants which are common to Ig of other classes (subclasses), i.e., to determinants of light chains and to common heavy chain determinants. Antibodies to non-Ig components may appear due to trace contaminants present, but not detected in the immunogen preparation. The immune response is an extremely sensitive recognition technique!

Absorption of unwanted antibody specificities from an antiserum by corresponding soluble antigens is still being done in a careful, stepwise procedure, but only for antisera used in some qualitative immunodiffusion techniques. Potentially disturbing effects which may result from absorption with soluble antigen, leading to the presence of a soluble excess of antigen or soluble immune complexes, must be particularly avoided in antisera intended for use in immunoselection, radioisotope-, enzyme-labeled antibody assays, and immunofluorescence techniques. Absorption by affinity chromatography on columns consisting of insolubilized antigens is a great improvement in this respect. They can be used in two ways, either for removing antibodies of unwanted specificity, or for the isolation of pure specific antibodies.

Two types of immunoadsorbents are used in our laboratories. The method of Avrameas and Ternynck[20] and Ishizaka et al.[21] is used with a slight modification if a large amount of easily available antigens (e.g., sera from individuals with selective Ig deficiencies) is at hand; the cross-linking of proteins with glutaraldehyde is accomplished in the presence of microfibrilar cellulose powder. The ratio of protein (g): acetate buffer (mℓ): cellulose powder (g): 2.5% glutaraldehyde (mℓ) is 1:80:2:20, respectively.

Immunoadsorbents prepared in this way consist of small particles which can be conveniently used in the column procedure. Antibodies absorbed on the column are eluted quickly by an 0.1 M glycine-HCl buffer, pH = 2.4, and, if immediately neutralized, they retain their activity.

If only a small amount of an antigen or a valuable preparation is available, preference is given to a more costly, but highly efficient immunoadsorbent preparation. The antigens are coupled covalently to Sepharose 4B beads by the cyanogen-bromide method[3] or to the activated beads (Pharmacia, Sweden) according to the instructions of the producer. The elution of absorbed antibodies from the column is achieved by 2 M KSCN in 0.1 M borate buffer, pH = 7.9, or by 1 M NaI in a 0.05 M TRIS buffer, pH = 9.0. Should these antibodies be preserved, a tandem column with Sephadex G 25 is used. The separation of the antibodies from the KSCN or NaI salt is monitored by a flow photometer at 280 nm and by drop reactions of the individual fractions with 1% $FeCl_3$ solution or in the case of NaI elution, with 1% $HgCl_2$. This procedure is a very mild one for the eluted antibodies, and is definitely superior to the elution with an acid buffer or 3 M urea. Moreover, in our hands, elutions of Sepharose 4B columns at low pH (2.4) are ineffective.

Immunoadsorbents prepared in both ways are kept at 4°C with addition of merthiolate (1:10,000) and can be used repeatedly for several years.

4. Testing of the Antisera

Because the quality and properties of antisera are decisive for the outcome of all techniques in which they are used, the investigator should have a good knowledge of each of them before he starts any investigation. Therefore, a reliable test system should be available in every laboratory, even in those where antisera from exclusively commercial sources are used. Such a test system has to be built up gradually, because a complete set of different antigens representing all Ig specificities is not commercially available. For the present, an exchange of purified antigens among different laboratories offers a temporary solution.

Suitable techniques to test antisera to be used in immunoprecipitation are the Ouchterlony (double-radial immunodiffusion) test and immunoelectrophoresis.[22] In the Ouchterlony plate, the tested antisera are reacted with H-Ig (paraproteins) representing all various classes and subclasses, also in their kappa and lambda combinations, with isolated Bence Jones proteins of both types, with Fab fragments of heterogeneous IgG and with normal serum. The antisera are tested undiluted, the purified antigens at a concentration of 1 mg/mℓ. If the precipitin line appears only with the corresponding homologous antigen, the antiserum is further tested in different dilutions against a known standard preparation by the technique in which it will be used. When additional unwanted ("nonspecific") reactions occur, immunoelectrophoretic analysis may help to identify the impurity and to select a suitable material for an additional absorption of the antiserum.

Antisera designated for more sensitive techniques (e.g., immunofluorescence) can be monitored during absorption by the same procedure; however, they should be performed in agar containing 3% polyethylene glycol 6000 (PEG).[23] Under these conditions, many otherwise-nonprecipitating antibodies will be revealed in the native plate: after washing of the plate, the precipitin lines may disappear (Figure 5). Some antigens (e.g., idiotypic, allotypic, or conformational determinants) seem to elicit a response of a very narrow specificity involving mainly nonprecipitating antibodies.[11] In such cases, all of the immunodiffusion tests should be performed in PEG plates and recorded by photography of the native plates. The final testing of antisera for, e.g., immunofluorescence, should be performed by that technique on monoclonal bone-

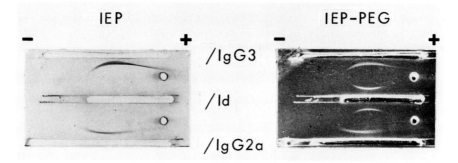

IEP   IEP-PEG

/IgG3

/Id

/IgG2a

FIGURE 5.   Demonstration of an IgG3 paraprotein in the serum of a (DBA/2 × C57BL/
Rij)F₁ mouse by immunoelectrophoresis. The serum was reacted with antiserum specific for
mouse IgG (/IgG3) and IgG2a (/IgG2a) subclasses and with an antiserum directed against
the idiotypic determinant of the paraprotein (/Id). Note that the paraprotein is precipitated
by the antiidiotypic serum only in the native 3% PEG agar plate (IEP-PEG) and not in the
normal or the PEG plate after the washing and staining procedure (IEP). (From Radl J., de
Glopper, E., and de Groot, G., *Vox Sang.*, 35, 10, 1978. With permission.)

marrow cells derived from patients suffering from myeloma, Waldenström's macroglobulinemia,[19] or chronic lymphatic leukemia. Alternatively, antisera can be tested
by using the defined-antigen-substrate spheres (DASS) system.[17,24]

5. IgG Fractions and Antibody Preparations of the Antisera

The use of whole antisera is usual and presents no problems in most of the immunoprecipitation techniques. In certain complex situations, however, where several different antisera are used in relatively high concentrations in one agar plate (e.g., the
immunoselection technique), the use of isolated Ig fractions from specific antisera can
be recommended. For techniques where enzyme-, radioisotope-, and fluoresceine-la-
beled antisera are applied, removal of serum proteins other than Ig from the antiserum
is a necessity. These proteins when labeled cause serious difficulties by increasing the
background staining or by interacting nonspecifically with other proteins or substances. Therefore, IgG fraction from an antiserum isolated by ion-exchange chromatography on DEAE cellulose,[25] or pure antibodies isolated by affinity chromatography
as described above, are the substances of choice for preparation of conjugates. The
labeled, purified-antibody preparations may have some advantage over the IgG fraction by giving less background staining, but their preparation is more costly and their
preservation in active form for longer periods of time still presents some problems.
Promising results in this respect were obtained by stabilization of the labeled-antibody
preparation with serum albumin of the species to which the antiserum is directed in a
final concentration of 0.5%.

III. IMMUNOGLOBULIN LEVELS DURING AGING

Investigations in humans and experimental laboratory animals have demonstrated
that the immune functions decline with aging (reviewed by Adler et al.[26]). This should
accordingly be reflected in the Ig serum spectrum. However, cross-sectional studies in
aging man on the levels of the three major Ig classes demonstrated no substantial
change in IgM and an increase in IgG and IgA.[27-32] In a longitudinal study by Buckley,
Buckley, and Dorsey,[23] about two thirds of the aging subjects studied showed increasing levels of IgG and IgA, and only in a smaller part of the group under investigation
were the Ig decreased.

Our study in 73 volunteers older than 95 years extended this information.[31] Apart from the quantitation of the Ig levels in this and a control group (young adults and healthy blood donors between 41 and 65 years of age), qualitative aspects of the Ig spectra were also carefully investigated. The concentration of IgG and IgA in the over-95-years-old individuals showing no H-Ig in their sera was increased. The average levels of IgM and IgD were lower but not significantly different from those of individuals of younger groups. The quantitation of IgG subclasses demonstrated significantly increased values of the IgG1 and IgG3 subclasses when compared to a control group of young adults. The IgG2 and IgG4 subclasses do not seem to contribute substantially to the increased total concentration of IgG in the aged.

Analysis of the data also showed that the variation among the Ig levels of different individuals clearly increases with age. Statistical comparison of variance showed a significant difference for IgM and IgG1, IgG2 and IgG3 subclasses between the old and the young. Similar results, as in humans, were obtained in the aging CBA/Rij[34] and C57BL/KaLwRij (unpublished results) mice. Also in these animals, no decrease in Ig levels, and an increasing variation of Ig values among individual mice, was observed with age.

IV. IMMUNOGLOBULINS OF RESTRICTED HETEROGENEITY AND TRANSIENT HOMOGENEOUS IMMUNOGLOBULINS

When investigating sera of humans older than 95 years[31] and those of aging mice[35,36] with a special attention to the Ig heterogeneity, several deviations from the normal pattern were observed. In 19% of the aged humans, an idiopathic paraproteinemia was found. In another 14% of the cases, the Ig showed changes compatible with the pattern of restricted heterogeneity. An imbalance in the kappa/lambda ratio was found in 40% of the investigated samples. Follow-up studies performed in aging mice substantially enriched our experience with these kinds of Ig abnormalities. Depending on the mouse strain investigated, similar changes appeared with lower or higher, but always increasing, frequency during aging of the animals. Minimal numbers of transient or permanent H-Ig, and minimal restriction of the Ig heterogeneity was seen in the aging CBA and BALB/c mice. The highest frequency of these abnormalities was found in mice of the C57BL strain[36] and in the thymusless nude mouse (in preparation) (Figure 2). Neonatal thymectomy performed in either high or low frequency strains further increased the frequency of the changes and shifted their onset to a younger age (in preparation).

These findings indicate that the extent of the antibody repertoire, as reflected in the heterogeneity of the serum Ig, becomes altered during aging. In accord with this postulation is the observation of Goidl et al.[37] and Doria et al.,[16] on a progressive decrease in the heterogeneity of the plaque-forming cell response in the aging mice. There are several reasons for an assumption that most of the Ig abnormalities observed are only a secondary consequence of an impairment of the T-immune system. It has been demonstrated in a number of clinical and experimental studies that a restriction in the heterogeneity of the immune response and the appearance of H-Ig accompany situations with diminished T-cell functions (reviewed by Radl[38]). These include some forms of severe combined immunodeficiency, Nezelof syndrome, Di George syndrome, Wiskott-Aldrich syndrome, and the reconsitution period after bone-marrow transplantation in children with combined immunodeficiencies, as well as in patients with aplastic anemia and leukemia who receive immunosuppressive pretreatment. Similar findings were obtained in experimental animal bone-marrow transplantations. It has been shown that during the reconstitution, which is a gradual process, the T cells mature more slowly than the B cells. This results in temporary imbalanced T-B interactions, in an immune response of restricted heterogeneity and in the appearance of H-Ig. Finally, the above-mentioned high incidence of these Ig aberrations in the aging thymusless-nude and thymectomized-normal mice, adds further evidence for the importance of the role which the T-immune system plays in the regulation of the heterogeneity of the Ig.

During aging, a similar situation may be encountered; a decline of T-cell functions was shown to precede a decrease in B-cell functions and the onset of most aging phenomena.[26] Involution of the thymus and decline in thymic hormone(s) known to occur with age may be of basic importance in this process.[39] As a consequence, cooperation with, and control of, the B cells by the T cells becomes impaired. The question as to what extent the malfunction of different T-cell subpopulations contributes to this B system aberration cannot be answered at present. Theoretically, a defect in the helper-T-cell population or an increase in the suppressor-cell activity is expected to restrict the numbers of the responding B-cell lines. Deficient function of suppressor-T cells may allow overshoot reactions of B-cell clones to thymus-dependent, but also to some "thymus-independent" antigens (the response to which is independent of T-cell help but under control of suppressor-T cells). Both subpopulations were demonstrated to be altered or to decline with age.[25,37,40]

A further question is the role of other factors that contribute to the development of this age-related immunodeficiency. The differences in the onset, extent, and the progression of the changes among animals of different strains clearly indicate genetic influences. Some other extrinsic factors such as environment, chronic antigenic stimulation, and virus infection must also be seriously considered.

V. IDIOPATHIC PARAPROTEINEMIA (BENIGN MONOCLONAL GAMMAPATHY)

A. Idiopathic Paraproteinemia in Humans

In the previous section, restricted heterogeneity of serum Ig and a transient appearance of H-Ig of usually low concentration were described as a rather frequent finding in aging individuals. Much more spectacular, however, is another Ig abnormality which has been repeatedly reported in the literature under different names, but most often as idiopathic paraproteinemia (IP) or benign monoclonal gammapathy. It was first observed by Waldenström in 1944,[41] who described three patients with myeloma-like proteins in their sera, but with no symptoms of myeloma during a follow-up period of more than 10 years. Since then, several hundreds of similar cases have been reported,[42-45] but only after large population studies[31,46-48] was the relationship of IP with aging properly recognized. The frequency of IP increases from 0% in the third decade up to 19% in the tenth decade of life. This condition is regarded as essentially "benign", because the development of IP into a B-cell malignancy was observed in only a few cases, despite the large number of cases followed up over long periods. An approximate rate of the incidence of IP to its malignant counterpart, i.e., paraproteinemia due to a B-cell malignancy, is about 100:1. The paraprotein level in IP is generally constant and usually below 2 g/100 mℓ; with small fluctuations, the paraproteinemia persists over many years, often until the individual's death. It is mainly this feature that distinguishes IP from paraproteins of other origin.[49] The class distribution of the paraproteins is approximately 60, 20, and 20% for IgG, IgA, and IgM, respectively. Paraproteins of IgD class and Bence Jones proteinuria in IP are very rare. Ig of classes other than that of the paraprotein remain within the normal limits or are only slightly decreased. Increased numbers of plasma cells in the bone marrow of individuals with IP are a frequent finding; however, these cells do not show morphological signs of a malignancy. This is also reflected in normal results of an X-ray examination of the skeleton. Family studies indicate a genetic predisposition for IP.

In spite of the large body of laboratory and clinical data on several aspects of IP, the etiology, pathogenesis, and significance of this phenomenon of aging remained obscure. It seemed that any new clues for their elucidation could only be obtained by experimental studies in an animal model. Results of some recent investigations confirm this assumption.

B. Idiopathic Paraproteinemia in Mice

1. Experimental Model—the Aging C57BL/KaLwRij Mouse

A search for a suitable model for studies on IP showed that an age-dependent increase in the appearance of H-Ig in serum was present in all mouse strains investigated[36] (Figure 6). However, the onset, frequency, and class distribution of the H-Ig in each of the strains were different. Follow-up studies in the CBA/Rij, BALB/c, and C57BL/KaLwRij mice demonstrated that only small portions of the H-Ig were transient paraproteinemias (10 to 20%) or paraproteinemias due to a B-cell malignancy (0 to 2%). The majority of the H-Ig were permanent paraproteinemias. The C57BL mouse, presenting the highest incidence of H-Ig, was chosen for further studies in order to determine to what extent this mouse paraproteinemia can be regarded as an analogue of the human IP. Results of this study demonstrated that, except for some quantitative aspects, most of the features of human and C57BL mouse IP were essentially the same (Table 1).

2. Idiopathic Paraproteinemia is an Intrinsic B-Cell Abnormality

The question as to whether factors intrinsic or extrinsic to the immune system and to the paraprotein-producing cell clone are responsible for the origin of IP was studied by transplantation experiments.[48] It was shown that an IP-producing clone from an old animal can be further propagated not only in young, lethally irradiated mice, but also equally as well in nonirradiated, young, healthy recipients by bone-marrow or spleen-cell transfer. The original paraprotein appeared in the sera of recipients after a period varying in different experiments between 1 and 9 months after transplantation; its concentration increased slowly and finally leveled off, never exceeding the level found in the donor. With subsequent transplantations, the "take" frequency gradually decreased. Propagation of IP for more than four generations was not successful. No detrimental influence of the IP transplantation on the survival or on the appearance of lymphoreticular malignancies in the recipients was observed.

These findings were in sharp contrast with those obtained in other experiments, where transplantation of cells from mice with a B-cell lymphoma or a myeloma led to continuous propagation of the tumors, with a high take frequency, progressive development of the paraproteinemia, and a shortened survival time of the recipients.

Results of this study indicate that IP represents, in its final stage in the aging C57BL mice, an intrinsic cellular abnormality which is manifested as a continuous but not "immortal" excess clonal proliferation. The defect is different by several criteria from that causing a B-cell malignancy. This conclusion regarding intrinsic factors as responsible for the origin of IP is valid only for the last phase in the development of IP. Further experiments indicate that some extrinsic factors may play an important contributing role in the early stages of the development of IP.

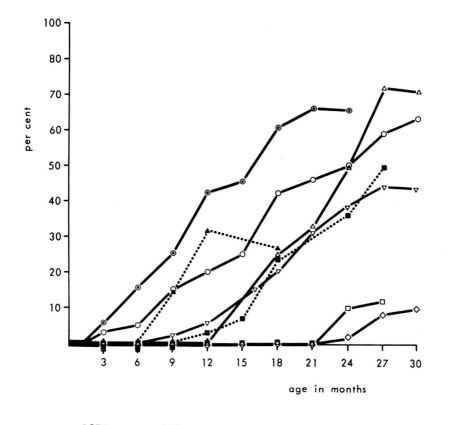

FIGURE 6. Frequency of homogeneous immunoglobulins in the sera of mice of different strains during aging. (From Radl, J., Hollander, C. F., van den Berg, P., and de Glopper, E., *Clin. Exp. Immunol.*, 33, 395, 1978. With permission.)

3. Extrinsic Factors Contribute to the Development of Idiopathic Paraproteinemia

As mentioned above (Section IV), thymectomy performed in young adult mice, but even more clearly, thymectomy in neonatal mice, substantially increased the frequency of the Ig pattern of restricted heterogeneity, of transient H-Ig, as well as of IP which appeared during aging of these animals (in preparation). This effect of thymectomy was obtained not only in mice with high incidence of spontaneous IP (C57BL strain), but also in a low-IP frequency strain, the CBA/Rij mouse.

Other studies are under way in order to determine possible contributing influences of factors extrinsic to the immune system on the development of IP. Preliminary results indicate that chronic and excessive antigenic stimulation may also increase the frequency with which IP will appear during aging in mice of the C57BL strain.

C. Three-Stage Hypothesis on the Development of Idiopathic Paraproteinemia

On the basis of clinical studies and experiments in animals, an hypothesis on the development of IP in three stages has been worked out.[50] This can be summarized as follows:

Table 1
COMPARISON BETWEEN IDIOPATHIC PARAPROTEINEMIA (IP) IN MAN AND THE MOUSE

Idiopathic paraproteinemia	Human	C57BL/KaLwRij
Frequency increases with age	Up to 19% in 10th decade	Up to 60% at 30 months ($\male$)
Essentially "benign"	Yes	Yes
Frequency of IP/malignant paraproteinemia	About 100/1	Probably > 100/1
Persistent at a steady level	Yes	Yes
Usually during rest of life	Yes	Yes
Serum paraprotein concentration	About < 2g%	< 0.4g%
Criteria for monoclonal Ig fulfilled	Yes	Yes
Class distribution of paraprotein	IgG $\geqslant$ IgM $\cong$ IgA	IgG $\geqslant$ IgM > IgA
Excess production of Bence Jones protein	Exceptionally	Not yet found
Number of paraproteins	Usually 1	Often > 1
Level of other Ig	Normal or slightly decreased	Normal
Antibody activity of IP known	Exceptionally	2 out of 300 (tested against 35 different antigens)
Genetic predisposition	Probably	Most likely

After Radl, J., Hollander, C. F., van den Berg, P., and de Glopper, E., *Clin. Exp. Immunol.*, 33, 395. 1978. With permission.

Stage 1. During aging, involution of the thymus and a genetically determined selective gradual decay of certain T-cell subpopulations lead to an impairment of the T cell functions. The progress and the extent of these changes are under the influence of some extrinsic factors.

Stage 2. Consequently, cooperation with, and a control of B cells by the T cells becomes impaired. Restriction of heterogeneity of the immune response and excessive clonal proliferations with an overshoot production of H-Ig and antibodies, occur as a result of this imbalance in the immune system network.

Stage 3. The repeated mono- or oligoclonal expansions result in a higher probability for either spontaneous or a virus-induced mutation of the regulatory genes within a given B-cell clone. This clone, turned on originally by an antigenic stimulus, will further continue to proliferate and secrete its Ig product, even after that stimulation has disappeared. This intrinsic defect in cell regulation is different from that in B-cell malignancies. IP can be considered to represent a benign tumor of a B-cell line.

SUMMARY

Using conventional and some refined techniques, quantitative and qualitative aspects of serum Ig were investigated in the aging-human and laboratory-animal populations. Some particular phenomena reflecting changes in the immune system were revealed. The average concentrations of IgG and IgA in man increase, those of IgM and IgD show only a nonsignificant decrease. Increased levels of IgG1 and IgG3 subclasses were found to be responsible for the elevated values of the IgG class. Increased variations with age among the Ig levels of different individuals were a general finding in both human and mouse species.

Qualitative changes in the Ig spectrum during aging are characterized by increasing frequency of the appearance of Ig of restricted heterogeneity, transient H-Ig, and persistent paraproteinemias, the so-called idiopathic paraproteinemias or benign monoclonal gammapathies. While the former changes seem to reflect imbalances in the immune system network due to a gradual decline in the helper-and control-T-cell functions, the IP was shown to represent an intrinsic defect within one B-cell clone.

REFERENCES

1. Mancini, G., Carbonara, A. O., and Heremans, J. F., *Immunochemical quantitation of antigens by single radial immunodiffusion, Immunochemistry,* 2, 235, 1965.
2. Voormolen-Kalova, M., van den Berg, P., and Radl, J., Immunoglobulin levels as related to age in nonhuman primates in captivity. I. Chimpanzees, *J. Med. Primatol.,* 3, 335, 1974.
3. Haaijman, J. J. and Brinkhof, J., A microfluorometric assay for immunoglobulin class and subclass levels in murine serum, *J. Immunol. Methods,* 14, 213, 1977.
4. Morell, A., Skvaril, F., Steinberg, A. G., van Loghem, E., and Terry, W. D., Correlation between the concentrations of the four subclasses of IgG and Gm allotypes in normal human sera, *J. Immunol.,* 108, 195, 1972.
5. de Bruyn, A. M. and Klein, F., The validity of the radial immunodiffusion method for the quantitative determination of human IgM, *J. Immunol. Meth.,* 11, 311, 1976.
6. Rowe, D. S., Grab, B., and Anderson, S. G., An international reference preparation for human serum immunoglobulins G, A and M: content of immunoglobulins by weight, *Bull. W. H. O.,* 46, 67, 1972.
7. Cejka, J. and Kithier, K., A simple method for the classification and typing of monoclonal immunoglobulins, *Immunochemistry,* 13, 629, 1976.
8. Wieme, R. J., *Studies on Agar Gel Electrophoresis, Techniques-Applications,* Arscia, Brussels, 1959.
9. Radl, J., Light chain typing of immunoglobulins in small samples of biological material, *Immunology,* 19, 137, 1970.
10. Radl, J., Immunoselection technique and its applications, in *Protides of the Biological Fluids,* Vol. 19, Peeters, H., Ed., Pergamon Press, Oxford, 1972, 541.
11. Radl, J., de Glopper, E., and de Groot, G., A rapid, simple and reliable technique for preparation of antisera against idiotypes of paraproteins, *Vox Sang.,* 35, 10, 1978.
12. Williamson, A. R., Isoelectric focusing of immunoglobulins, in *Handbook of Experimental Immunology,* Vol. 1, Weir, D. M., Ed. Blackwell Scientific, Oxford, 1973, 8.
13. Radl, J., Dooren, L. J., Eijsvoogel, V. P., van Went, J. J., and Hijmans, W., An immunological study during post-transplantation follow-up of a case of severe combined immunodeficiency, *Clin. Exp. Immunol.,* 10, 367, 1972.
14. Radl, J., van den Berg, P., Voormolen, M., Hendriks, W. D. H., and Schaeffer, U. W., Homogeneous immunoglobulins in sera of rhesus monkeys after lethal irradiation and bone marrow transplantation, *Clin. Exp. Immunol.,* 16, 259, 1974.
15. Skvaril, F. and Barandun, S., A simple method for the simultaneous detection of human immunoglobulins of both light chain types., *J. Immunol. Methods,* 3, 127, 1973.
16. Doria, G., D'Agostaro, G., and Pontti, A., Age-dependent variations of antibody avidity, *Immunology,* 35, 601, 1978.
17. Bloemmen, F. J., Radl, J., Haaijman, J. J., van den Berg, P., Schuit, H. R. E., and Hijmans, W., Microfluorometric evaluation of the specificity of fluorescent antisera against mouse immunoglobulins with the Defined Antigen Substrate Spheres (DASS) system, *J. Immunol. Methods,* 10, 337, 1976.
18. Radl, J., de Glopper, E., Schuit, H. R. E., and Zurcher, C., Idiopathic paraproteinaemia. II. Transplantation of the paraprotein-producing clone from old to young C57BL/KaLwRij mice, *J. Immunol.,* 122, 609, 1979.
19. Hijmans, W., Schuit, H. R. E., and Klein, F., An immunofluorescence procedure for the detection of intracellular immunoglobulins, *Clin. Exp. Immunol.,* 4, 457, 1969.
20. Avrameas, S. and Ternynck, T., The cross-linking of proteins with glutaraldehyde and its use for the preparation of immuno-adsorbents, *Immunochemistry,* 6, 53, 1969.

21. **Ishizaka, T., Ishizaka, K., Orange, P., and Austen, K. F.,** The capacity of human immunoglobulin E to mediate the release of histamine and slow-reacting substance of anaphylaxis (SRS-A) from monkey lung, *J. Immunol.,* 104, 335, 1970.

22. **Ouchterlony, O. and Nilsson, L. A.,** Immunodiffusion and immunoelectrophoresis, in *Handbook of Experimental Immunology,* Vol. 1, Weir, D. M., Ed., Blackwell Scientific, Oxford, 1973, 19.

23. **Harrington, J. C., Fenton, J. W., and Pert, J. H.,** Polymer-induced precipitation of antigen antibody complexes: precipiplex reactions, *Immunochemistry,* 8, 413, 1971.

24. **Knapp, W., Haaijman, J. J., Schuit, H. R. E., Radl, J., van den Berg, P., Ploem, J. S., and Hijmans, W.,** Microfluorometric evaluation of conjugate specificity with the defined antigen substrate spheres (DASS) system, *Ann. N.Y. Acad. Sci.,* 254, 94, 1975.

25. **Fahey, J. L. and Terry, E. W.,** Ion exchange chromatography and gel filtration, in *Handbook of Experimental Immunology,* Vol. 1, Weir, D. M., Ed., Blackwell Scientific, Oxford, 1973, 7.

26. **Adler, W. H., Jones, K. H., and Nariuchi, H.,** Ageing and immune function, in *Recent Advances in Clinical Immunology,* Thompson, R., Ed., Churchill Livingstone, Edinburgh, 1977, 77.

27. **Haferkamp, O., Schlettwein-Gsell, D., Schwick, H. G., and Störiko, K.,** Serumproteine im hohen Lebensalter unter besonderer Berücksichtigung der Immunglobuline und Antikörper, *Klin Wschr.,* 44, 725, 1966.

28. **Grundbacher, F. J. and Schreffler, D. C.,** Changes in human serum immunoglobulin levels with age and sex, *Z. Immun.-Forsch.,* 141, 20, 1970.

29. **Kalff, M. W.,** A population study on serum immunoglobulin levels, *Clin. Chim. Acta,* 28, 227, 1970.

30. **Finger, H., Emmerling, P., and Hof, H.,** Serumimmunglobulin-Spiegel in Senium, *Dtsch. med. Wschr.,* 98, 2455, 1973.

31. **Radl, J., Sepers, J. M., Skvaril, F., Morell, A., and Hijmans, W.,** Immunoglobulin patterns in humans over 95 years of age., *Clin. Exp. Immunol.,* 22, 84, 1975.

32. **Riesen, W., Keller, H., Skvaril, F., Morell, A., and Barandun, S.,** Restriction of immunoglobulin heterogeneity, autoimmunity and serum protein levels in aged people, *Clin. Exp. Immunol.,* 26, 280, 1976.

33. **Buckley, C. E., Buckley, E. G., and Dorsey, F. C.,** Longitudinal changes in serum immunoglobulin levels in older humans., *Fed. Proc., Fed. Am. Soc. Exp. Biol.,* 33, 2036, 1974.

34. **Haaijman, J. J., van den Berg, P., and Brinkhof, J.,** Immunoglobulin class and subclass levels in the serum of CBA mice throughout life, *Immunology,* 32, 923, 1977.

35. **Radl, J. and Hollander, C. F.,** Homogeneous immunoglobulins in sera of mice during aging, *J. Immunol.,* 112, 2271, 1974.

36. **Radl, J., Hollander, C. F., van den Berg, P., and de Glopper, E.,** Idiopathic paraproteinaemia. I. Studies in an animal model — the aging C57BL/KaLwRij mouse, *Clin. Exp. Immunol.,* 33, 395, 1978.

37. **Goidl, E. A., Innes, J. B., and Weksler, M. E.,** Loss of IgG and high avidity plaque-forming cells and increased suppressor cell activity in aging mice, *J. Exp. Med.,* 144, 1037, 1976.

38. **Radl, J.,** The influence of the T immune system on the appearance of homogeneous immunoglobulins in man and experimental animals, in *Humoral Immunity In Neurological Disorders,* Karcher, D., Lowenthal, A., and Strosberg, A. D., Eds., Plenum Press, New York, 1979, 517.

39. **Weksler, M. E., Innes, J. B., and Goldstein, G.,** Immunological studies of aging. IV. The contribution of thymic involution to the immune deficiencies of aging mice and reversal with thymopoietin, *J. Exp. Med.,* 148, 996, 1978.

40. **Barthold, D. R., Kysela, S., and Steinberg, A. D.,** Decline in suppressor T cell function with age in female NZB mice, *J. Immunol.,* 112, 9, 1974.

41. **Waldenström, J. G.,** Incipient myelomatosis or essential hyperglobulinemia with fibrinogenopenia — a new syndrome?, *Acta Med. Scand.,* 117, 216, 1944.

42. **Hällen, J.,** Discrete gammaglobulin (M-) components in serum, *Acta Med. Scand. Suppl.,* 462, 1, 1966.

43. **Zawadzki, Z. A. and Edwards, G. A.,** Nonmyelomatous monoclonal immunoglobulinemia, in *Progress in Clinical Immunology,* Vol. 1, Schwartz, R. S., Ed., Grune & Stratton, New York, 1972, 105.

44. **Waldenström, J. G.,** Benign monoclonal gammapathies, in *Multiple Myeloma and Related Disorders,* Vol. 1, Azar, A. and Potter, M., Eds., Harper & Row, New York, 1973, 247.

45. **Kyle, R. A. and Bayrd, E. D.,** The monoclonal gammapathies, multiple myeloma and related plasma-cell disorders, in *Benign Monoclonal Gammathy,* I. N. Kugelmass, Ed., Charles C. Thomas, Springfield, Ill., 1976, 284.

46. **Axelsson, U., Bachman, R., and Hällen, J.,** Frequency of pathological proteins (M-components) in 6995 sera from an adult population, *Acta Med. Scand.,* 179, 235, 1966.

47. **Axelsson, U.,** An eleven-year follow-up on 64 subjects with M-components, *Acta Med. Scand.,* 201, 173, 1977.

48. **Englisova, M., Englis, M., Kyral, V., Kourilek, K., and Dvorak, K.,** Changes of immunoglobulin synthesis in old people, *Exp. Gerontol.,* 3, 125, 1968.
49. **Radl, J.,** Immune system disorders in man and in experimental models accompanied by the production of homogeneous immunoglobulins — paraproteins, in *Protides of the Biological Fluids,* Vol. 23, Peeters, H., Ed., Pergamon Press, Oxford, 1976, 405.
50. **Radl, J.,** Idiopathic paraproteinemia. — A consequence of an age-related deficiency in the T immune system. Three stage development — a hypothesis, *Clin. Immunol. Immunopathol.,* 14, 251, 1979.

Chapter 9

IMMUNOFLUORESCENCE

W. Hijmans, J. J. Haaijman, and Henrica R. E. Schuit

TABLE OF CONTENTS

I. INTRODUCTION

The development of the technique of immunofluorescence, which was introduced by Coons et al. in 1941,[1] shows the characteristics of a biological growth curve. A lag period, due to the fact that the first author was understandably called upon to perform other duties, was followed by a lag period which started with the paper of Coons and Kaplan in 1950.[2] The method then became operational. Milestones in the further development were the replacement of the carbon arc by less cumbersome light sources and of the fluorescein isocyanate as the fluorochrome by the isothiocyanate (FITC) compound, which does not require biochemical dexterity. The use of tetramethylrhodamine isothiocyanate (TRITC) as the second fluorochrome considerably widened the scope of immunofluorescence.[3] Standard diaillumination was superseded by the dark-field condensor, and the final step was the introduction of epiillumination, first described by Brumberg,[4] and developed by Ploem.[5] This approach provided a major stimulus to the optical industry for research and development, which was specifically directed towards fluorescence. It is gratifying to note that many wishes expressed in a previous review[6] have been fulfilled. It now seems safe to state that the technique of immunofluorescence has entered the third stage, that of the stationary phase, in which one can hope for and expect continuous improvements, but no major changes. It is therefore an opportune moment for a methodological review. In accordance with the scope of this book, it will be geared to research methods. The authors are well aware that, especially in routine diagnostic procedures, much can be achieved by simple means. They are also convinced that immunological changes which are pertinent to the process of aging are likely to be of a subtle and perhaps diverse nature. Optimal techniques are therefore essential. It is for this reason that this review will be highly selective and focus on details which are sometimes seemingly trivial, but which have been applied successfully in gerontological and other research programs. The emphasis on particular aspects is the result of personal experience, but this does not exclude the existence of equally satisfactory alternatives. Experience also shows that, although most investigators have no direct interest in the technical aspects of microscopy, some insight into these matters may help to considerably improve the quality of the results. Some parts of this chapter therefore provide background information, while others are written in a more imperative style.

The principle of the method is simple: antibodies are coupled to fluorescent dyes and these conjugates can then react with the corresponding antigen *in situ*. The presence and localization of the antigen can then be detected by exposing the substrate to the exciting light source and observing the fluorescent light emitted by the fluorochrome. There are many modifications of this scheme. The most widely used is the indirect test in which the substrate is first exposed to the antiserum and then incubated with a fluorescent anti-immunoglobulin preparation.

Other modifications and comprehensive information on this technique in general can be found in Nairn's standard text (now in its fourth edition[7]), in publications on immunological methods,[8,9] in a practical instruction manual,[10] and in the proceedings of special conferences.[11-14]

II. FLUORESCENCE

A few words on the physical basis of fluorescence will suffice for an adequate understanding of this aspect of fluorescence microscopy. A large number of organic molecules absorb light and then transform it to light of a longer wavelength — this is, light which carries less energy. Stoke's law, which, in accordance with the energy conservation principle, states that the wavelength emitted by fluorescent material is longer than that used to excite the fluorescence, is derived from this phenomenon. The time between excitation and emission is in the order of nanoseconds, as opposed to periods ranging from milliseconds to seconds in phosphorescence. In general, the excitation spectrum can be considered to be equal to the absorption spectrum, of which the emission spectrum forms a mirror image. From a quantitative point of view, the emission is a direct function of the amount of light absorbed. The conclusion can be immediately drawn from this statement that fluorescence microscopy should be more sensitive than classical absorption microscopy for the detection of specific components. Absence of such a fluorescent component results in a totally dark image and, when present, emission has, in principle, no upper limit, since it is dependent on the amount of excitation energy with a maximum infinite image contrast. Absence of the object in absorption microscopy with transmitted light gives a field with maximum illumination and, at a given concentration, all light will be absorbed, which means a totally dark field. In immunofluorescence, the fluorochrome is coupled to an antibody, which adds to the property of high sensitivity, immunological specificity, and the possibility of localization of antigens in the specimen.

In practice, there is the choice between two fluorochromes. FITC has a maximum absorption in the blue region and a maximum emission in green; TRITC transforms green light into red (Figure 1).

III. THE MICROSCOPE

For reasons mentioned in the Introduction, this description will be limited to the system of epiillumination as introduced by Ploem.[5] In more than one respect, it is superior to the conventional type of immunofluorescence microscope with diaillumination, even when the latter is equipped with a wide-angle darkfield condensor and interference-excitation filters. Epiillumination is therefore indicated in any gerontological research, especially since relatively simple systems have now become available commercially, following the trend towards single-purpose microscopes. More elaborate equipment can be used for quantitative fluorescence and this approach has been applied to assess the relative efficiency of different variables which determine the final outcome, such as the light sources, filters, optics, reagents, and the different immunological systems. For these microfluorometric readings, aminoethyl-Sephadex beads are conjugated with either fluorescein or rhodamine, and these beads of microscopic size then serve as standards.[15]

A. The Principle of Epiillumination

In this system, the excitation light is directed towards the interference dividing plate, which acts as a chromatic beam splitter. It is inserted above the objective at an angle of 45°, so that the excitation light enters through the back entrance of the objective, which thus functions as a condensor (Figure 2). Additional filters are placed in the excitation and emission pathways. The system can be adapted to different fluorochromes. A number of separate filter blocks, each of which contains the complete set of excitation and emission filters with the corresponding dichroic mirror, and selected for one fluorochrome, can now be purchased.

B. Quantitative Evaluation of the Equipment

1. Light Sources

Full information on the comparative investigations of the different light sources has been presented elsewhere[16] and a summary is given in Table 1. The determination of

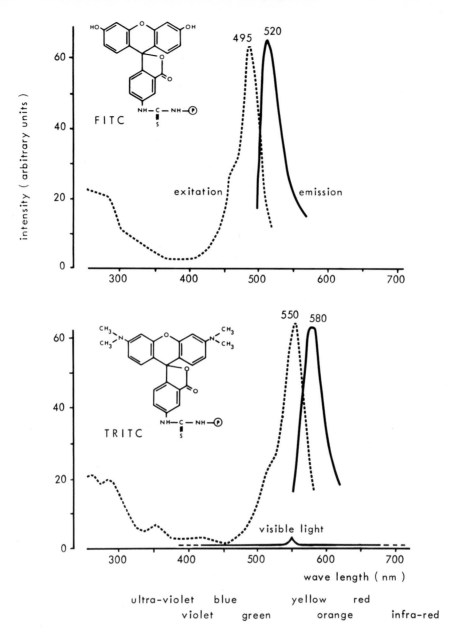

FIGURE 1.   Excitation (———) and emission (———) spectra of FITC and TRITC.

the performance of a light source is a hazardous undertaking because of variables which are difficult to control, such as variations within one type of light source, differences among collector designs, and the length of the optical pathways. The results, however, are so unambiguous that it is justified to draw the following conclusions. The 100-Watt high-pressure mercury lamp is superior by far to any of the other five light sources tested and the 12-Volt halogen lamp is the poorest. The HBO 50 Watt and the HBO 200 Watt are remarkably comparable in their performance, which makes the low cost 50-Watt lamp with its small size and high stability a good second choice. A disadvantage of the 100-Watt mercury lamp is the need for a highly stabilizing DC power supply, which makes it much more expensive than the AC-operated mercury

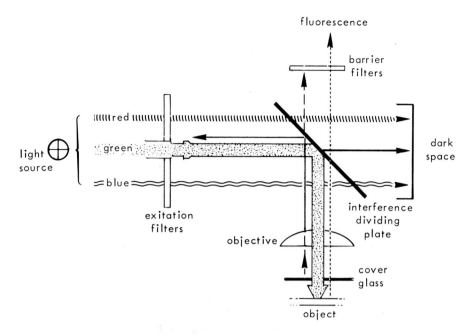

FIGURE 2.   Principle of the fluorescence microscope with epiillumination according to Ploem.[5]

Table 1
THE INFLUENCE OF THE LIGHT SOURCE ON THE FLUORESCENCE YIELD OF AMINOETHYL-SEPHADEX BEADS STAINED WITH EITHER FITC OR TRITC

Light source	FITC	TRITC
50 Watt mercury	10	32
100 Watt mercury	80	150
150 Watt mercury	5	14
200 Watt mercury	10	30
75 Watt xenon	4	2
100 Watt, 12 Volt halogen	1	1

Note: The fluorescence intensity was measured quantitatively with the value for the halogen light source as the unit. For full details, see Reference 16.

arcs. However, neither the pay-off in terms of savings by the use of more diluted conjugates, nor the price paid for better fluorescence images has been assessed. The superiority of TRITC over FITC in terms of fluorescence yield under these conditions[17] is confirmed in these determinations, but the expectation of a need for a separate xenon source for FITC is not borne out by these data.

From a theoretical point of view, the laser beam deserves attention, because the beam is monochromatic and very homogeneous with a high energy yield. In practice, however, the situation is more complex and this light beam has not been placed in operation.

2. Filters

Filter systems are used in immunofluorescence to prevent the fluorescent image from being dominated by unwanted excitation light from the light source, and to select that part of the emission spectrum which can be registered as a specific signal. Primary or excitation filters are designed to allow passage of only the wavelengths that are necessary to stimulate fluorescence. Secondary or emission (barrier) filters remove excitation irradiation not absorbed by the object, and they should allow passage of a large part of the fluorescent light emitted by the fluorochrome.

There seem to be two major causes of difficulties in the understanding of problems which are associated with filters. First, there is the question of their efficacy. Most filters transmit the major part of the light at the wavelength they are designed to transmit, and peak transmittance of 90% can often be expected. It is not generally appreciated, however, that filters often also transmit some light in the wavelength they are supposed to block. The permissable transmission in these regions may have to be as low as 10^{-8} in highly efficient fluorescence systems.[18,19]

The second cause of problems is the often-confusing terminology. A brief survey is therefore presented here. There are two main types of filters:

(A) **Colored glass** — these filters consist of glass mixed with different inorganic salts and are manufactured in two forms:
   1. Filters transmitting certain wavelength bands. These filters are mostly known under an abbreviation indicating their color properties, followed by a number which represents the factory code (for Schott filters, see Reference 20). Much in use are the red-suppressing BG 38 (German: Blauglas) and the near ultraviolet-transmitting UG 1 (German: Ultraviolettglas). The transmission bands of these filters are mostly broad, and they are often used in combination with the interference filters to be discussed below.
   2. Filters which transmit light above a certain wavelength. These filters are alternatively termed:
      - K filters (German: Kantenfilter), followed by a number indicating the wavelength in nm of 50% transmission of 3 mm thickness (examples are: K 510 and K 580);
      - GG, OG, and RG filters (German for, respectively, Gelbglas, Orangeglas, and Rotglas), followed by the 50% transmittance value. The names indicate the color properties of the filters. Examples of these filters are the much used GG 455, GG 475, OG 515, and RG 610;
      - LP (Long-Pass) filters; an example is the LP 520, in which the number stands for the 50% transmission wavelength. The LP 520 functions in the same way as the OG 515 and the K 510, in that they all transmit most wavelengths above about 525 nm.
(B) **Interference filters** — these filters consist of a glass base on which multilayers of dielectric materials are vacuum deposited. The interference filters may be divided into two classes:
   1. Narrow-band interference filters; these filters transmit wavelength bands typically 15 to 25-nm in width at 50% transmission. The peak transmission of these filters can be of the order of 80%. Narrow-band filters of this type are now known as BP (Band-Pass) filters, followed by the peak transmission wavelength and the band width at 50% transmission, which is given after the dash sign, e.g., BP 525/20.
   2. Interference filters which transmit wavelengths shorter than a given wavelength. These filters are mostly termed KP (German: Kurzpass) filters. The abbreviation SP for short pass is sometimes used. The transmittance values of these filters can be as high as 90%.

In principle, any excitation and emission specification can be met by a careful combination of different filters. The combination of an LP filter with a KP filter can again be designated as a BP filter, but this code is then followed by the two half-power points (50% transmission), separated by a hyphen, e.g., BP 530-560.

The question of which filters should be used is often asked. There is no simple answer, as it will depend on, among other things, the material to be studied, the light source, and the goal of the study. For this reason, the following annotated suggestions are given. Some of these filter sets can be obtained as such, others can be easily assembled. Costs of filters are often mentioned as a factor in their selection. This is not valid, since there is no known upper limit with respect to their lifetime, and they contribute to obtaining results which can stand critical assessment.

In double-wavelength IF methods where two fluorescent dyes are present in the same preparation, special measures are necessary to visualize both fluorochromes selectively. Combinations of LP and KP filters, constituting a wavelength window, are the best choice for this purpose at present. In Figure 3, the method of selective filtering is shown for FITC and TRITC. Stylized filter characteristics have been superimposed on the excitation and emission spectra of these dyes.

A heat-protective filter (KG 1 or Calflex®) and a red-suppression filter, such as a 4-mm-thick BG 38, can be inserted in the excitation beam next to the light source. The heat-protective filter is optional with the 50-Watt mercury lamp and the red-suppression filters can be part of the excitation filter combination.

FITC

a. Excitation filters — the KP 490 has a high transmittance in the wavelength region of the absorption peak, but also a considerable transmittance in the red light region. It is therefore marketed in combination with a red suppressive filter such as the BG 38. Furthermore, this filter is open to the left, which means that the specimen is subjected to short wavelength blue light. The ensuing autofluorescence can be prevented by adding an LP 450 or even an LP 470. The latter combination has the characteristics of a narrow band-pass filter with very high transmittance (Figure 4), but also less excitation energy in comparison with the band filter BP 450-490.

b. Interference dividing plate — this type of filter reflects part of the spectrum and transmits light of the other wavelength areas. For FITC, the 510 dichroic mirror should be selected. It is a delicate filter and should only be factory handled.

c. Emission filters — on this level there are three options: i. LP 520, which transmits practically all light of a wavelength longer than 530 nm and has a 50% transmission at 520 nm, as indicated by the code number. It is open to the right and should therefore not be used in combination with TRITC; ii. LP 520 + KP 560. This combination means a wide window in the emission spectrum of FITC with exclusion of orange and red light and is the first choice in the double-wavelength method with TRITC; iii. BP 525. This forms a narrow window which transmits only green light, thus providing a highly specific gate for FITC emission, but the intensity is somewhat less than with the wider window.

TRITC

a. Excitation filters — the combination of an LP 520 with a KP 560 presents an excellent window for almost the whole range of the absorption (excitation) peak of this dye. The addition of a 1-mm-thick BG 36 filter, which blocks

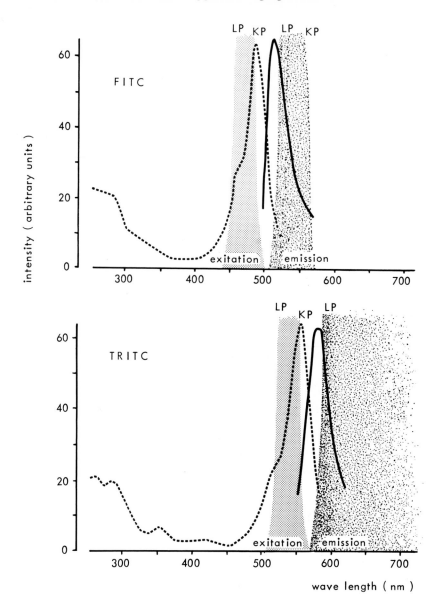

FIGURE 3.   Examples of selective filtering for FITC and TRITC.

most light of a wavelength of 580 nm, provides an extra barrier between the excitation and the emission spectra.

b.   Interference dividing plate — the code number of the filter for this dye is 580, and this filter also should not be handled by the customer.

c.   Emission filters — the LP 580 takes over where the excitation filter KP 560 ends. There is no need for a short-wavelength pass filter, as the cut-off in the red region is provided by nature: the eye becomes insensitive to wavelengths beyond 700 nm (Figure 1).

3. Optics

a. **Objectives** — In the system of epiilumination, the light beam enters the objective from above; the objective therefore functions as a condensor. An objective is charac-

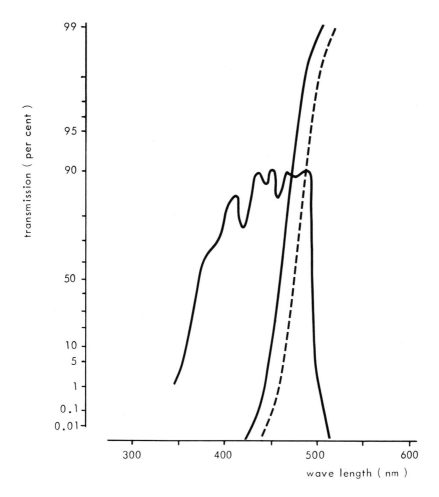

FIGURE 4. The KP 490 filter in combination with a LP 450 filter (———) results in a wide band filter combination, to be used for excitation for FITC. The combination of the KP 490 filter with a LP 470 filter (– – –) functions as a narrow band filter. Note the log scale on the ordinate.

terized by its magnification and its numerical aperture (N.A.). The value of the N.A. is a measure for its collecting power; the excitation energy should therefore be related to the N.A. The same applies to the light which is emitted by the specimen: the larger the N.A., the more fluorescence is collected (Figure 5).

For a quantitative evaluation of objectives with different magnifications and N.A. values, microfluorometric measurements were performed with FITC-conjugated Sephadex microbeads. The results (Table 2 and Figure 6) confirm the theoretical considerations and the experience in practice: there is an increase in the fluorescence intensity with just over the fourth power of the N.A. Classically, only objectives with a high magnification had a large N.A. Medium-power objectives with high N.A. values have been recently constructed for maximum fluorescence without maximum magnification.

b. **Eyepieces** — The influence of eyepiece magnification has also been studied by microfluorometry. These studies have confirmed the expectation that eyepieces with high magnification collect less energy per surface area than the low power ones. They simply spread the image over a larger surface. Results (Table 3 and Figure 7) clearly

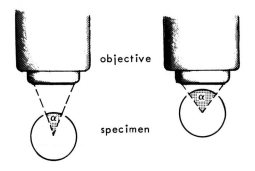

FIGURE 5.   An objective with a high numerical aperture (N. A. = ½ α) collects more light than an objective with a low numerical aperture.

Table 2
INFLUENCE OF OBJECTIVE ON FLUOR/PL OF AMINOETHYL-SEPHADEX BEADS STAINED WITH FITC

Type	Magnification	Phase contrast	Immersion	N.A.	Fluor/pl[a]
	10×	+	−	0.22	5
	10×	−	−	0.25	7
	20×	−	−	0.40	15
	20×	+	+	0.45	60
	22×	−	O + W	0.65	965
PLAN	25×	−	−	0.45	80
	25×	−	−	0.50	133
APO	25×	−	−	0.65	1,016
	25×	−	W	0.60	277
	40×	+	+	0.75	292
APO	40×	−	O	1.00	608
PLANAPO	40×	−	O	1.00	573
FL	40×	−	O	1.30	7,487
	50×	−	W	1.00	2,910
	54×	−	O	0.95	4,925
	63×	+	O	1.30	8,818
FL	70×	−	O	1.30	10,855
	90×	+	O	1.15	3,701
NPL	100×	+	O	1.30	6,260

Note: Each fluor/pl value is the average of fifteen individual bead measurements. Bead diameters were measured with an eyepiece micrometer which was recalibrated with an objective micrometer for each objective. The light source (100W mercury arc) was adjusted to optimally fill the entrance pupils of the different objectives.

[a]   Fluorescence per picolitre.

show that the fluorescence per unit of surface will decrease with the square root of the eyepiece magnification. This magnification should therefore be as low as possible.

Since improved light sources, filters, and optics have become standard equipment, it is no longer necessary to resort to the monocular tube. Indeed, in spite of its inherent loss of light, a binocular tube should be regarded as an improvement in itself, because it entails much more than combining the images projected on the two retinas. There may be a different color sensitivity between the eyes, and the correction of disparity may add to obtaining clearer images with less background noise, which is especially welcome in membrane fluorescence of cells in suspension.

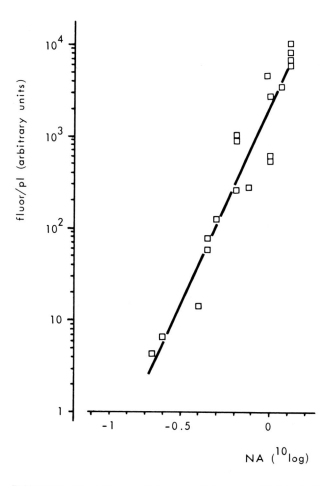

FIGURE 6. The influence of the numerical aperture (N.A.) of objectives on the fluorescence per picolitre of aminoethyl-Sephadex beads stained with FITC. The fluorescence/picolitre data from Figure 5 are plotted versus the logarithm of the numerical aperture of the objectives. The drawn line represents the least squares fit with the equation: $y = 3.34 + 4.25x$, in which the fluorescence/picolitre and x stands for the logarithm of the numerical aperture. Each value represents the average of 15 individual bead measurements. Eyepiece: 6.3 ×.

c. **Multiple Wavelength Illuminators** — These types of illuminators contain two or more sets of filters, together with the corresponding dichromic beam splitters, each selected for a given fluorochrome. The switch from one set to another is simple and rapid, i.e., within a fraction of a second. This is essential because of the fact that the human eye has a very short memory for the exact position of an object. If two different images are presented to an observer within a very short time, the two observations can still be combined. He can then decide whether a cell is negative or positive and, in the latter case, whether it is positive for one or both fluorochromes. This modification also offers the possibility of an often very welcome control by adding, for instance, a nonrelated conjugated protein to the substrate to investigate the occurrence of nonspecific uptake of protein, which is a prominent feature of eosinophilic cells. Additionally, blank controls should be a starting point of any new system, in order to obtain information on the autofluorescence of the tissues or cells.

d. **Phase Contrast** — Another advantage of epiillumination is the possibility to com-

Table 3
INFLUENCE OF EYEPIECE
MAGNIFICATION ON
FLUORESCENCE OF TRITC
STAINED AMINOETHYL-SEPHADEX
BEADS

Type	Magnification	Fluorescence
	5.0×	430
C	5.0×	480
MOBIMI	5.0×	455
B	6.0×	284
PERIPLAN	6.3×	233
B	8.0×	125
KPL	8.0×	101
PERIPLAN	10.0×	60
PERIPLAN GF	10.0×	52
PERIPLAN	12.0×	33
KPL	12.5×	25

Note: Each fluorescence value is the average of 15 individual bead measurements. The apparent diameter of the beads was measured with an eyepiece micrometer.

plete such a system with darkfield, and especially, with phase-contrast illumination, so that immunological information can be related to morphological criteria. Although the phase-contrast condensor is definitely not difficult to handle, experience shows that investigators often have problems, especially with centering, and this results in either inadequate morphological detail or neglecting to use this most valuable accessory equipment. Although — to quote Goldman[21] — "It is almost embarrassing to speak in public about some of the simple things," there is a simple solution; it consists of mounting the correct phase ring in the standard condensor. This limits its application to one magnification, but this is almost always sufficient.

If a degree of orientation in the tissue section which is not provided by filter sets used for immunofluorescence is needed, one can resort to excitation with short wavelength blue-light. This causes autofluorescence of small blood vessels, such as in, e.g., kidney and skin sections. Another method to obtain gross orientation, suggested by Ploem,[22] consists of staining the nuclei by low concentrations of ethidium bromide, which gives red fluorescence with blue excitation light.

The results of the investigations presented in these paragraphs may serve as a general guideline for choosing the optimal equipment for IF microscopy. Our investigations have been by no means exhaustive, nor have they led to the description of *the* fluorescence microscope. Rather, the aim has been to draw the attention of the IF microscopist to the improvement in image contrast and the increase in fluorescence intensity which may result from a careful choice of the available microscope components. Neither can this information serve as an excuse for not applying basic principles such as the need for clean and well-aligned optics.

IV. PREPARATION OF ANTISERA AND THEIR PURIFICATION

Elsewhere in this volume, Radl[23] has described many details which have been shown to be extremely useful in the preparation of the reagents. A minimum requirement is

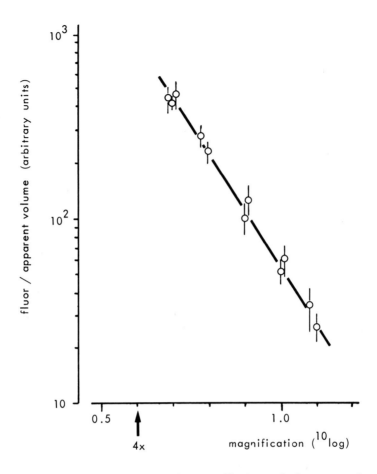

FIGURE 7. The influence of eyepiece magnification on the fluorescence of aminoethyl-Sephadex beads stained with TRITC. The fluorescence and diameter of individual beads were measured with different eyepieces. The apparent volume of the beads was used. Each point is the average of fifteen individual bead measurements. Bars indicate standard deviations. The drawn line represents the least squares fit. The position of the 4 × wide-angle eyepieces is indicated on the abscissa with an arrow. Objective: 25 ×/ 0.60 W.

an IgG fraction prepared by column chromatography from an antiserum, which has been absorbed over solid phase immune absorbents. If cells are used for absorption, unexpectedly large amounts are needed, and also, repeated cycles are necessary to obtain the desired specificity.[24] It is not generally known that only in exceptional cases do more than half of the number of immunoglobulin molecules represent the desired antibodies. Purified antibody preparations are therefore superior and, in the actual tests, they also give rise to less background staining. They are not always easy to prepare and the yield is often low. Another disadvantage is their lability, which makes it necessary to add stabilizing substances, usually homologous serum components such as albumin or gamma globulin. The antibodies obtained by the technique of somatic cell hybridization offer promising possibilities, although no comparative studies are yet available. In this method, an antibody-forming cell is fused with a malignant cell from a plasma cell tumor. The latter will, by definition, grow autonomously, and at the same time synthesize and secrete the monoclonal antibody of the former cell.

With the standard types of antisera, the animal source is not important. The infor-

Table 4
ANTISERA AND CONJUGATES: BASIC INFORMATION REQUIRED

1. The species of animal immunized
2. The source and method of preparation of the antigen
3. The immunizing schedule, route, and adjuvant
4. The absorbent and absorption procedure and evidence of specificity before and after absorption
5. The immunoglobulin separation process or other chemical treatment, particularly the preservative used and any other dilutions or additions such as proteins used for stabilization
6. Specificity as determined by standard, reproducible tests
7. Some expression of the potency of the antiserum with a guideline for a working dilution
8. Fluorochrome used with F/P ratio
9. The lot number

mation should be available, however, and it is essential to have this knowledge when two antisera are being mixed for use in the double-staining technique. Other useful items which should be available to the investigator are given in Table 4. What is important is that the specificity and the sensitivity of any fluorescence procedure are no better than the antiserum employed.

The relevant physio-chemical information on the two most widely used fluorescent dyes, FITC and TRITC, has already been mentioned, except for the question of purity. In the United States, FITC is a certified dye, but the situation is less satisfactory with regard to TRITC. It is possible to check its purity by thin-layer chromatography, however in practice, few laboratories are willing to do this. It is absolutely necessary to take proper precautions to prevent deterioration once a dye which gives good results has been purchased. Both dyes should be stored in the dark in a dessicator, and TRITC also in the freezer. Before opening a bottle, its contents should be brought to room temperature to prevent condensation of water on the cold dye.

In spite of these precautions, the dye may lose its activity after a long period of storage, and this will lead to loss of fluorescence of the conjugated protein. If the latter preparation is highly valuable, relabeling with an active batch is worth attempting. Fluorescent conjugates should have a fluorochrome-to-protein ratio within a certain range, where it can be assumed that each antibody molecule has a statistical probability of carrying a few fluorochrome molecules. This is accomplished by carefully and slowly adding, under constant stirring, one part of the dye in solution to one hundred parts of protein, with a continuous pH monitoring. For the preparation of conjugates on a laboratory scale, the following scheme (described in detail previously[25]) has proved to be easy to follow and gives highly reproducible results.

The temperature of the reagents is brought to 4°C and all procedures are carried out at this temperature. To 2 mℓ of the IgG fraction is added 0.2 mℓ of a 0.5 M carbonate-bicarbonate buffer (pH 9.0). The dye solution is prepared by dissolving 0.01 mg of the dye per mg protein to be conjugated in 2 mℓ freshly prepared 2% bicarbonate solution with a pH of 8.2. For TRITC, prolonged shaking (e.g., with a supermixer) for several hours at room temperature is necessary. The fluorochrome solution is added dropwise to the protein solution under continuous stirring lasting for 30 min after the dye has been added. The mixture is then left overnight. Despite this careful processing, a small amount of free dye is always present; this is removed by dialysis or preferably by the use of molecular sieves such as Sephadex G 25 or G 50. Merthiolate is added to a final concentration of 1:10,000. The sample is divided into aliquots of about 0.5 mℓ and stored at −70°C.

The central question is the specificity of the conjugate. The information supplied by the producer is to be regarded as an indispensible guideline, but it should always be kept in mind that reagents are biological products and therefore subject to deterioration, and that a given product is not necessarily optimal for all substrates or micro-scopes. A number of tests should be performed. We have a preference for immuno-diffusion techniques, performed in PEG 6000 plates.[23] Model systems have also been shown to be useful; particularly good results have been obtained by microfluorometry of antigens coupled to Sepharose beads, which have been reacted with the test conju-gate. These results can be expressed quantitatively to reference background readings and also to beads which carry other antigens. An example is given by Bloemmen et al.[26] working with antimouse antisera. They determined the highest permissible per-centage of impurity, and a large number of conjugates failed to meet these critera. Neither these model systems nor chemical specification can substitute for performance testing in which the reactions of a conjugate or antiserum with different specified bio-logical substrates are evaluated under the same conditions as in the eventual system in which the conjugate is to be applied. It is the best way to circumvent all problems related to standardization of equipment, experimental conditions, etc., if the relevant biological substrates of sufficient purity are available. However, it has two weak as-pects. The first is that it is based on circular reasoning. A system is called monoclonal or said to be carrying determinants of single specificity if it reacts only a with certain antisera, which are then called monospecific. New and unknown antisera may then be tested for specificity by assuming monoclonality of the cells or monospecificity of the substrate. The second weak point is a consequence of the fact that only those reactivi-ties which are present in the antiserum and which are directed against antigens con-tained within the target cells or tissues are appraised. Other reactivities in the antiserum may go unnoticed.

A final point concerns the choice between the direct technique in which the antibody preparation is labeled, and the indirect technique which makes use of unlabeled anti-body preparations as the first layer. From a theoretical point of view, the latter should lead to an increase in fluorescence intensity on the basis of amplification, and this is indeed often the case. Another advantage is that not every antiserum has to be labeled separately, but that one labeled anti-immunoglobulin preparation will suffice. A major drawback of all multilayer techniques is the time which is required for the extra incu-bations. Moreover, the number of controls which are necessary to establish the speci-ficity of a given reaction increases almost exponentially with the number of reagents used, also because an increase in nonspecific staining can be expected. It is for these reasons that we prefer the direct technique, although not maximally sensitive, for its simplicity and unambiguous results.

V. THE SPECIMEN

Best results, in terms of image contrast and morphological details of the individual cells, are obtained with suspensions. These can be washed; background values are then negligible, but the obvious drawback is the loss of histological localization. If infor-mation about membrane - associated antigens is desired, the suspended cells are incu-bated with the reagents. Storage problems of lymphocytes have been largely overcome by the diluted formaldehyde-fixation technique,[33] full details of which are given in the Appendix A. When intracellular antigens are being studied, a cytocentrifuge is indis-pensable for the preparation of slides, because enriched slides and well-preserved cells are obtained with this instrument. (For details, see Appendix B.)

Cryostat sections of tissues are the obvious choice if there is a need for histological localization of the antigen under investigation. If these are also present in large amounts in the serum, they may be difficult to distinguish from background fluores-cence, even in spite of thorough washing of the specimen.

Classical fixation techniques with formalin and paraffin embedding are not compatible with the high quality requirements one must demand in most gerontological research where more than subtle changes cannot be expected.

VI. CONTROLS

Evaluation of the results of immunofluorescence is based on visual observation, and to some extent it is therefore subjective, but the many possibilities for controls outweigh this disadvantage. Once the immunochemical tests are satisfactory, performance testing should be carried out with the determination of optimal dilution of conjugates in a system which is as closely related to the system in which the reagents are going to be applied as possible. Chess board titrations are essential in the indirect method, which requires additional controls at the level of the middle layer and of the conjugate. Classical immunological controls consist of absorption of the conjugate or the antiserum with the specific antigen prior to their application in the test, which then should be negative. Where possible, the specific antigen should be coupled to erythrocytes or other particulate carriers to prevent formation of soluble immune complexes. The specificity of the staining reaction should also be monitored by inhibition or blocking procedures by first exposing the specimen to the unconjugated antiserum. Pretreatment time should be in excess of the staining time and a ratio of 8:1 is generally thought to be adequate. Usually, however, the inhibition is not complete, perhaps due to the fact that there may occur a continuous exchange between labeled and unlabeled antibodies.

The two-wavelength system of epiillumination offers many other possibilities for control tests, which are often crucial. Nonrelated conjugated antisera or nonantibody proteins can be tested simultaneously with a specific reagent as well as with reagents with assumedly the same specificity, but from a different animal or a different animal species. Problems of nonspecific uptake of immunoglobulins can often be solved by incubating the cells with the conjugate at 37°C for one to two hours; this will release exogenous immunoglobulins. Specificity can also be revealed in the case of membrane-associated immunoglobulins by checking their light chain type. If synthesized by the cells, these immunoglobulins should be either of the kappa or the lambda light-chain type, but not of both. Independent capping after application of two different conjugates is another indicator of specificity (See Figure 8.)

Especially when working with cell suspensions is the phase contrast equipment invaluable, because it adds morphology to fluorescence. By combining the different modifications, we have been able to distinguish five different categories of mononuclear cells in blood: B and T cells, mature monocytes, null cells, and a fifth category which we have provisionally called "undefined cells".

If all results are according to expectation, the investigator is entitled to assume that his reagents are specific. If the unexpected arises, he may blame the conditions of his experiment, but he may also have made a new discovery. It is not within the scope of this contribution to provide guidelines for these occasions.

VII. PHOTOGRAPHY

The quality of the specimen to be recorded is particularly important. It is convenient and also illustrative to have a field containing sufficient cells which are evenly distributed. The morphology of the cells should be easily distinguishable; for the morphological evaluation of vitally stained cells in phase contrast microscopy, embedding in 90% glycerol is of paramount importance. For the recording of cytoplasmic fluorescence, the magnification obtained with a 40× or 54× immersion objective lens is sufficient.

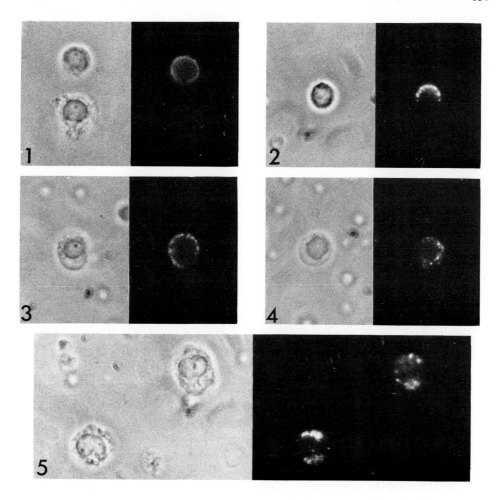

FIGURE 8. Phase contrast microscopy and immunofluorescence. 1. Small lymphocyte, typical, membrane associated, confluent pattern in immunofluorescence with a rhodamine T-cell specific antiserum (IgG fraction). 2. Small lymphocyte, typical membrane associated, finely speckled pattern in immunofluorescence with capping after incubation with a fluorescein labeled anti Fab antiserum (F(ab')2 fraction). 3. Larger lymphocyte, incubation and fluorescence pattern as sub 2, no capping. 4. Undefined mononuclear cell, atypical, not clearly membrane associated, irregular pattern in immunofluorescence after incubation as sub 2. 5. Mature monocytes, fluorescence pattern as sub 4 after treatment as indicated sub 2.

For membrane fluorescence, we use the Leitz® equipment with the 63× phase contrast objective. It has a very high N.A. (1.30) and, when combined with a 6.3 × eyepiece magnification, excellent results can be obtained, especially if a 100-Watt light source substitutes for the standard 50 Watt.

It is very difficult to judge the required exposure time by eye. An automatic camera such as the Leitz Orthomat® guarantees reproducible results, provided that the "detail" or point-measurement is used. The adjustment of the apparatus has to be established empirically for each type of film by making a test series with different DIN-ASA settings. The values on the film itself then only serve as an approximation. It is therefore not possible to give exposure times here, but they are so short that fading presents no problem. Correct exposure time is particularly important for the recording of membrane fluorescence, because by overexposure the delicate fluorescence pattern of the membrane will be lost.

The Ilford HP5 film developed in Promicol and printed on Agfa Brovira® Speed paper gives excellent black and white prints. Kodak Ektachrome® 200 ASA daylight film is presently best suited for color diapositives; the sensitivity can be considerably enhanced by the processing at higher ASA values. Exposure of the vitally stained cells using the FITC filter combination in the vertical illuminator without actual excitation, gives the best results for the recording of the phase contrast image on both films. Integrating measurement should then be used.

VIII. RESULTS AND CONCLUSIONS

The aging immune system follows the same pattern as other systems with aging, with its decrease in function and increase in variability. This is an overall pattern which needs specification and some of our attempts to define these changes in more detail with the technique of immunofluorescence will be summarized here.

The appearance of idiopathic paraproteins with age has been dealt with elsewhere in this volume.[23] The probe of choice for individual paraproteins is the anti-idiotype antiserum. If applied in immunofluorescence, the presence of paraproteins can be detected within the plasma cells or on the membrane of B cells. Preliminary results suggest that these B cells originate in the spleen, and that the actual secretion of these immunoglobulins takes place in the bone marrow.

It is generally accepted that, after intravenous administration of the antigen, the first antibodies will be formed in the spleen. For the secondary response, the bone marrow becomes the major site of antibody formation.[27] As part of an investigation on the humoral immune response in relation to aging, the number of immunoglobulin-containing cells was determined in the spleen, mesenteric lymph nodes, bone marrow, and Peyer's patches of CBA mice of different ages. The total number remained constant, but the relative contribution of the bone marrow increased with age, possibly due to a gradual shift in the individual animal from primary-type responses to a pattern of secondary-type responses.[28] There was, however, also a diminished reaction at the level of the bone marrow to sheep red blood cells as a specific antigenic stimulus.[29] An unexpected finding was the virtually complete absence of positive cells in the Peyer's patches and in the mesenteric lymph nodes of the aged animals.

The same experimental design was used in the study of the congenitally athymic nude mice.[30] The results clearly indicated that the thymus is not responsible for the shift of the immunoglobulin-containing cells to the bone marrow compartment. In protected surroundings, these mice can reach the age of two years, and the age-related deterioration of the thymus-dependent limb of the immune system can therefore not be the cause of aging, but should rather be regarded as a consequence of it.

The numbers of B and T cells in mice during aging have been determined by the membrane-staining technique. Results depend on the strain, the housing condition, the organ of the animal, and its age. The number of B, T, and null cells tends to decrease with aging, but the number of T cells in the spleen and B and T cells in the bone marrow remains remarkably constant. The most striking phenomenon was the steady increase in the numbers of non-T, non-B cells with age (unpublished observations).

These and related studies have made it clear that results obtained so far should be regarded as an approximation in the definition of the immunological defect of the aging individual because of the complexity of the immune system. This can be exemplified by the fact that several subpopulations of T cells can now be distinguished, and recent studies[31,32] with the technique of membrane immunofluorescence have shown that any isotype combination can occur on B cells, although their frequencies depend on the source of lymphocytes.

It has also become clear that new techniques or new modifications of existing methods are urgently required for further analysis. For the technique of immunofluorescence, a third fluorochrome would be most welcome.

APPENDIX A

Fixation Procedure With Diluted Formaldehyde

Reagents
1.   5% EDTA disodium (Titriplex III®, E. Merck, Darmstadt, W. Germany) in PBS
     Lymphoprep® - (Nyegaard, Oslo, Norway)

     Washing solution containing 5% BSA and 0.1% EDTA:
     • 25 ml of 20% BSA (Poviet, Amsterdam)
     • 75 ml of PBS, pH 7.2 to 7.4
     • 4 ml of 5% EDTA
     • adjust pH to 6.8 with 20% NaOH
     Washing solution containing 1% BSA: 5% BSA solution is diluted with PBS

2.   0.04% Formaldehyde: commercial formalin — 37% — is diluted 10 times with PBS and kept as stock solution at +4°C. Shortly before use, the solution is diluted 100 times with PBS.
3.   Buffered glycerol: 9 parts glycerol p.a. (Merck, store at +4°C) 1 part PBS, pH 7.8

Method
1.   ±9 ml of blood is mixed with 1 ml of 5% EDTA (a).
2.   Leucocytes are counted and a blood smear is prepared for staining.
3.   The blood is diluted with an equal volume of PBS and 5 ml are layered on 2 ml of Lymphoprep and centrifuged for 13 min at $1000 \times g$.
4.   The interphases are collected, washed once with 5% BSA solution and centrifuged at +4°C for 15 min at $300 \times g$.
5.   The cell pellet is resuspended in 1 ml of the 1% BSA solution; 0.025 ml of the suspension is fixed with 3 ml of 0.04% formaldehyde (b) in disposable plastic tubes for 10 min at room temperature.
6.   The cells are centrifuged in a serofuge and washed twice with 1% BSA.
7.   The cell pellet is resuspended in 0.05 ml of 1% BSA; 0.025 ml of conjugate is added, incubated for 30 min at room temperature with gentle shaking every 10 min.
8.   The cells are washed once with 1% BSA and centrifuged in a serofuge.
9.   The *supernatant is removed as completely as possible* (c) and the cell pellet is resuspended on a vortex mixer.
10. The cells are deposited in a small drop of *buffered glycerol* (d) on a cover glass (24 × 32 mm) which is then covered with an object glass.
11. The cover glass is sealed with *paraffin* (e).

a.	Titriplex III® as anticoagulant	— Not toxic for cells
b.	Fixation with formaldehyde	— Preserves morphological and immunological properties
c.	Embedding in glycerol	— Gives an optimum phase contrast image
d.	Complete removal of supernatant	— To prevent dilution of glycerol
e.	Sealing with paraffin	— Does not diffuse into cell suspension like the acetone in nail polish.

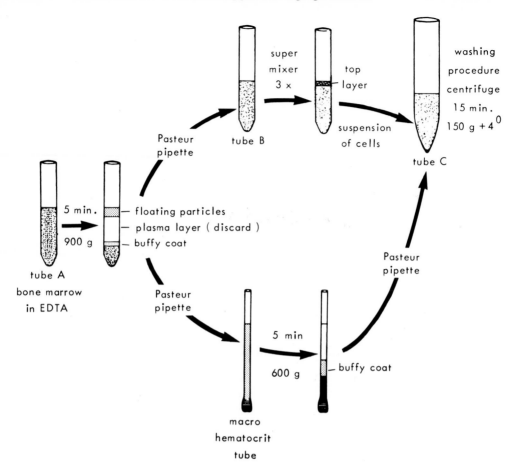

FIGURE 9. Schematic presentation of procedures, used in the preparation of slides for cytoplasmic staining. For details, see text.

APPENDIX B

Preparation Of Slides For Cytoplasmic Staining[25,34]

Bone marrow — In man, up to 1 mℓ of marrow is drawn in the usual way with a dry or moistened syringe and quickly transferred to a 10-mℓ centrifuge tube (A) containing 0.5 mℓ of a 5% EDTA solution in PBS (Figure 9). In the mouse, bone marrow cells are obtained by flushing the femurs with the EDTA solution in PBS. For the preparation of the conventional smears, the suspension of marrow is poured into a small petri dish and a few particles are collected by use of a Pasteur pipette, smeared onto a slide and stained by the May-Grünwald-Giemsa method. To the remaining suspension is added 3 mℓ of 5% BSA solution and this diluted suspension is returned to the tube (A) and centrifuged (900 g) for 5 min at room temperature. The floating particles of bone marrow are collected, transferred to another centrifuge tube (B) containing 2 mℓ of the washing solution and the cells shaken out on a supermixer. The suspension beneath the top layer, containing the tissue particles is then transferred to a 30-mℓ centrifuge tube (C). This procedure is repeated twice.

The plasma layer in tube A is drawn into a Pasteur pipette and discarded. The white cell layer is transferred to a macrohematocrit tube made from a 1-mℓ graduated pipette cut at 10-cm length and sealed at one end in a bunsen flame by means of a pair of pliers. The buffy coat is centrifuged (600 g) for 5 min at room temperature and the concentrated white cells are removed and transferred to a tube (C), to which washing solution is added to a final volume of approximately 30 mℓ. The tube (C) is centrifuged (150 g) for 15 min at 4°C and the deposit is resuspended in the washing solution to a final concentration of 4×10^6 cells/mℓ.

Slides are prepared in a cytocentrifuge. To moisten the filter papers, the cups are filled with one drop of the BSA solution and centrifuged for 1 to 2 min. Then 0.05 mℓ of the suspension is added and centrifuged for approximately 4 to 7 min.

Peripheral blood — The Lymphoprep technique as described in Appendix A is used.

Tissues — Pieces of tissue with a total volume of about 1 cm³ are ground with a borel type mincer and suspended in about 30 mℓ washing solution in a beaker. In the mouse cell suspensions of the spleen, mesenteric lymph nodes and Peyer's patches are obtained by mincing the tissues with scissors and sieving through a nylon gauze filter with phosphate buffered saline (PBS) supplemented with 1% (w/v) bovine serum albumin. For further processing, see under "Bone marrow" (Tube C).

Remarks — One milliliter of bone marrow is sufficient: if more is aspirated, unwanted mixing with peripheral blood occurs. Because plasma cells are difficult to recognize in the counting chamber, it is impossible to count the immunologically active cells in the bone marrow suspension accurately; this count is therefore omitted. It may be useful for the lymphocytes in peripheral blood and tissues. The washing procedure is an essential step for removal of interfering extracellular immunoglobulins.

The use of hard filter paper such as Green 602 or Schleicher & Schull 602/hard is required. It is very convenient that the cells can stand storage in the EDTA solution at 4°C for at least 24 hr, so that long-distance transport presents no problems. If unfixed, the slides, wrapped in cellophane, keep well at −70° for many years.

Fixation — For convenience in locating the cell preparation on the slide, a circle is drawn around this area with a diamond pencil. The slides are also numbered in the same way. Fixation is accomplished by means of an acetic acid-ethanol (5/95, v/v) solution for 15 min at −20°C. This solution should be renewed frequently, e.g., every 2 weeks.

The cells must not be allowed to dry after fixation. The slides are washed for 1 hr at 4°C in PBS with three changes of the buffer. The washing procedure is performed most effectively by putting the slides in a bottomless histological staining box in a 1-ℓ beaker containing PBS and placing the beaker on a magnetic stirrer.

Under the conditions mentioned above, the procedure was found to be very efficient for immunoglobulins and definitely superior to methanol and acetone, because it gives a striking contrast between the nucleus and cytoplasm. It should not be regarded as a universal fixative, however, and other fixatives may be necessary for other substrates.

The washed slides are dried outside the encircled area, placed in a moist chamber and covered with one drop of the conjugate. Care should be taken that the cells do not dry. After incubation for 30 min at room temperature, the slides are placed for 15 min in separate beakers containing PBS. They are then dried again around the encircled areas, mounted in buffered glycerol (9 parts glycerol, 1 part PBS) and sealed with paraffin wax.

The fixed and stained slides can be stored at −20°C for many years if proper precautions are taken to prevent damage to the cover glasses and the sealing is kept intact.

ACKNOWLEDGMENT

The authors dedicate this publication to the memory of Dr. A. H. Coons, who laid the foundation and pioneered many advancements in the field of immunofluorescence.

REFERENCES

1. **Coons, A. H., Creech, H. H., and Jones, R. N.,** Immunological properties of an antibody containing a fluorescent group, *Proc. Soc. Exp. Biol. Med.,* 47, 200, 1941.
2. **Coons, A. H. and Kaplan, M. H.,** Localization of antigens in tissue cells. II. Improvements in a method for the detection of antigen by means of fluorescent antibody, *J. Exp. Med.,* 91, 1, 1950.
3. **Hiramoto, R., Engel, K., and Pressman, D.,** Tetramethyl-rhodamine as immunohistochemical fluorescent label in the study of chronic thyroiditis, *Proc. Soc. Exp. Biol. Med.,* 97, 611, 1958.
4. **Brumberg, Y. M.,** Concerning fluorescent microscopes, *Z. Obshchey Biologii,* 16, 222, 1955.
5. **Ploem, J. S.,** The use of vertical a illuminator with interchangeable dichroic mirrors for fluorescence microscopy with incident light, *Z. Wiss. Mikrosk.,* 68, 129, 1967.
6. **Faulk, P. W. and Hijmans, W.,** Recent developments in immunofluorescence, *Prog. Allergy,* 16, 9, 1972.
7. **Nairn, R. C.,** *Fluorescent protein tracing,* Churchill Livingstone, Edinburgh, 1976.
8. **Coons, A. H.,** Fluorescent antibody, in *Methods in Immunology and Immunochemistry,* Vol. 5, Williams, C. A. and Chase, M. W., Eds., Academic Press, New York, 1976, 424.
9. **Johnson, G. D. and Holborow, E. J.,** Immunofluorescence, in *Handbook of Experimental Immunology in Three Volumes,* Vol. 1., Weir, D. M., Ed., Blackwell Scientific, Oxford, 1973, 18.
10. **Wick, G., Baudner, S., and Herzog, F.,** *Immunofluorescence,* Die Medizinische Verlagsgesellschaft, Marburg/Lahn, Germany, 1978.
11. *Standardization in Immunofluorescence,* Holborow, E. J., Ed., Blackwell Scientific Publications, Oxford, 1970.
12. *Defined Immunofluorescent Staining,* Beutner, E. H., Ed., New York Academy of Sciences, New York, 177, 1971.
13. *Fifth International Conference on Immunofluorescence and Related Staining Techniques,* Hijmans, W. and Schaeffer, M., Eds., New York Academy of Sciences, New York, 254, 1975.
14. *Immunofluorescence and Related Staining Techniques,* Knapp, W., Holubar, K. and Wick, G., Eds., Elsevier/North Holland, Amsterdam, 1978.
15. **Haaijman, J. J. and Hijmans, W.,** Essentials of Immunocytochemistry with fluorochrome markers with emphasis on the double staining techniques, in *Pulse-cytophotometry,* Lutz, D., Ed., European Press, Ghent, Belgium, 1978, 215.
16. **Haaijman, J. J.,** Quantitative Immunofluorescence Microscopy, Methods and Applications, Ph.D. thesis, Leiden University, The Netherlands, 1977.
17. **Hijmans, W., Schuit, H. R. E., Yamashita, T., and Schechter, I.,** An immunofluorescence study on the specificity of antibodies synthesized in separate cells after the administration of an immunogen with double specificity, *Eur. J. Immunol.,* 2, 1, 1972.
18. **Ploem, J. S.,** A study of filters and light sources in immunofluorescence microscopy, in *Defined Immunofluorescent Staining,* Beutner, E. H., Ed., New York Academy of Sciences, New York, 177, 1971, 290.
19. **Ploem, J. S.,** General Introduction, in *Fifth International Conference on Immunofluorescence and Related Staining Techniques,* Hijmans, W. and Schaeffer, M., Eds., New York Academy of Sciences, New York, 1975, 4.
20. *Farb and Filter Glass,* Schott, Jenaer Glaswerk Schott & Gen., Mainz, West Germany.
21. **Goldman, M.,** Fluorescence microscopy, in *Defined Immunofluorescent Staining,* Beutner, E. H., Ed., New York Academy of Sciences, New York, 177, 1971, 407.
22. **Ploem, J. S., Tanke, H. J., Al, I., and Deelder, A. M.,** Recent developments in immunofluorescence microscopy and microfluorometry, in *Immunofluorescence and Related Staining Techniques,* Knapp, W., Holubar, K., and Wick, G., Eds., Elsevier/North Holland, Amsterdam, 1978, 3.
23. **Radl, J.,** Immunoglobulin levels and abnormalities in aging humans and mice, in *Immunological Techniques Applied to Aging Research,* Adler, W. and Nordin, A. A., Eds.
24. **Asma, G. E. M., Schuit, H. R. E., and Hijmans, W.,** The determination of numbers of T and B lymphocytes in the blood of children and adults by the direct immunofluorescence technique, *Clin. Exp. Immunol.,* 29, 286, 1977.
25. **Hijmans, W., Schuit, H. R. E., and Klein, F.,** An immunofluorescence procedure for the detection of intracellular immunoglobulins, *Clin. Exp. Immunol.,* 4, 457, 1969.
26. **Bloemmen, F. J., Radl, J., Haaijman, J. J., van den Berg, P., Schuit, H. R. E., and Hijmans, W.,** Microfluorometric evaluation of the specificity of fluorescent antisera against mouse immunoglobulins with the defined antigen substrate spheres (DASS) system, *J. of Immunol. Methods,* 10, 337, 1976.
27. **Benner, R., van Oudenaren, A. and de Ruiter, H.,** Antibody formation in mouse bone marrow. IX. Peripheral lymphoid organs are involved in the initiation of bone marrow antibody formation, *Cell. Immunol.,* 34, 125, 1977.

28. **Haaijman, J. J., Schuit, H. R. E. and Hijmans, W.,** Immunoglobulin-containing cells in different lymphoid organs of the CBA mouse during its life-span, *Immunology,* 32, 427, 1977.

29. **Blankwater, M. J. and Benner, R.,** in preparation.

30. **Haaijman, J. J., Slingerland-Teunissen, J., Benner, R. and van Oudenaren, A.,** The distribution of cytoplasmic immunoglobulin containing cells over various lymphoid organs of congenitally athymic (nude) mice as a function of age, *Immunology,* 36, 271, 1979.

31. **Vessière-Louveaux, F. M. Y. R., Hijmans, W. and Schuit, H. R. E.,** Presence of multiple isotypes on the membrane of human tonsilar lymphocytes, to be published, *Eur. J. Immunol.,* 10, 136, 1980.

32. **Vessière-Louveaux, F. M. Y. R., Hijmans, W. and Schuit, H. R. E.,** Multiple heavy chain isotypes on the membrane of the small B lymphocytes in human blood, *Clin. Exp. Immunol.,* 1981.

33. **Schuit, H. R. E., Hijmans, W. and Asma, G. E. M.,** Qualitative and quantitative data on surface markers after formaldehyde fixation of the cells, *Clin. Exp. Immunol.,* 41, 559, 1981.

34. **Vossen, J. M. J. J., Langlois van den Bergh, R., Schuit, H. R. E., Radl, J., and Hijmans W.,** The detection of cytoplasmic immunoglobulins by immunofluorescence: improvements in techniques and standardization procedures, *J. of Immunol. Methods,* 13, 71, 1976.

Chapter 10

THE STUDY OF IMMUNE FUNCTION IN AGED HUMANS

J. M. Hefton and M. E. Weksler

TABLE OF CONTENTS

I. INTRODUCTION

It has been established that lymphocytes from persons over 65 years of age incorporate less thymidine than do cells from young subjects when cultured with plant lectins.[1-5] This defective response may be due either to fewer mitogen-responsive cells in mononuclear preparations from old people and/or a failure of initially responding lymphocytes to expand into a pool of proliferating cells.

The studies described in this chapter were undertaken to characterize at the cellular and cytokinetic levels the cause of the defective thymidine incorporation observed with lymphocyte preparations from old subjects. In agreement with other workers,[6] we have found that there was no decrease in the concentration of blood lymphocytes from old persons. We have characterized the nature of this defect by determining the number of initial responding units and the kinetics of proliferation after stimulation. The number of responding units was determined by limiting dilution analysis, the vesicular stomatitis virus (VSV) plaque assay, and kinetic analysis of lymphocyte proliferation. The kinetics of the proliferative expansion of the initially stimulated cells were studied by colchicine-block experiments, bromodeoxyuridine (BrdU) labeling of sister chromatids, and cell-cycle measurements. It was concluded from these studies that the defect in the lymphocyte preparations from older human subjects is due to both a decrease in the number of mitogen-responsive units and a deficiency in the expansion of those responsive cells which are present.

II. SELECTION OF SUBJECTS FOR STUDY

Blood was taken from healthy laboratory personnel between the ages of 20 and 35 years and from older persons between the ages of 65 and 97. Old persons were selected from volunteers who were free of debilitating disease and not taking any drugs known to affect the reactivity of lymphocytes in culture. Many of the older subjects had symptoms of atherosclerotic cardiovascular disease and related disorders. None of the older subjects was acutely ill. This use of human volunteers had been approved by the Human Rights in Research Committee of the New York Hospital-Cornell Medical Center.

III. PREPARATION OF LYMPHOCYTE CULTURES

A. Preparation of Lymphocyte Suspensions

Venous blood obtained from healthy volunteers was drawn into a plastic syring containg 10 units of heparin (Riker Laboratories Inc., Northridge, Calif.) per mℓ of blood. The blood was diluted with an equal volume of calcium- and magnesium-free Hank's Balanced Salt Solution (HBSS Microbiological Associates, Bethesda, Md.). The blood (35 to 40 mℓ) was layered over 12 mℓ of a mixture of Ficoll® (Pharmacia Fine Chemicals, Piscataway, N.J.) and Hypaque® (sodium diatrizoate, Winthrop Laboratories, N.Y.) in sterile 50-mℓ screw-cap centrifuge tubes (# 25330, Corning Glass Works, Corning, N.Y.).

Ficoll®-Hypaque® mixtures were prepared by mixing one part of 50% Hypaque® with four parts of 8% (wt/vol) Ficoll® in water. The density of the Ficoll®-Hypaque® mixture was adjusted to a specific gravity of 1.078 to 1.080 with distilled water and passed through a 0.45 μm Millipore® filter.

The tubes containing the diluted blood layered on Ficoll-Hypaque® were centrifuged at 400 × g for 40 min at 20°C. The cells removed from the resultant interface were washed three times with HBSS in 16 × 125 mm sterile screw-cap tubes (#2037, Falcon Plastics, Oxnard, Calif.) and collected by centrifugation at 150 × g for 10 min at 20°C. Cells were then resuspended in a small volume of culture medium (RPMI-1640, Microbiological Associates), enriched to 20% with heat-inactivated pooled human AB sera, and with 2mM L-glutamine (Microbiological Associates), 100 units/ml penicillin and 100 g/ml streptomycin (Grand Island Biological Company, Grand Island, N.Y.). Cells were counted in a haemocytometer chamber and diluted to 2×10^6 lymphocytes per ml in complete culture medium (RPMI-1640 plus additives as above).

Lymphocytes isolated according to this schedule were routinely 85 to 95% viable when tested by trypan blue exclusion. When the viability of such lymphocyte preparations was estimated by flow cytometry measurement of nucleic acids stained with Acridine orange, 85 to 95% viability could only be achieved by reducing the time of centrifugation from 40 min to 25 min and increasing the g force from 400 to 600. The usual recovery of lymphocytes by this method was 10^6 cells per ml of whole heparinized blood. Some individuals consistently gave fewer (5×10^5 cells per ml) or more (2×10^6 cells per ml) lymphocytes. This range of variation was observed in both the young and old populations studied.

Some investigators enrich the resultant suspension for lymphocytes by permitting the monocytes present to adhere to a plastic surface, following one hour incubation at 37°C, or to adhere to nylon wool, during passage through a 30×10 column. Monocytes have been reported to enhance the response of T lymphocytes to plant lectins.[7] Removal of monocytes was therefore not effected in the preparations used in these studies since T-lymphocyte proliferation was being measured.

B. Lymphocyte Proliferation Stimulated by PHA

Unfractionated lymphocytes were cultured in triplicate in sterile multiwell round-bottom plates (Linbro IS-MRC-96-TC, Linbro Chemical Co., New Haven, Conn.) in a total volume of 0.2 ml complete culture medium (as above). These cells were incubated in the presence and absence of purified PHA (Burroughs-Wellcome Co., Research Triangle Park, N.C.) at a dose found to stimulate maximal thymidine incorporation. Cultures were incubated in a 5% CO_2/95% humidified air environment. DNA synthesis during the final 24 hr of culture was assessed by thymidine incorporation. One μCi of methyl (^{3}H) thymidine (sp act 2 Ci/mM, Amersham/Searle Corp., Arlington Heights, Ill.) in 1 μl was added to each culture well. At the end of the incubation period, the lymphocytes were aspirated from the wells, transferred to glass fiber filter paper (Reeve-Angel, Inc., Clifton, N.J.) and washed with water and methanol using a Titertek Cell Harvester (Flow Laboratories. Rockville, Md.). The glass fiber discs were placed into 15×45 mm vials and 2.5 ml of Aqueous Counting Scintillant (Amersham/Searle Corp) were added. These mini-vials were counted in a Delta® 300, 6890 Liquid Scintillation System (Searle Analytic Inc., Des Plaines, Ill.). The results were expressed as the average thymidine incorporation in counts per minute of the replicate cultures. Thymidine incorporation, expressed as $\overline{cpm}$, ranged from 6,900 to 91,200 in lymphocyte suspensions from 48 old people as compared to a range of 19,900 to 118,400 for cells cultured from 48 young people. 35 out of the 48 of these lymphocyte suspensions from old people had lower $\overline{cpm}$ values than the control cultures from young people.

A dose-response curve was established for each batch of purified PHA to determine the amount necessary for maximal stimulation of thymidine incorporation by lymphocytes in culture. Batches of PHA prepared by Burroughs-Wellcome usually produced maximal stimulation at a final concentration of 5 μg/1 ml. Although thymidine incorporation by lymphocytes stimulated with PHA is routinely measued after 24 hr incubation with tritiated thymidine there is evidence[8] this may induce alterations in the cell cycle of the dividing cells. Cultures of human lymphocytes stimulated with PHA incubated with tritiated thymidine for 18 hr contained increased numbers of cells in the

G_2 and M phases of the cell cycle and a reduced proportion of cells in the S phase. This effect may be the result of intranuclear incorporation of tritium with qualitative differences in various populations of human lymphocytes.

IV. DETERMINATION OF THE NUMBER OF LYMPHOCYTES RESPONDING TO BLASTOGENIC STIMULI

The impaired response to PHA of lymphocytes from old persons is not the result of decreased numbers of T lymphocytes in the mononuclear cell preparations. Old and young people do not differ significantly in the numbers of monocytes or T lymphocytes in their mononuclear suspensions. The frequency of mitogen-responsive units in such lymphocyte preparations from young and old subjects can be established by several methods, including: limiting dilution analysis of the fluctuation of the PHA response; Vesicular Stomatitis Virus (vsv) plaque assay to enumerate the number of lectin-activated T lymphocytes in a population; incubation with colchicine to isolate cells dividing for the first time from those undergoing subsequent divisions.

A. Limiting Dilution Analysis

Twenty-four replicate cultures each containing the same number of lymphocytes were established. One half of the lymphocyte cultures were incubated with PHA and one half without PHA. A series of 24 such replicate cultures was set up, each with a different number of lymphocytes ranging from 10^3 to 10^4 cells per well. The samples were cultured with PHA and harvested as described above. An individual culture was considered to have a positive response to PHA when thymidine incorporated was greater than two standard deviations above the mean of thymidine incorporated by the 12 cultures containing the same number of lymphocytes incubated without PHA. The percent negative responses at each lymphocyte level was determined and least squares regression analysis used to obtain the plot relating the percentage of negative responses to the number of lymphocytes in the cultures. The percentage of negative responses depends on the frequency of responding units and the size of the aliquot as given by the formula $P = e^{-fa}$ (P = percent negative responses; f = frequency of responsive units; a = number of lymphocytes in culture). When f = a, the percentage of negative responses would equal 37%.

The frequency of responsive units equals the reciprocal of the number of cells which in replicate cultures gives 37% negative responses, as determined from a semilog plot relating the percent of negative responses to the number of cells cultured (Figure 1). The percentage of negative responses at several lymphocyte concentrations from nine young and from ten old persons was determined and the number of responding units calculated from the semilogarithmic plot of the data. From the cumulative data illustrated in Figure 1, it can be seen that the frequency of PHA responsive units is 1 per 1.400 mononuclear cells from young persons and 1 per 2.950 mononuclear cells from old persons.

B. Enumeration of Concanavalin A (Con A)-Responsive Lymphocytes by Virus Plaque Assay

Resting lymphocytes are refractory to Vesicular Stomatitis Virus (vsv) infection, while activated T lymphocytes support the multiplication of vsv. The numbers of Con A responsive cells in populations from young and old people were enumerated by counting the number of lytic foci on an L-cell monolayer produced by a lymphocyte preparation infected with vsv as described by Jiminez and Bloom[9] and Sutcliffe et al.[10] Thirty ml of venous blood from both old and young donors was defibrinated and

FREQUENCY OF PHA-RESPONSIVE UNITS IN LYMPHOCYTE PREPARATIONS FROM YOUNG AND OLD PERSONS

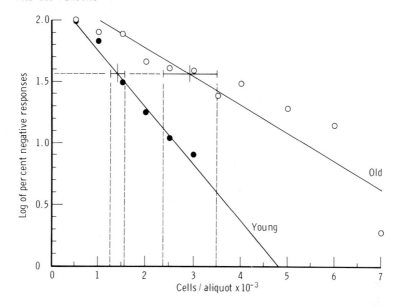

FIGURE 1.   Fluctuation analysis was performed on limiting dilutions of lymphocytes from nine young and ten old subjects. Replicate cultures containing a range of lymphocyte concentrations were cultured in the presence or absence of PHA. The percent of negative responses at each lymphocyte concentration for young and old populations was determined. The mean response of the old or young populations at each cell concentration is shown. Thus, the total number of positive responses in cultures from all young or from all old persons was divided by the total number of cultures with PHA established at this cell concentration. Least squares regression analysis was used to obtain the linear plot shown which relates the percent of negative responses to lymphocyte number. The 95% confidence interval on the reciprocal of the aliquot size at which 37% of the cultures were unresponsive is given for each population.

mixed with a 3% solution of gelatin (Difco Laboratories, Detroit, Mich.) in 0.15 M NaCl and allowed to sediment for 1 hr at 37°C. Th gelatin-serum-lymphocyte mixture obtained was incubated in a nylon wool column (Associated Biomedic Systems, Buffalo, N.Y.) which had been prewet with RPMI-1640 containing 15% fetal bovine serum (FBS, Microbiological Associates) for 30 min. The effluent cells were treated with 0.83% ammonium chloride 0.17 M Tris to lyse erythrocytes,[11] were washed three times with HBSS, and were collected by centrifugation at 50g for 10 min at 20°C. After the third wash, the cells were resuspended in RPMI 1640 containing 6% heat-inactivated FBS, 100 units penicillin per ml, 100 g streptomycin/ml, and 2 mM 1-glutamine. The incubation of 2×10^6 cells was carried out in 2 ml of culture medium in the presence or absence of 20 g of Con A (Sigma Chemical Co) in loosely capped plastic 12 × 75 mm tubes (Falcon Plastics) at 37°C in a 5% CO_2/95% humidified air environment for 72 hr.

VSV harvested from chicken embryo fibroblasts was added to the lymphocytes at the end of the culture period at a multiplicity of approximately 20 to 1. The infected cultures were incubated for 2 hr at 37°C. After incubation the cultures were centrifuged and free virus neutralized by incubation in a potent guinea pig anti-vsv serum for one hour at 4°C. The cells were then washed extensively in minimal essential medium (MEM) supplemented with 6% FBS to remove antibody and antibody-virus com-

Table 1

VIRUS PLAQUE FORMATION BY YOUNG AND OLD
LYMPHOCYTES CULTURED IN MEDIUM WITH OR
WITHOUT CON A

Experiment number	Age of donor	PFU/10^6 lymphocytes Con A		ΔPFU per 10^6 lymphocytes	Old PFU/ young PFU
		Absent	Present		
1	22	3,402	297,845	294,443	0.134
	86	4,253	43,667	39.414	
2	24	67	16,518	16,451	0.004
	75	68	138	70	
3	38	525	25,683	25,158	0.190
	75	870	5,654	4,784	
4	25	393	5,849	5,456	0.510
	84	1,502	4,288	2,786	
5	28	73	139,617	139,554	0.053
	65	144	7,501	7,357	
6	23	1,782	28,603	26,847	0.450
	65	3,634	15,725	12,091	
Mean					0.224

Note: Lymphocytes from young and old individuals were incubated for 72 hr
with or without Con A. These cells were exposed to vesicular stomatitis
virus, washed, and exposed to anti-VSV antibody. Aliquots of the virus-
infected cell suspension were poured over an L-cell monolayer. Lytic foci
in the monolayer were enumerated after 48 hr of incubation. The number
of lytic foci (plaques) per 10^6 lymphocytes plated are reported.

plexes. Viable counts were obtained on each culture using trypan blue exclusion before
plating.

Indicator monolayers were prepared from mouse L cells. The infected lymphocytes
were plated in MEM supplemented with 6% FBS, antibiotics and glutamine, in 1%
agar above the L-cell monolayer in 60-mm Petri dishes. Three log dilutions of lymphocytes, each in duplicate, were made for each culture. The plates were then incubated
in humidified air in 5% CO_2 at 37°C for 36 hr, fixed in 10% formalin in saline, and
stained with crystal violet. Plaques are counted and the number of plaque-forming
cells per million lymphocytes calculated.

The number of activated lymphocytes per million viable cells from old or young
persons was compared at the end of a 72-hr culture period in the presence or absence
of Con A (Table 1). Six experiments were performed. In the absence of Con A, the
number of virus-producing cells in cultures from old persons was greater than in cultures from young persons. Six experiments were performed using six different preparations of virus. In each of the six experiments similar results were obtained. The survival of cells from old or young persons in culture without Con A was comparable:
74% of young lymphocytes and 72% of old lymphocytes were viable by trypan blue
exclusion after 72 hr in culture. Although there was an increased number of activated
lymphocytes in cultures from old subjects without mitogen, Con A activated fewer
lymphocytes in cultures from old persons. In each of the six experiments performed,
Con A activated more lymphocytes in cultures from young than in cultures from old
subjects. This difference was statistically significant (P < 0.04). The number of Con
A-activated lymphocytes from old persons was approximately one-fifth the number of

Con A-activated lymphocytes from young persons. In the presence of Con A, the survival of lymphocytes from old persons (46%) was significantly less than the survival of cells from young persons (67%). Consequently, if the results had been expressed as the number of activated lymphocytes per initially cultured cells, the difference between young and old persons would be even greater.

C. Kinetic Analysis of T-Lymphocyte Proliferation Stimulated by PHA

It was observed that thymidine incorporated by T lymphocytes from old people when incubated with PHA for 96 hr was less than that incorporated by T cells from young subjects (Figure 2). In each of seven experiments, PHA-induced thymidine incorporation by T lymphocytes from old persons was less than that by T lymphocytes from young persons. Thymidine incorporation by T lymphocytes from old subjects cultured without colchicine (unblocked) averaged 42% of that of lymphocytes from young subjects. This difference is statistically highly significant (P < 0.003).

To assess the number of lymphocytes initially responding to PHA, thymidine incorporation was measured 24 hr after the addition of colchicine[12] to prevent cells from entering a second round of thymidine incorporation. In these experiments, T lymphocytes were cultured as described above. 0.02 ml of 5 μg/ml colchicine (Sigma Chemical Co., St. Louis, Mo.) was added to the cultures at the outset of the incubation period or at 24-hr intervals thereafter. (³H) thymidine was added 24 hr after the addition of the colchicine and harvested 24 hr later. Incubation periods ranged from 48 to 168 hr. T lymphocytes assessed in this manner were also cultured in the standard fashion with PHA. Other cultures were incubated with colchicine medium from the outset and thymidine incorporation measured during the last 24 hr of incubation which ranged from 120 to 192 hr.

Under these conditions[12] the (³H) thymidine incorporation measured during the first 96 hr of culture reflects activation of cells newly triggered into DNA synthesis. Thus, it was found (data not presented) that the amount of thymidine incorporated by lymphocytes during each 24-hr period after a 24-hr incubation with colchicine was identical to that incorporated during the same 24-hr pulse when colchicine was present from the initiation of the culture. It is clear that if one assumes that nucleotide transport and pool size are comparable, thymidine incorporation under these conditions, in the presence of colchicine, reflects the number of first generation responding cells passing through the S phase of the cell cycle during the labeling period. Based upon colchicine block and thymidine pulse experiments (Figure 2), it was found that first generation responding T lymphocytes from old or from young persons entered DNA synthesis at the same time. In all seven experiments, maximal thymidine incorporation by first generation responding T lymphocytes occurred between 48 and 72 hr. The rate of entry of first generation responders into DNA synthesis was not altered over a 50-fold range of PHA concentrations. Thymidine incorporation by T lymphocytes from young subjects was significantly greater (P < 0.005) during the first two 24-hr labeling periods (24—48 and 48—72-hr). The greatest difference between young and old T cells with regard to first generation responding lymphocytes was between 48 and 72 hr of culture. There was no difference in thymidine incorporation by lymphocytes from old and young donors during the 72- to 96-hr period.

To estimate the total number of first generation responding T lymphocytes, thymidine incorporated during each of the 24-hr labeling periods between 24 and 96 hr of colchicine-blocked cultures were summed. In each of the seven experiments, total thymidine incorporated by first generation responding T lymphocytes from old individuals was less than that by T lymphocytes from young individuals. The summated thymidine incorporation by T lymphocytes from old persons averaged 57% of that

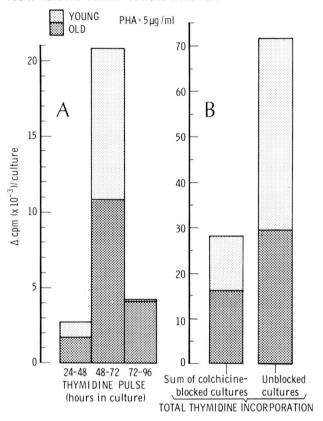

THYMIDINE INCORPORATED BY LYMPHOCYTES FROM OLD AND YOUNG PERSONS DURING CULTURE WITH PHA

FIGURE 2.   PHA-induced thymidine incorporation by lymphocytes from young or old subjects was measured in culture. In all cases thymidine incorporation was measured during a 24-hr period. In the absence of colchicine unblocked cultures, thymidine incorporation was measured during the fourth day of lymphocyte culture. In colchicine-blocked cultures, colchicine was added to achieve a final concentration of 0.5 μg/ml 24 hr before the addition of thymidine. Total thymidine incorporated by colchicine block cultures was calculated by adding the amount of thymidine incorporated on the second, third, and fourth day of culture.

incorporated by T lymphocytes from young donors. This difference is statistically highly significant ($P < 0.008$). The conclusion that there are fewer first generation responding lymphocytes in T-lymphocyte preparations from old persons is in accord with the results of limiting dilution analysis and the vsv plaque assay.

Although the amount of thymidine incorporated by first generation responding lymphocytes from old persons is less than that incorporated by first generation responding lymphocytes from young persons, this difference is not as great as that observed in cultures without colchicine. Thus, total thymidine incorporated by lymphocytes from old persons cultured with colchicine was 57% of that incorporated by lymphocytes from young persons, while in the absence of colchicine, lymphocytes from old persons incorporated only 39% as much as was incorporated by lymphocytes from young persons. In unblocked cultures, thymidine incorporation by second and third generation cells contribute to the total thymidine incorporated. These results imply that in cultures from old persons, the response of second or third generation lymphocytes to PHA is even more markedly impaired than is the response of first generation lymphocytes to PHA.

V. PROLIFERATIVE CAPACITY OF RESPONDING LYMPHOCYTES

It was hypothesized that the difference in thymidine incorporation by lymphocytes from young and old persons increased with each division in culture. This was tested for, and quantitated, by comparing the thymidine incorporation of increasing numbers of lymphocytes from young and old people, by searching for a second wave of thymidine incorporation in colchicine-treated cultures of lymphocytes from young and old persons, and by incubating cells in the presence of Bromodeoxyuridine (BrdU) to quantitate their proliferative capacity.

A. Thymidine Incorporation by Increasing Numbers of Cells in Culture

To measure the response to PHA of lymphocytes derived from first generation PHA-responding cells, increasing numbers of lymphocytes were placed into culture with PHA. The amount of thymidine incorporated per culture was measured and related to the number of cells in culture (Figure 3). Colchicine was added at a final concentration of $0.5~\mu g/m\ell$ to some of the cultures from young persons.

Lymphocytes from young persons showed an exponential increase in thymidine incorporation as the number of cells in culture increased, suggesting that positive interaction (synergy) among the increasing numbers of cells in culture contributes to the total thymidine incorporated. A linear rise in thymidine incorporation with increasing cell number was observed in cultures of lymphocytes from young persons when colchicine was present.

This supports the interpretation that exponential rise in thymidine incorporation observed in cultures of lymphocytes from young subjects results from recruitment of an expanding pool of proliferating cells. In contrast to the behavior of cells from young subjects, thymidine incorporation by lymphocytes from old persons in the absence of colchicine showed a linear rise as the number of cells in culture increased. This would imply a failure to recruit cells into a proliferating pool of cells. The observation is consistent with the fact that cell cooperative interactions in the immune responses are impaired in old subjects.

B. Observation of a Second Peak of Thymidine Incorporation by Cochicine-Treated Lymphocytes

In view of the increased proliferative capacity of lymphocytes from young subjects, a search for a second wave of thymidine incorporation in culture was made. When thymidine incorporation was measured during consecutive 24-hr periods from 24 to 168 hr, a second peak of thymidine incorporation was observed in cultures from young persons but not in cultures from old persons (Figure 4). The late peak of thymidine incorporation was separated from the first peak by a valley. The time at which the second peak was seen varied in different individuals from the fifth to the seventh day of culture. As noted earlier, the sum of thymidine incorporation between 24 and 96 hr expressed as a percent of the unblocked cultures is greater in the old subject. For example, in the experiment illustrated in Figure 4, the colchicine-blocked thymidine incorporation was 42% of thymidine incorporation by unblocked cultures from old persons. In cultures from young persons the colchicine-blocked thymidine incorporation was 32% of thymidine incorporation by unblocked cultures.

The late peak of thymidine incorporation did not occur when colchicine was added

THYMIDINE INCORPORATED BY INCREASING NUMBERS OF LYMPHOCYTES
FROM OLD AND YOUNG PERSONS

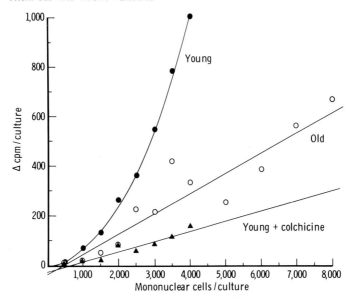

FIGURE 3.   PHA-induced thymidine incorporation by lymphocytes from
ten old and nine young persons was measured in culture. Increasing numbers
of lymphocytes were placed into culture with PHA and the relationship between the amount of thymidine incorporated per culture, and the number of
cells in culture was determined. Some cultures of lymphocytes from young
persons contained colchicine at a final concentration of 0.5 μg/mℓ.

at the initiation of the culture. This implies that the late peak reflected DNA synthesis
by cells derived from the proliferation of first generation responding cells. The failure
to see a second peak of thymidine incorporation with cells from old subjects provides
additional support for the hypothesis that with old persons the response of progeny
of the initial responding cell is more impaired than is the response of the initially responsive lymphocytes.

C. Analysis of Proliferative Capacity of Lymphocytes from Young and Old Persons by BrdU Labeling of Sister Chromatids

The impaired proliferative capacity of lymphocytes from old persons was quantitated in cells cultured with PHA for 72 hr.

Lymphocytes suspended in 5 mℓ of complete culture medium (as above), at a concentration of 10^6 per mℓ, were diluted with 5 mℓ of media containing 50 μg of purified
PHA. Bromodeoxyuridine (BrdU) (Sigma Chemical Co., St. Louis, Mo.) was added
to lymphocyte preparations after 24, 48, and 72 hr in culture. The final concentration
of BrdU was 75μM per culture. Control cultures received identical doses of complete
culture medium.

Colcimid (Grand Island Biological Co., Grand Island, N.Y.) was added (0.1 μg/mℓ)
to lymphocytes (cultured as described above) for two hours. To prepare metaphase
chromosomes, cells were trypsinized, and pelletted at 150g × 10 minutes. The cells were
resuspended in 0.075 M KCl at room temperature for 15 min. They were fixed in three
washes of a glacial acetic acid: methanol (3:1) solution. The fixed cells were gently
dropped onto pre-cleaned slides. These slides were dried, stained for ten minutes with
10^{-4} M 33258 Hoechst stain, rinsed with demineralized water, mounted in pH 7 sodium

THYMIDINE INCORPORATED BY LYMPHOCYTES CULTURED
WITH PHA

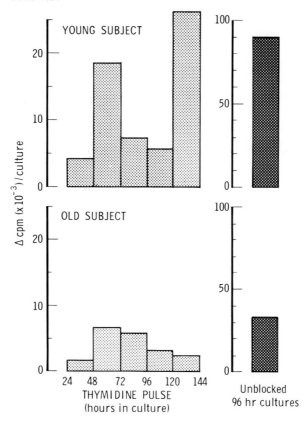

FIGURE 4. PHA-induced thymidine incorporation by lymphocytes from an old and young person during the second to sixth day
of colchicine-blocked cultures and during the fourth day of unblocked cultures was measured. In all cases, thymidine incorporation was measured during the 24 hr period indicated. In the colchicine-blocked cultures, colchicine was added 24 hr before the
addition of thymidine.

citrate buffer and sealed with rubber cement. After 6.5 hr exposure to a 150-Watt
Durolite lamp, the coverslips were removed and the slides were rinsed with demineralized water. The slides were then stained with Harleco®-Wright Giemsa for 15 min,
rinsed with demineralized water and air-dried prior to mounting with permount.

In the presence of BrdU the addition of colcimid three hours prior to the termination
of the cultures permitted observation of changes in the fluorescence of metaphase chromatids stained with Hoechst 33258.[13] In this way the number of PHA responsive cells
completing one, two or three divisions were quantitated. Lymphocyte cultures from
old people contained only one-half the number dividing for the second time and less
than one-quarter of the cells dividing for the third time as cultures from young persons.

VI. CELL CYCLE KINETICS OF LYMPHOCYTES IN CULTURE

The findings presented above are compatible with a reduced capacity of lymphocytes
from old people to proliferate in culture. However, these observations might also re-

flect a delay in time of entry into the division cycle, or a prolongation of the length of the cell cycle, or both.

A. Establishment of Time of Entry into Cell Cycle

Cells cultured with PHA were incubated with colchicine to determine if lymphocytes from old people entered cell division at the same time after stimulation as did lymphocytes from young people. Lymphocyte suspensions, with 1 μg/mℓ colchicine in the medium, were cultured (as described above) for 28 to 36 hr. At hourly intervals the cells were harvested and prepared on slides (as described above) for examination of metaphase chromosomes. The lymphocyte cultures from old people revealed metaphase structures as early (30 to 32 hr) as lymphocyte cultures from young people.

The rate of entry into mitosis of first generation responding lymphocytes from young and old subjects was measured in the presence of colchicine (as above) during the first 75 hr in culture with PHA. Cells, in the presence and absence of colchicine, were seeded in Linbro microtiter plates at 10^5 cells per well. Cells were cultured for various lengths of time, and thymidine incorporation measured during the final three hours of culture. Thymidine incorporation by first generation responding lymphocytes increases to a maximum between 48 and 60 hr, and then decreases in cultures from both young and old subjects. Thus, the activation of initially responding lymphocytes in cultures from old people is neither delayed in its onset, or time of maximal response.

B. Establishment of Cell Cycle Times in Lymphocytes Cultured from Young and Old People

To determine whether responding lymphocytes from old people take longer to complete one cycle of cell division than lymphocytes from young, the interval between peaks of thymidine incorporation in synchronized cell cultures may be measured.

Lymphocyte suspensions were cultured for 72 hr with PHA (as described above). Hydroxyurea was then added to a final concentration of 2mM and the cultures incubated for an additional 15 hr. Cells were then washed twice with HBSS to effect hydroxyurea removal. These lymphocytes were then resuspended at 10^6 cells per mℓ in complete culture medium (as described above). Cells were plated (0.2 mℓ of lymphocyte suspension per well) in triplicate in Linbro round-bottom microtiter plates, and cultured for various lengths of time. Each well was pulsed with 1 μCi (methyl-^{3}H) thymidine (Amersham, Arlington Heights, Ill.) for a 1-hr period.

The mean cell cycle time observed was 15 hr ($\pm$1 hr) in cultures from both young and old individuals. Thus, those lymphocytes from old individuals which are responsive to PHA stimulation initiate cell division as soon as lymphocytes from young people, and accomplish that division in the same length of time.

It thus appears that the age-associated defect in the response to PHA of lymphocytes from humans is the result of a reduced number of cells able to respond. It also appears that those lymphocytes from old people which are mitogen responsive divide with kinetics similar to those of cells from young people. These mitogen-responsive lymphocytes from aged people, however, appear to have reduced capacity to undergo successive divisions following mitogen stimulation.

DISCUSSION

This study investigated the basis of the impaired thymidine incorporation by lymphocytes from old persons. Two mechanisms of this defect were considered: 1. a deficiency of mitogen-responsive lymphocytes in old persons, and 2. a failure of these mitogen-responsive lymphocytes to expand into a pool of proliferating cells. The methods discussed showed that lymphocyte preparations from old people had fewer cells capable of responding to mitogenic stimulation than did preparations from young people. The percentage of mitogen-responsive lymphocytes from old persons relative to preparations from young persons was 22% by VSV plaque assay, 47% with limiting dilution analysis, and 55% by the assessment of first generation responding lymphocytes. This defect does not appear to be due to a relative deficiency of lymphocytes in cell preparations from old people since no decrease was found in the number of lymphocytes in such mononuclear preparations. Although there is no reduction in the number of lymphocytes, the functional capacity of a lymphocyte subpopulation appears to be impaired. The level of thymic hormone has been reported to decline with age[14]. The capacity of thymic hormones to facilitate differentiation of functionally active lymphocytes[15] suggests that the decline of thymic hormone during aging may be the basis for the loss of the mitogen-responsive subpopulation of lymphocytes.

The age-associated impairment of thymidine incorporation by lymphocytes cultured with PHA is greater in the absence of colchicine than in the presence of colchicine. This suggests that mitogen-responsive lymphocytes from old donors fail to expand normally into a pool of proliferating cells. Increasing numbers of cells from old donors incorporated thymidine in the same pattern as did cells from young donors which had been cultured in the presence of PHA. This suggested a failure of progeny cells from old donors to enter the proliferating pool. Consistent with this suggestion is the lack of a second peak of thymidine incorporation in cultures from old donors since the second peak reflects thymidine incorporation by progeny cells. This impairment in proliferative capacity was quantitated by culturing cells in the presence of bromodeoxyuridine. Under these conditions, in relation to lymphocytes from young people, only 44% of the lymphocytes from old people divided for a second time, and only 14% divided for a third time, or more. These data support the interpretation that fewer lymphocytes from old people can undergo two or three proliferative cycles in the presence of PHA. These results could be explained by Hayflick's hypothesis[16] that normal cells have a limited proliferative capacity.

Cell cycle kinetics of lymphocytes in culture were examined in order to explain the failure of many lymphocytes from old persons to undergo subsequent rounds of division. Observations of metaphase cells in suspensions of lymphocytes cultured with and without colchicine revealed that in cultures from old people there was no delay in the time of onset of cell division, or time of maximal division, for those lymphocytes capable of response. The measurement of cell cycle time for lymphocytes cultured with PHA showed no difference in durations of the cycle for responsive lymphocytes from old or young individuals.

It thus appears that the age-associated defect in the response to PHA of lymphocytes from humans is the result of a reduced number of cells able to respond. Our results indicate that those lymphocytes from old people which are mitogen-responsive divide with kinetics similar to those of cells from young people. These mitogen-responsive lymphocytes from aged people, however, appear to have a reduced capacity to undergo successive divisions following mitogen stimulation.

REFERENCES

1. **Pisciotta, A. V., Westring, D. W., De Prey, C., and Walsh, B.,** Mitogenic effect of phytohemagglutinin at different ages, *Nature,* 215, 193, 1967.
2. **Hallgren, H. M., Buckley, C. E., Gilbersten, V. A., and Yunis, E. J.,** Lymphocyte phytohemagglutinin responsiveness, immunoglobulins and autoantibodies in aging humans, *J. Immunol.* 4, 1101, 1973.
3. **Weksler, M. E. and Hutteroth, T. H.,** Impaired lymphocyte function in aged humans, *J. Clin. Invest.* 53, 99, 1974.
4. **Foad, B. S. I., Adams, Y., Yamaguchi, Y., and Litwin, A.,** Phytomitogen responses of peripheral blood lymphocytes in young and older subjects, *Clin. Exp. Immunol,* 17, 657, 1974.
5. **Diaz-Jouanen, E., Strickland, R. G., and Williams, R. C.,** Studies of human lymphocytes in the newborn and the aged, *Am. J. Med.,* 58, 620 1975.
6. **Fernandez, L. A., MacSween, J. M., and Lancey, G. R.,** Lymphocyte responses to phytohemagglutinin: age-related effects, *Immunology,* 31, 583, 1976.
7. **Hansen, G. S., Rubin, B., and Sørensen, S. F.,** Human leucocyte responses in vitro. I. Transformation of purified T lymphocytes with and without addition of partially purified monocytes, *Clin. Exp. Immunol,* 29, 295, 1977.
3. **Pollack, A., Bagwell, C. B., and Irwin, G. L.,** Radiation from tritiated thymidine perturbs the cell cycle progression of stimulated lymphocytes, *Science,* 203, 1025, 1979.
9. **Jiminez, L. and Bloom, B. R.,** Virus plaque assay for antigen-sensitive in delayed hypersensitivity. in *In Vitro Methods in Cell Mediated Immunity,* Bloom, B. R. and Glade, P. R., Eds., Academic Press, New York, 1971, 553.
10. **Sutcliffe, S., Kadish, A. S., Stoner, G., and Bloom, B. R.,** Application of the virus plaque assay to studies of human lymphocytes, in *In Vitro Methods in Cell-Mediated and Tumor Immunity,* Bloom, B. R. and David, J. R., Eds., Academic Press, New York, 1976, 319.
11. **Boyle, W.,** An extension of the ^{51}Cr-release assay for the estimation of mouse cytotoxins, *Transplantation,* 6, 761, 1968.
12. **Lohrmann, H. P., Graw, C. M., and Graw, R. G.,** Stimulated lymphocyte cultures, responder recruitment, and cell cycle kinetics, *J. Exp. Med.* 139, 1037, 1974.
13. **Tice, R., Schneider, E. L., and Rary, J. M.,** The utilization of Bromodeoxyuridine Incorporation into DNA for the analysis of cellular kinetics, *Exp. All. Research,* 102, 232, 1976.
14. **Bach, J. F., Dardene, M., and Salomon, J. C.,** Studies on thymus products, *Clin. Exp. Immunol.,* 14, 247, 1973.
15. **Basch, R. S. and Goldstein, G.,** Thymopoietin-induced acquisition of responsiveness to T-cell mitogens, *Cell. Immunol.,* 20, 218, 1975.
16. **Hayflick, L.,** The cell biology of human aging, *N. Engl. J. Med.,* 295, 1302, 1976.

Chapter 11

HOMING TECHNIQUES AND THEIR APPLICATION TO THE STUDY OF LYMPHOID CELL AGING

R. W. Gillette

TABLE OF CONTENTS

I. INTRODUCTION

For the purpose of this discussion, the lymphoreticular system may be regarded as an organic unit populated by a variety of lymphoid cells that are in a constant state of dynamic flux. Movement appears to be a fundamental property of most lymphocytes; cells in many cases move freely from one anatomic location to another. For example, T lymphocytes are produced in the bone marrow, mature in the thymus, and function in the peripheral lymphoid organs. Indeed, in the case of the long-lived T lymphocyte, the distinguishing characteristic of these cells is their ability to recirculate through the vascular system. The predilection of lymphocytes to migrate through specific anatomical locations has been termed "homing" or lymphocyte "migration".[1,2]

Alteration in homing patterns occurs when an immunologic stimulus is superimposed upon the normal dynamic states of the various lymphoid subpopulations contained in a lymphoid organ.[3] Such changes represent a part of the normal response of the animal to stress. As an example, lymph nodes of mice draining an area within which an immune response exists, such as to sheep erythrocytes,[4] or a progressing neoplasm.[5] prevent the normal exit of lymphocytes from the lymph node and thus increase dramatically the cellular content of the organ. This process is termed "trapping"[6] and has been shown to be an integral part of the animal's response to noxious stimuli.

Table 1 lists some of the factors that influence the normal distribution of lymphoid cells within the lymphoreticular system. The list is not intended to be all-inclusive. Advantage may be taken of the ability of such factors to modify the normal homing of lymphocytes, to study the types and subpopulations of lymphocytes that become involved in the cellular immune response under the various conditions.

Homing of lymphoid cells may be most efficiently studied using radioactively labeled lymphocytes. The most widely used isotope is ^{51}Cr. ^{51}Cr as sodium chromate may be purchased from nearly any distributor of radioisotopes and at a wide variety of specific activities. A number of other radiolabels such as isotopes of iodine,[7] hydrogen,[8] carbon,[9] technetium,[10] and indium,[11] can also be utilized to tag lymphocytes.

II. METHOD FOR LABELING LYMPHOID CELLS WITH ^{51}Cr

The method most extensively relied upon is a modification of that first described by Bainbridge and Gowland.[12] Cell suspensions are prepared by gently teasing of spleen, thymus or Peyer's patches of the small intestine. Bone marrow cells are most easily obtained by aspiration of long bones with media delivered by a small gauge needle. Lymph node cells are brought into suspension by passing a pool of nodes such as the mesenterics, inguinals, brachials, and axillaries through a fine nylon mesh. Suspensions of peritoneal cells may be obtained by flushing the peritoneal cavity with saline containing heparin to prevent clotting. The yield of peritoneal cells may be increased by inducing an exudate by intraperitoneal inoculation with thioglycollate,[13] proteose peptone,[14] or adjuvant.[15]

Regardless of the type of lymphoid cell under consideration, the labeling of cells is accomplished by following the steps outlined below. The cell suspensions are washed twice with a medium such as RPMI-1640 containing 5 to 10% fetal bovine serum. A final cell count is taken and the cell suspension adjusted to 10^8 viable cells per mℓ. Twenty-five μCi of ^{51}Cr/10^8 cells are then added and the mixture is incubated at 37°C for 30 min. The lymphoid cells are then centrifuged at $100 \times$ g for 15 minutes and the supernatant removed from the cell pellet. The cells are gently resuspended and washed an additional three times to remove unbound ^{51}Cr. The labeled cells are prepared at a

Table 1
FACTORS THAT ALTER THE NORMAL TRAFFIC OF
LYMPHOID CELLS

	References
Presence of Infection	21, 22, 23, 24
Presence of Tumors	25, 26, 42
Age of Cell Recipient or Donor	28, 43
Treatment with Immunopharmacologic Agents - Steroids	43, 44
- Antilymphocyte Serum	20,45
Irradiation	18, 45
Genetics	46
Immune Stress	47, 48, 49, 50

concentration of 10^8 viable cells in medium. 0.2 ml of suspension is inoculated intravenously in the caudal tail vein or intraperitoneally. We have observed that identical homing patterns emerge over a wide range of injected numbers of labeled lymphocytes; therefore, the volume or number of injected cells may be adjusted if so desired.

III. VALIDITY OF THE CHROMIUM LABEL

The utility of the ^{51}Cr label rests upon three considerations. First, ^{51}Cr labels only viable cells in vitro. If lymphocytes are killed prior to labeling, uptake of ^{51}Cr by the dead cells is minimal. Only those cells demonstrated to be viable by the Trypan blue exclusion method will label. Second, ^{51}Cr has been shown to be a stable label at least for the purposes outlined above. [51]Cr is thought to bind weakly to cellular proteins and that the bulk of the loss with time occurs because of the natural turnover of proteins by the cell.[16] Finally and perhaps most importantly, ^{51}Cr is not reutilized in vivo despite the fact that the uptake of chromate by lymphocytes appears to be energy independent[17]. Lymphoid cells are labeled only in vitro while label lost in vivo is soon excreted by the kidneys.

IV. DATA

We have established that 24 hr is sufficient time for a stable migration pattern to develop[16]. For most experiments, this provides sufficient time for all necessary experimental manipulation of recipient animals. With the exception of the liver, the percent recovery of label from individual lymphoid organs remains nearly stable for another 48 hr. The percent recovery from the liver falls quickly due to destruction of dead or damaged cells that represent the most significant part of the accumulation of radiolabeled cells to that organ.

Table 2 contains a list of the individual lymphoid structure that may be conveniently removed from injected recipient animals and assayed for content of [51]Cr. The results are expressed as mean and standard deviation of values derived from panels of four or more experimental animals. Data generally are analyzed for statistically significant differences using Students' t test.

For most experiments, it is unnecessary to examine the extensive list of lymphoid organs itemized in Table 2. Generally, the lymph node samples are composed of a pool of inguinal, brachial, axillary, and mesenteric nodes. Also, the organ survey may be limited to spleen, liver, and pooled lymph nodes for most preliminary experiments.

Table 2
TOTAL ORGAN SURVEY OF THE
DISTRIBUTION OF ^{51}CR-LABELED
INTRAVENOUSLY INOCULATED
LYMPH NODE AND SPLEEN
CELLS IN SYNGENEIC BALB/C
RECIPIENTS[a]

Organ surveyed	Lymph node	Spleen
Lymph Nodes		
Inguinal	1.1 ± 0.1	0.4 ± 0.2
Brach. + Axill.	1.8 ± 0.2	0.7 ± 0.3
Mesenteric	3.1 ± 0.5	5.3 ± 0.9
Cervical	2.7 ± 0.9	2.4 ± 0.2
Deep Cervicals	0.7 ± 0.4	1.0 ± 0.2
Mediastinal	0.5 ± 0.1	0.3 ± 0.1
Total Lymph Nodes	9.9[b]	10.1
Spleen	26.0 ± 2.7	20.4 ± 1.4
Liver	20.6 ± 0.8	34.0 ± 0.6
Lungs	1.6 ± 0.1	2.0 ± 0.8
Bone Marrow	9.7 ± 1.2	6.7 ± 0.9
Small Intest.	3.3 ± 0.7	2.9 ± 0.2
Total Percent Recovery	71.1	76.1

[a]   Normal lymph node or spleen cells were inoculated intravenously.

[b]   Note that while the total recovery of label was equivalent in either type of recipient, percent distribution within individual lymph nodes varied significantly.

V. TYPES OF HOMING EXPERIMENTS

There are two basic kinds of protocols that may be used in the majority of experiments employing homing techniques.

The first type of homing experiment utilizes injection of labeled lymphoid cells from donors that have been experimentally manipulated. Since the recipient is assumed to be in a normal physiological state, alteration in the percentage migration to host lymphoid organs correlates with changes in the cellular composition of donor lymphoid organs caused by the experimental procedures. Controls for this type of protocol consist of normal lymphoid cells inoculated into age matched normal recipients. This last provides evidence that the reagents and labeling conditions did not influence the results. In addition, comparison can then be made between the control and pooled normal data derived from a large number of experiments. From a statistical viewpoint, there should be no difference between pooled data and control values.

In the second kind of homing protocol, labeled cells from normal syngeneic donor mice are inoculated into experimental (treated) recipients. Comparison is then made to the percent organ distribution of aliquots of lymphoid cells injected into normal, age-matched recipients. This procedure has a distinct advantage in that both experimental and control animals are inoculated with aliquots of the identical lymphoid cell preparation. Differences in organ distribution reflect recruitment of normal cells by host lymphoid organs that result from the experimental procedures. Such changes in percent migration to recipient lymphoid organs may be caused either by depletion of specific subpopulations of lymphoid cells or changes in the requirements for specific lymphocytes within lymphoid organs that are mediated via the trapping mechanism.

VI. VARIATION IN DISTRIBUTION AS A FUNCTION OF ORGAN SOURCE

Table 3 lists the mean percentage recovery of ^{51}Cr-labeled lymphocytes from various organ sources in the lymphoid organs of normal syngeneic recipients. As can be seen, the patterns of distribution are uniquely different depending upon the source of the inoculated cells. The differences in distribution reflect the relative content within specific lymphoid organs of distinct subpopulations of lymphocytes. For example, the principle lymph node seeking subpopulation has been shown to be composed in the main of long-lived recirculating T lymphocytes.[19] Treatment with antilymphocyte serum specifically deletes this population of lymphocytes while its influence upon the spleen-seeking population is minimal.[20] As can be seen in the table, long-lived lymphocytes are less numerous in the spleen while thymus and bone marrow are nearly devoid of such cells.

VII. PITFALLS

A number of important factors that can greatly influence the results of experiments that use homing techniques must be taken into consideration.

Of great importance is the viability of the cell suspension to be labeled with [51]Cr. As pointed out above, dead cells do not absorb Cr; therefore, the number of CPM in the inoculum is directly proportional to the number of viable cells incubated with the label. When the percent of Trypan blue excluding lymphocytes is below ninety, viability becomes a very significant factor. Therefore, it is good practice to discard any preparations with more than 10% nonviable cells. If care is taken in preparing lymphocyte suspensions, viability counts in excess of 95% are easily attained.

The purity of the ^{51}Cr is another important consideration. Vanadium is a decay product of radiochromium. Vanadium and its salts are extremely toxic to lymphocytes; therefore, the number of half lives through which the labeling preparation passes becomes an important factor. Toxicity of the labeling solution can be detected by taking viable cell counts after incubation at 37°C. Cell damage during labeling is usually reflected in excessive recovery of label in recipient livers. If the percent recovery of ^{51}Cr from the liver is consistently above 25%, toxic levels of vanadium in the ^{51}Cr are usually the cause.

The health of either the donor or recipient is of obvious concern. Infectious agents[21-24] as well as neoplasia[25,26] have been clearly demonstrated to greatly influence the homing patterns of lymphocytes. Therefore, it is important to use mice purchased from a reliable source. In addition, all animals should be rested after shipment. The stress associated with travel may also modify the cellular content of lymphoid organs, probably through the elevation of corticosteroid secretion associated with adrenal stimulation.

The donors and recipients must be syngeneic. Zatz et al.[27] have convincingly demonstrated that when lymphoid cells that are histoincompatibel are inoculated, the homing patterns are significantly altered. Histoincompatibility at other than the major H-2 locus or differences in allo-antigens such as thy, appear unimportant.

There are small but significant genetically determined differences in the cellular composition of lymphoid organs. Therefore, it is important that the same strain of mouse

Table 3

DISTRIBUTION OF ⁵¹CR-LABELED LYMPHOID CELLS FROM NORMAL BALB/C DONOR MICE IN NORMAL SYNGENEIC RECIPIENTS[a]

	Cell source					
Organ surveyed	Lymph node	Spleen	Bone marrow	Thymus	Peyer's patches	Peritoneum
Spleen	15.2 ± 1.6[b]	17.9 ± 1.5	13.1 ± 1.0	25.0 ± 4.6	8.4 ± 1.7	7.8 ± 1.4
Lymph Node Pool	11.3 ± 2.0	5.2 ± 0.6	0.3 ± 0.1	1.2 ± 0.4	1.5 ± 0.4	0.3 ± 0.1
Liver	20.1 ± 2.6	19.1 ± 2.6	20.7 ± 0.6	18.1 ± 1.9	28.2 ± 3.9	25.1 ± 2.4
Bone Marrow[c]	4.6 ± 0.5	5.5 ± 0.8	13.4 ± 3.2	8.1 ± 1.6	5.2 ± 1.3	0.4 ± 0.1
Small Intestine	3.1 ± 0.4	1.4 ± 0.2	0.9 ± 0.2	0.5 ± 0.1	1.4 ± 0.4	2.1 ± 0.3
Thymus	0.1 ± 0.1	0.3 ± 0.1	0.1 ± 0.1	0.1 ± 0.1	0.2 ± 0.1	0.1 ± 0.1
Kidney	1.1 ± 0.2	1.4 ± 0.2	1.4 ± 0.4	2.1 ± 0.2	1.8 ± 0.6	1.8 ± 0.3
Lungs	1.2 ± 0.1	2.9 ± 0.4	5.6 ± 0.9	0.7 ± 0.1	3.1 ± 1.2	3.1 ± 0.5
Blood[d]	3.4 ± 0.2	7.4 ± 0.9	36.8 ± 3.5	12.4 ± 0.2	8.6 ± 2.2	1.0 ± 0.6

[a]   Represents pooled results obtained from control normal to normal transfers used in approximately 50 different experiments.

[b]   ± one standard deviation.

[c]   Assumes that the radioactivity in the femur represents 10% of the total marrow pool.

[d]   Assumes that the radioactivity in the blood sample represents 20% of the total blood pool.

be used in any given experiment. Direct comparisons should only be made between results obtained from experimental protocols using syngeneic animals.

Age of either donor or recipient is critical.[28] Fortunately, there is a period of about two months after weaning during which the age of the recipient is not a factor. Therefore, when physiologic manipulation of the donor is attempted, the recipients should be less than three months of age. If experimentally manipulated donors must be carried in excess of three months, then it is imperative that age-matched control animals be included in the experimental protocol. The use of homing techniques in studies of aging will be further discussed later in this chapter.

VIII. DEMONSTRATION THAT PATTERNS OF LYMPHOID CELL MIGRATION ARE A FUNCTION OF VIABILITY

An unfounded criticism of the use of homing methods to study the distribution of lymphocyte subpopulations is that the patterns of migration encountered after labeled cell transfer are random. A control that may be added to show that this is not true is the use of heat-killed lymphocytes. Table 4 provides typical data showing that lymphocytes killed after labeling distribute much differently than viable cells. The bulk of the ⁵¹Cr inoculate with heated lymphocytes was recovered from the liver.

IX. HOMING IS DETERMINED BY CELL MEMBRANE COMPONENTS

Specific subpopulations of lymphocytes home to definite anatomical locations within lymphoid organs.[29-32] Ability to home normally is related to specific chemical structures carried on the cell membrane. For example, if lymph node cells are treated with neuraminidase[33] or trypsin[34,35] before inoculation, their capacity to migrate to the lymph nodes is greatly reduced. Also, when mitogens such as concanavalin A are coupled to the lymphocyte membrane, lymph node-seeking subpopulations are transformed into spleen-seeking cells.[36]

Table 4
CHANGES IN THE HOMING
PROPERTIES OF LYMPH NODE
CELLS AFTER HEAT KILLING

Recipient organ	Lymph node cells	
	Normal	Heat killed[a]
Lymph Nodes	15.1 ± 1.4[b]	<.01
Spleen	17.8 ± 2.0	2.2 ± 0.6
Liver	18.7 ± 2.5	40.1 ± 4.4
Small Intestine	2.9 ± 0.4	<.01

[a] Heated to 56° for 30 min.
[b] ± One standard deviation.

Table 5
HOMING PATTERNS OF TRANSFORMED
LYMPHOCYTES

Lymphoma	Type	Percent recovery of ^{51}Cr			
		Spleen	Lymph nodes	Liver	Small intestine
YAC	T[a]	5.4[b]	<0.1	31.8	0.6
YC8	T	13.6	<0.1	18.6	1.6
LSTRA	T	8.7	<0.1	28.9	2.1
P388	-[c]	20.2	0.1	37.4	0.6
NS1	B	4.0	<0.1	36.4	0.3
MOPC31C	B	12.1	0.3	26.3	0.5
MPOC195	B	8.6	0.2	23.1	0.4
AKR	T	11.5	0.2	25.7	2.6

[a] Determined by the ability of anti thy serum of the appropriate specificity to cause release of ^{51}Cr from labeled target lymphoma cells in the presence of guinea pig complement.
[b] Standard deviation: 10% of less
[c] Not tested.

Lymphocytes transformed either by RNA virus infection or chemical carcinogens also distribute uniquely when compared to normal T or B lymphocytes. In addition, significant differences in homing have been observed between established lines of transformed lymphocytes (Table 5). This occurred despite the fact that some of the lymphoma could be demonstrated to be of T or B lineage. The data suggest that important membrane antigens are absent or modified on transformed lymphocytes.

X. APPLICATION OF HOMING TECHNIQUES TO AGING

As pointed out previously, the age of either donor or recipient is highly critical to migration assays. It is for this reason that the technique of homing may be applied very effectively to the study of lymphoid organ and cell aging. Most studies of age-associated changes in the lymphoid cell subpopulations within different lymphoid organs have been performed by labeling lymphocytes from various aged donors and analyzing the homing patterns of such cells in normal recipients of a standard 6 to 8 weeks of age. By using standard-age recipients, it is possible to eliminate the variation in results caused by the age level of the recipient.

Table 6
CHANGES WITH AGE OF
THE SPLEEN-SEEKING
POPULATIONS IN THE
SPLEENS OF NORMAL
BALB/C AND AKR MICE

Age in weeks	Percent recovery in spleen	
	BALB/c	AKR
8	19.2[a]	23.1
15	20.1	21.0
20	21.5	15.9
25	24.6	12.8
30	24.8	12.9
35	26.6	11.3
40	30.8	9.5

[a]   Standard deviations did not exceed 6% in any case.

Homing technique is particularly useful for detecting age-related changes in lymphocyte subpopulations that may be associated with increased risk of some forms of malignancy. For example, Table 6 compares the levels of spleen-seeking cells in the spleens
of BALB/c and leukemia-prone AKR mice. BALB/c display the pattern of change
similar to that of most lower incidence strains, i.e., a continual modest increase in the
spleen-seeking population as the animal ages. In contradistinction, AKR spleen-seeking populations exhibit a continual decline over the same time span until by the time
AKR animals reach the pre-leukemia stage, the spleen-seeking population is less than
half that of young animals. The data suggest that depletion of part of the spleen-seeking subpopulation in the spleen may be directly related to the diathesis of AKR mice
for leukemia. A similar reduction in spleen-seeking cells from the lymph nodes was
also observed.

Perhaps of greater significance were the changes observed in the levels of spleen-
seeking cells in AKR bone marrow (Table 7). BALB/c age-matched mice exhibited a
slow decline with age of a spleen-seeking population within the bone marrow compartment, AKR donor bone marrow contained progessively increasing numbers of spleen-
seeking cells. Again, the data suggest that such changes may be fundamental to the
leukemogenic process in AKR.

XI. AGE-ASSOCIATED CHANGES IN NORMAL MICE

A variety of functional changes attributed to aging have been reported to occur in
subpopulations of lymphocytes from different lymphoid organs. These include increased suppressor cell activity,[37] induction of autoimmunity,[38] changes in cellular[39]
and humoral[40] immunity, and failure of normal lymphocyte maturation.[41] Many of
these changes are reflected in the relative representation of various subpopulations of
lymphocytes in lymphoid organs. Further, most of such alterations may be detected
early in the aging process by the application of homing methods. A summary of the
most significant changes in lymphocyte distribution with time are outlined in Table 8.
The alterations of greatest magnitude were those found with the spleen-seeking populations. It seems likely that many of the changes in this subpopulation relate to increases in the levels of suppressor-cell activity found in aged spleen.

Table 7
CHANGES WITH AGE OF
THE SPLEEN-SEEKING
POPULATIONS IN THE
BONE MARROW OF
NORMAL BALB/C AND
AKR MICE

Age in weeks	Percent recovery in spleen	
	BALB/c	AKR
8	14.1[a]	6.5
15	13.5	9.6
20	11.9	10.0
25	10.5	14.1
30	9.4	13.8
25	9.5	16.2
40	5.6	18.6

[a] Standard deviations did not exceed 10% in any case.

Table 8
SUMMARY OF GENERAL CHANGES IN
THE HOMING PATTERNS ASSOCIATED
WITH AGING

Cell source	Subpopulation	Change with age
Lymph Node	Lymph Node-Seeking	Declines Late
Spleen	Lymph Node-Seeking	Unchanged
Lymph Node	Spleen-Seeking	Increases
Spleen	Spleen-Seeking	Increases
Bone Marrow	Spleen-Seeking	Declines

Homing methods may also be applied directly to problems relating to aging on the cellular level. In general, experiments of this type require the use of a donor that is unable to adequately regenerate a particular subpopulation of lymphocytes. As an example, thymectomy destroys the ability of mice to properly regenerate the long-lived recirculating T-cell population without effecting those T-2 lymphocytes that are peripheral to the thymus.[28] When lymph node cells from thymectomized donors are migrated in normal mice, there is a time associated decline in the lymph node-seeking population. By three months, the percentage of such cells reaches fifty percent of normal and by six months reaches a stable level and no further decrease occurs. The data may be interpreted to mean that by six months, the youngest T-2 lymphocytes at the time of thymectomy have died. Therefore, the maximum age of long-lived murine lymphocytes was estimated to be 5 to 6 months. This figure correlates well with estimates obtained using other methods.

REFERENCES

1. **Austin, C. M.,** Patterns of migration of lymphoid cells, *Aust. J. Exp. Biol. Med. Sci.,* 46, 581, 1968.
2. **Zatz, M. M. and Lance, E. M.,** The distribution of chromium-51-labeled lymphoid cells in the mouse, *Cell. Immunol.,* 1, 3, 1970.
3. **Zatz, M. M. and Lance, E. M.,** The distribution of ^{51}Cr-labeled lymphocytes into antigen-stimulated mice, *J. Exp. Med.,* 134, 224, 1971.
4. **Zatz, M. M. and Gershon, R. K.,** Thymus dependence of lymphocyte trapping, *J. Immunol.,* 112, 101, 1974.
5. **Ogura, T. and Yamamura, Y.,** Distribution of ^{51}Cr-labeled lymphoid cells in the lymph node draining the inoculated tumor in the rat, *Gann,* 64, 433, 1973.
6. **Zatz, M. M. and Lance, E. M.,** Lymphocyte trapping in tolerant mice, *Nature (London) New Biol.,* 234, 253, 1971.
7. **Glllette, R. W.,** Kinetic studies of macrophages 1. Distributional characteristics of radiolabeled peritoneal cells, *J. Reticuloendothel. Soc.,* 10, 223, 1971.
8. **Durkin, H. G., Caparale, L., and Thorberke, G. J.,** Migratory patterns of B Lymphocytes 1. Fate of cells from central and peripheral lymphoid organs in the rabbit and its selective alteration by anti-immunoglobulin, *Cell Immunol.,* 16, 285, 1975.
9. **Rici, M., Romagnani, S., Passadena, A., and Biliotti, G.,** Lymphocyte transformation and macrophage migration in guinea pigs immunized with Freund's complete adjuvant, *Clin. Exp. Immunol.,* 5, 659, 1969.
10. **Barth, R. F. and Singla, O.,** Migratory patterns of technetium-99m-labeled lymphoid cells 1. Effects of antilymphocyte serum on the organ distribution of murine thymocytes, *Cell Immunol.,* 17, 83, 1975.
11. **Frost, P. and Smith, J.,** The radiolabeling of lymphocytes with ^{111}indium 1. Elucidation of optimal labeling conditions, *Proc. Exp. Biol. Med.,* 1977.
12. **Bainbrudge, D. R. and Gowland, G.,** Detection of homograft sensitivity in mice by the elimination of chromium-51-labeled lymph node cells, *Ann. N. Y. Acad. Sci.,* 129, 257, 1966.
13. **Feedman, M. and Gallily, R.,** Cell interactions in the induction of antibody formation, *Cold Spring Harbor Symp. Quant. Biol.,* 32, 415, 1967.
14. **Fishman, M. R.,** Antibody formation in vitro, *J. Exp. Med.,* 114, 337, 1961.
15. **Gillette, R. W. and Lance, E. M.,** Kinetic studies of macrophages II. The effect of specific antisera on radiolabeled peritoneal cells, *Cell Immunol.,* 4, 207, 1972.
16. **Ronai, P. M.,** The elution of ^{51}Cr from labeled leukocytes - a new theory, *Blood,* 33, 408, 1969.
17. **Sanderson, C. J.,** The uptake and retention of chromium by cells, *Transplantation,* 21, 526, 1976.
18. **Gillette, R. W. and Lance, E. M.,** Kinetic studies of macrophages II. The effect of specific antisera on radiolabeled peritoneal cells, *Cell. Immunol.,* 4, 207, 1972.
19. **Lance, E. M. and Taub, R. N.,** Segregation of lymphocyte populations through differential migration, *Nature,* 221, 841, 1969.
20. **Taub, R. N. and Lance, E. M.,** Effects of heterologous anti-lymphocyte serum on the distribution of ^{51}Cr-labeled lymph node cells in mice, *Immunology,* 15, 633, 1968.
21. **Taub, R. N., Rosett, W., Adler, A., and Morse, S. I.,** Distribution of labeled lymph node cells in mice during the lymphocytosis induced by Bordetalla Pertusis, *J. Exp. Med.,* 136, 1581, 1972.
22. **Woodruff, J. J. and Woodruff, J. F.,** Virus-induced alterations of lymphoid tissues III. Fate of radiolabeled thoraic duct lymphocytes in rats inoculated with Newcastle Disease Virus, *Cell. Immunol.,* 5, 307, 1972.
23. **Woodruff, J. J. and Woodruff, J. F.,** Influenza A virus interaction with murine lymphocyte I. The influence of influenza virus A/Japan 305 (H2N2) on the pattern of migration of recirculating lymphocytes, *J. Immunol.,* 117, 852, 1976.
24. **Gillette, R. W. and Fox, A.,** Changes in the homing patterns of chromium 51-labeled lymphoid cells by Moloney Sarcoma Virus infection, *J. Natl. Cancer Inst.,* 58, 1621, 1977.
25. **Gillette, S. and Bellanti, J. A.,** Kinetics of lymphoid cells in tumor-bearing mice, *Cell Immunol.,* 8, 311, 1973.
26. **Gillette, R. W. and Boone, C. W.,** Changes in the homing properties of labeled lymphoid cells caused by solid tumor growth, *Cell Immunol.,* 12, 363, 1974.
27. **Zatz, M. M., Gingrich, R., and Lance, E. M.,** The effect of histoincompatibility antigens on lymphocyte migration in the mouse, *Immunology,* 23, 665, 1972.
28. **Gillette, R. W.,** Changes in the migration patterns of spleen and lymph node cells associated with thyrectomy and aging, *J. Reticuloendothel. Soc.,* 18, 204, 1975.
29. **Sprent, J.,** Circulating T and B lymphocytes of the mouse I. Migratory properties, *Cell Immunol.,* 1, 10, 1973.

30. **Stamper, H. B. and Woodruff, J. J.,** Lymphocyte homing into lymph nodes: in vitro demonstration of the selective affinity of recirculating lymphocytes for high endothelial venules, *J. Exp. Med.,* 144, 828, 1976.

31. **Cahill, R. N. P., Paskitt, D. C., Frost, J., and Trnka, Z.,** Two distinct pools of recirculating T lymphocytes: migratory characteristics of nodal and intestinal T lymphocytes, *J. Exp. Med.,* 145, 420, 1977.

32. **Guy-Grand, D., Griscelli, C., and Vassalli, P.,** The mouse gut T lymphocyte, a novel type of T cell, *J. Exp. Med.,* 148, 1661, 1978.

33. **Woodruff, J. J. and Gesmer, B. M.,** The effect of neuroaminidase on the fate of transfused lymphocytes, *J. Exp. Med.,* 129, 551, 1969.

34. **Woodruff, J. J. and Gesner, B. M.,** Lymphocytes: circulation altered by trypsin, *Science,* 161, 176, 1968.

35. **Ronnie, G. H., Smith, M. E., and Ford, W. L.,** Lymphocyte migration into cell-mediated immune lesions is inhibited by trypsin, *Nature,* 267, 520, 1977.

36. **Gillette, R. W., McKenzie, G. O., and Swanson, M. H.,** Effect of concanavalin A on the homing of labeled T lymphocytes, *J. Immunol.,* 111, 1902, 1973.

37. **Singhal, S. K., Roder, J. C., and Dawe, A. K.,** Suppressor cells in immunosenecence. *Fed. Proc., Fed. Am. Soc. Exp. Biol.,* 37, 1245, 1978.

38. **Naor, D., Bonavida, B., and Walford, R. L.,** Autoimmunity and aging: the age-related response of mice of a long-lived strain to trinitrophenylated syngeneic mouse red blood cells, *J. Immunol.,* 117, 2204, 1976.

39. **Meredith, P., Tittor, W., Gerbase-DeLima, M., and Walford, R. L.,** Age-related changes in the cellular immune response of lymph node and thymus cells in long-lived mice, *Cell Immunol.,* 18, 324, 1975.

40. **Makinoden, T. and Peterson, W. J.,** Secondary antibody-forming potential in mice in relation to age - its significance to senescence, *Dev. Biol.,* 14, 96, 1966.

41. **Friedman, D., Keiser, V., and Globerson, A.,** Reactivation of immunocompetence in spleen cells of aged mice, *Nature,* 251, 545, 1974.

42. **Elbovim, C. N., Reinisch, C. L., and Schlossman, S. F.,** T and B lymphocyte migration into syngeneic tumors, *J. Immunol.,* 118, 1042, 1977.

43. **Lance, E. M. and Cooper, S.,** Effects of cortisol and antilymphocyte serum on lymphoid populations, in *Hormones and the Immune Response,* Wolstenholme, G. E. W. and Knight, N., Eds., Ciba Foundation Study Group 36, 73, 1970.

44. **Gillette, R. W. and Lance, E. M.,** Kinetic studies of macrophages III. The effect of hydrocortisone upon the distribution of radiolabeled peritoneal cells, *J. Reticuloendothel. Soc.,* 12, 701, 1972.

45. **Zatz, M. M.,** Differential effects of ATS and irradiation on trapping in lymph nodes and spleen, *Immunology,* 30, 749, 1976.

46. **Zatz, M. M., Mellons, R. C., and Lance, E. M.,** Changes in lymphoid populations of aging CBA and NZB mice, *Clin. Exp. Immunol.,* 8, 491, 1971.

47. **Zatz, M. M.,** Effects of BCG on lymphocyte trapping, *J. Immunol.,* 116, 1587, 1976.

48. **Gillette, R. W. and Lance, E. M.,** Kinetic studies of macrophages: homograft response, *Transplantation,* 11, 95, 1971.

49. **Gillette, R. W. and Swanson, M. H.,** Kinetic studies of macrophages V. Effects of antigen and adjuvant stimulation, *J. Reticuloendothel. Soc.,* 13, 31, 1974.

50. **Gillette, R. W. and Boone, C. W.,** Effect of tumor immunity on the distribution of labeled lymphoid cells in tumor-challenged mice, *Cell Immunol.,* 14, 386, 1974.

51. **Sprent, J. and Basten, A.,** Circulating T and B lymphocytes of the mouse II. Lifespan, *Cell. Immunol.,* 7, 40, 1973.

Chapter 12

THE USE OF THE MITOGEN ASSAY IN RESEARCH ON AGING AND IMMUNE FUNCTION

William H. Adler

TABLE OF CONTENTS

INTRODUCTION

In 1959, Hungerford et al. observed that lymphocytes from the peripheral blood of humans, when exposed to a plant lectin, phytohemagglutinin (PHA), would, after a period of time, enter division cycles and continue dividing in culture for an extended period.[1] Based on that observation, many different culture techniques were developed and adapted for the culture of both human lymphocytes and lymphocytes from various species of animals. There were two major points brought out by these studies. One was that the degree of induced stimulation by PHA showed a great deal of individual variation amongst humans and animals;[2,3] second, that individuals suffering from various types of immune deficiency disease in which thymic development was negligible had lymphocytes which would not respond to PHA stimulation.[4] This observation, along with experimental work in animals,[5] determined that the T lymphocyte which depended upon thymic environmental factors in order to differentiate into an immunocompetent cell was the cell which responded to PHA stimulation. Because of that observation, the mitogenic response to PHA in vitro became a laboratory assay as a functional test for the T lymphocyte. The assay has been used in aging research for the same reason. The findings are that lymphocytes from humans, mice, and rats over an age span, lose their ability to enter into mitotic cycles when exposed to PHA.[6,7,8] (See Chapter 10.) This is one of the major findings which form the basis for the opinion that T-lymphocyte function decreases with the increasing age of the host.

It is the purpose of this presentation to explore the various culture techniques used for setting up the mitogen assay. It will also be important to consider some of the parameters of culture techniques. The points to be considered are (1) the factors which can lead to a normal mitogen response, (2) what constitutes a normal mitogen response, (3) what factors lead to a decrease in the mitogen response, and (4) the significance of the level of mitogen responsiveness when compared with other immune assays.

II. MATERIALS AND METHODS UTILIZED FOR THE PERFORMANCE OF THE MITOGEN RESPONSE IN VITRO

A. Culture Techniques

General considerations of culture techniques include the choice of a suitable culture medium for maintaining the viability of cells in culture while permitting proliferation in response to a mitogenic stimulant. Culture media in general consist of a salt solution and energy source combined with a serum preparation, and there are many choices for each component. Choices are influenced by the consideration of the source and type of cells used for culture. In general, the salt solution with an energy source and amino acids used for most in vitro culture systems consists of RPMI-1640 (GIBCO®). The serum preparation used in studies from this laboratory consists of fetal calf serum used at a 10% concentration for mitogen studies involving human cells and pooled human AB serum heated at 56° for 30 min and used in a 5% concentration for studies dealing with both mouse and rat lymphocytes. The choice of a serum preparation for cells from different species is crucial for maintaining both cellular survival and a high level of proliferative response. Different serum preparations will affect the ongoing level of background division in a cell population and also the degree to which that cell population can be pushed by a mitogenic stimulus. An ideal medium will allow virtually no ongoing background synthesis of DNA, yet will maintain 100% viability of cells in culture and permit all cells to go through unlimited division cycles once stimulated with a mitogen. There are synthetic media which have been described in other assay systems, but as yet have not been used for these studies, and may not be useful for all mitogens.[9] Most media preparations will also contain a source of antibiotic activity, such as penicillin and streptomycin, which have a negligible effect on mammalian cells, and gentamycin which, at the concentration utilized, has negligible effects also. It should be possible with careful culture techniques to avoid all use of antibiotics. Another consideration is the buffer system used to deal with the metabolic by-products of sustained cell proliferation in vitro. There are many choices in this regard, perhaps the most popular being a bicarbonate buffer system with a CO_2-air atmosphere. This buffer system can effectively be used in cultures with a high metabolic activity. Use of a bicarbonate buffer requires an incubator with an humidified CO_2 atmosphere. Cultures in a CO_2-humidified atmosphere cannot be enclosed in sealed containers, such as flasks or sealed culture plates. Other buffer systems such as HEPES and MOPS do not require an incubator with a CO_2 atmosphere since all cultures can be maintained in sealed containers. The results obtained with any of these buffer systems are approximately the same, although there may be differences in the density of cells able to be cultured.

B. Mitogenic Preparations

There are many preparations of mitogenic compounds available to the investigator. Perhaps the most-utilized compounds are phytohemagglutinin (PHA), concanavalin A (Con A) (both of which stimulate the T-lymphocyte population), and endotoxin lipopolysaccharide (LPS), which stimulates the splenic B lymphocyte population in mice. Other compounds such as pokeweed mitogen (PWM), can stimulate a combination of both T and B cells. These preparations are used at concentrations which are somewhat independent of the density of cells in the culture. In a standard mitogen response, the individual mitogen is added to the cells at the beginning of culture. Depending upon the mitogen utilized, the detection techniques for the degree of proliferative response will have variable application, which will be discussed below. The source of the mitogens is unimportant in most cases because most mitogens are fairly well characterized by each commercial source. The mitogen which does require a more careful choice is endotoxin lipopolysaccharide. In most cases a preparation which is non-antigenic and containing a high level of lipid A will be most appropriate. All mitogen preparations are relatively stable in storage. They can be kept in standard dilutions prior to the initiation of cultures and used as an addition to the culture in variable amounts depending upon the volume of culture media.

C. Techniques for the Detection of Cellular Proliferation

The detection of a proliferative response can rely on morphologic and objective assays such as measuring the incorporation of radioisotope-labeled precursors into DNA. The morphologic assays depend on the observation that dividing lymphocytes activated by mitogens have a different morphology than resting lymphocytes. These "blast" cells, which arise in response to mitogenic stimuli, can be identified under a microscope quite readily. The difficulty with utilization of a morphologic technique is that many of the mitogens cause clumping of cells and this makes it very difficult to count individual activated blast cells. A more objective technique utilizes radioisotope-labeled thymidine such as tritiated thymidine (3H-TdR). This technique measures the amount of radioactivity incorporated into newly synthesized DNA. The choice of isotope is up to the investigator and depends on several considerations. Most laboratories use tritiated thymidine for DNA labeling, and the considerations are the length of pulse and the specific activity of the tritiated thymidine. There should be enough label present in the cultures so that it is not a limiting factor in determining the proliferative response. Also, a very high specific-activity label can damage the cells which incorporate it and can cause a cessation of cell proliferation. Convenient labeling times vary from 4 to 24 hr, and by using low activity thymidine, one is able to obtain a good degree of incorporation in stimulated cultures which is much above background levels. The length of labeling time can be determined by the individual investigator, but usually very long pulse times will not offer a corresponding increase in level of incorporation. A reason for this could be the release of cold thymidine into the medium by cells which are dying throughout the culture period, or the release of enzymes which will destroy thymidine prior to its incorporation into new DNA. A cell harvester is used to collect the cells from the cultures, precipitate the DNA with trichloroacetic acid (TCA), and dehydrate the DNA with absolute methanol. The DNA on fiberglass filters is solubilized with NCS in the counting vials prior to the addition of scintillation fluid. After dark adaptation, the level of radioactivity is assessed with the use of a scintillation counter.

D. Preparation of Cells for Culture

Cellular preparations obtained from human peripheral blood utilize Ficoll®-Hypaque® at a density of 1.080 as a separating agent to acquire a lymphocyte population which is relatively free from red cells and granulocytes.[10] This is accomplished through standard procedures, and there is no difference in the separation of cells from older or younger individuals. The cells obtained from animal species may or may not require Ficoll®-Hypaque® separation. For separation of murine white cells from red cells it is necessary to use a Ficoll®-Hypaque® preparation at a density of 1.100. To obtain single cell suspensions from solid lymphoid organs, a variety of techniques have been developed. Most techniques utilize the mincing of tissue with subsequent pushing through a #60 stainless-steel mesh in tissue culture medium. Filtration through gauze will remove clumps of cells and debris. Experiments in our laboratory have shown no increase in susceptibility to damage of cells from old animals using these techniques. Therefore, there does not appear to be any selection of cells or cell types utilizing stainless-steel meshing and subsequent suspension of cells in tissue culture medium prior to culture. There is no advantage to keeping cells cold prior to initiation of cultures during the time they are being separated, counted, and the viability determined. The most expeditious handling of cells from the time of removal from the animal until the initiation of in vitro culture is perhaps the primary consideration in any tissue culture technique. This is especially true when using thymocytes as the source of cells since prolonged storage causes lysis of thymocytes. The number of cells available for culture is markedly affected by delays between the time the cell suspension is obtained and the time of initiation of in vitro culture. Another procedure which should be used minimally is centrifugation of cells. From the time the single cell suspension is obtained until the cells are placed in culture, the use of repeated centrifugation will cause increased cell clumping and death. This is especially true with cells from spleens of older mice. The cells from old mice are prone to clumping, and a great deal of cell loss is caused by repeated contrifugation of these preparations. This finding does not apply to peripheral blood lymphocytes from older humans.

E. Factors Which Can Influence the Degree of Mitogen Responsiveness of Lymphoid Cells in Culture

There are a variety of factors which can influence the degree of responsiveness of a particular culture to a mitogenic stimulus. The appreciation of the degree of mitogen responsiveness of a lymphocyte population is a complicated procedure. Each factor is interrelated, and the appreciation of the degree of mitogen responsiveness is the sum total of their negative and positive effects. In any system used by an investigator to

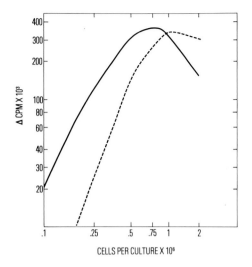

FIGURE 1. Spleen cells from 2-month-old
(——) and 24-month-old C57BL/6 mice (· · · ·)
were cultured at variable densities. The cultures
were stimulated with PHA and pulsed with 1 μCi
3H-TdR 16 hr prior to harvest at the end of a 3-
day culture period. The cells were grown in 0.2
mℓ volumes in RPMI-1640 with 5% human
serum. The results are expressed as the mean
CPMs in triplicate-stimulated cultures less the
mean CPMs in background cultures at each six
density groups tested.

determine mitogen responsiveness it is possible, knowingly or unknowingly, to manipulate the factors to obtain a result which is desired. With that realization it becomes
more important to understand these factors.

The first variable to be considered is the cell density used in the cultures. At the
extremes of cell density, it is possible to have too few cells to be detected with any
technique to determine responsiveness, or so many cells in culture that the metabolic
load will exceed the buffer capacity, and no response would be detected. Between these
two extremes, the investigator has a choice of densities. His choice will depend upon
the degree of discrimination that he wishes to obtain with a culture technique, the
availability of cells, and the degree of responsiveness that the cells can demonstrate.
The choice is complicated by the realization that cell populations from the young animals demonstrate a linear degree of responsiveness as the density is increased. However, cells from older animals may not demonstrate linearity in the degree of responsiveness related to the density of the cells in culture.[10,11] It is also possible, using high
numbers of cells in culture, to show that less responsive cells from an older animal
can perform "better" than the cells from younger animals. This discrepency, as shown
in Figure 1, is due to the buildup of metabolites in the cultures with subsequent low-
ering of the level of isotope incorporation into DNA. The cells from young mice
respond early with a greater proliferation, and the medium is exhausted sooner. The
cells from older animals will incorporate more isotope because the medium is able to
handle the early lower level of response. Another important effect of changing cell
densities is shown in Figure 2. In these experiments, cells were cultured at different
densities over a period of 4 days. Cells stimulated with Con A cultured at a low density
did not sustain proliferation over the entire period, whereas cells cultured at a higher

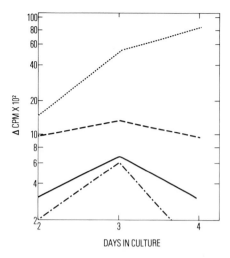

FIGURE 2.   Thymus cells from C57BL/6 mice were cultured for 2, 3, or 4 days at different densities. The cultures were pulsed with 1 μCi tritiated thymidine 16 hr prior to harvest. The cells were cultured in 0.2 mℓ volumes in RPMI-1640 with 5% human serum at the following densities: 10^5 cells per culture ($-\cdot-$); 2.5×10^5 cells per culture (——); 5×10^5 cells per culture (———); and 7.5×10^5 per culture (-·-··-), The results were expressed as the mean CPM of five replicate-stimulated cultures less the mean CPM of five replicate-background unstimulated cultures for each group at each day of the experiment.

density with the mitogen exhibited continued proliferation over the entire culture period. Therefore, continued cellular proliferation is dependent upon a certain minimum number of cells in the culture vessel. At lower densities, a low response is obtained because the cells do not continue to proliferate after the initial burst. On the other hand, at higher densities proliferation continues and a second problem is encountered. The second factor which must be considered is the choice of the period of culture time necessary to record a maximum response.

The period of time that cell cultures are maintained can influence the levels of response obtained. As shown in Figure 3, a cell population which exhibits a poor response may take a longer time in culture to reach its peak level, whereas a cell population which exhibits a good response will peak at an earlier time period. The reason for this relates back to the release of metabolites and exhaustion of culture medium. A slower and lower response can build up to a peak simply because media exhaustion is not a factor until later in the culture period. A large degree of proliferation which occurs rapidly can exhaust culture medium and build up metabolites, so there is a rapid falloff in isotope incorporation. Therefore, late in culture an actual lower response will have a level of isotope incorporation which is greater than that which is found in a culture with a higher response. The consideration of the density of cells to be cultured and the time they are to be cultured is crucial for the correct interpretation of results. When dealing with a T mitogen response of cells from older animals and humans under standard conditions, one can expect a lower level of response than seen with cells from the young. However, with inappropriate culture conditions, this lower response may not be appreciated.

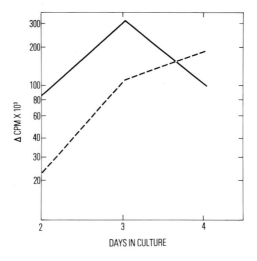

FIGURE 3. In these experiments spleen cells from 2-month-old C57BL/6 mice were divided into two groups. One group was X-irradiated with 80 R (–––) the other was not (——). Each group was then used to establish cultures using 5×10^5 viable cells per 0.2 ml media. The cultures were stimulated with Con A and groups were pulsed with 1 μCi 3H-TdR at variable periods of time 16 hr prior to harvest. Cell culture groups were harvested at the end of 2, 3, and 4 days of cultures. Results are expressed as mean CPMs of four replicate-stimulated cultures less the mean CPMs of background nonstimulated cultures.

There is another consideration in manipulation of cell densities in culture and the subsequent degree of mitogen responsiveness. In Figure 4 it can be seen that the degree of incorporation of the isotope in the DNA, although linear over many densities, usually exhibits a slope of four to five. As cell density is increased in culture, one obtains a disproportionately higher subsequent incorporation of isotope. What this suggests is that there is greater ability to proliferate as the number of cells in culture is increased. This may represent an interaction of cells or cellular growth factors which are released by the greater number of cells in culture and which encourage continued proliferative ability. The result of this density effect is that lower responses appear to be disproportionately lower than they actually may be. Even though half the number of cells are in culture, one may not obtain half the degree of proliferative incorporation of tritiated thymidine. This would cast serious doubt on the use of the mitogen assay as a quantitative tool to determine the number of cells in a particular organ or in peripheral blood which can respond to a mitogenic stimulus. Interestingly enough, the responsiveness to endotoxin LPS does appear to approach the slope of one (Figure 4). Why this may be is not apparent. Experiments have been performed to evaluate this disproportionate responsiveness. The data in Table 1 show that a constant density of X-irradiated spleen cells added to cultures of variable numbers of spleen cells will result in a better response of low densities of spleen cells than can be obtained in the absence of the X-irradiated population. The slope of responsiveness approximates one, and low densities of responding cells are able to respond two to three times better in the presence of an X-irradiated feeder population. The function of the X-irradiated population is not known, but the ability of the population to promote cellular proliferation varies in terms of the age of the cell donor for the X-irradiated population (Table 1). It is only

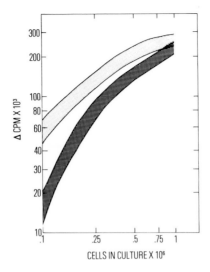

FIGURE 4. In these experiments C57BL/6 mouse spleen cells were cultured in 0.2 mℓ of media (RPMI-1640; 5% human serum) at different densities for 3 days. Tritiated thymidine (1 μCi) was added to the cultures for the first 16 hr. One set of cultures was stimulated with LPS ⬚⬚⬚ and another set with PHA ▩▩▩ . There were five cultures performed at each density, and the results are shown as the range of values of CPM s for each group. The results are shown as the CPM s in the stimulated cultures less the CPM s in background nonstimulated cultures.

when the feeder population is obtained from younger animals that augmentation can be seen. This would suggest that the slope of five seen in the absence of a feeder layer is due to an enhancing effect of increased cell density of a population of cells which in themselves do not respond to the mitogen, but which are able to promote the response of the appropriate cells. It may be possible, using feeder layer populations from young animals which are X-irradiated, to obtain some degree of quantitative measurement of numbers of cells responding in both young and old animals. It is also possible that the proliferative defect of cells from older animals is due to a lack or loss of function of these enhancing cells.

Another important consideration in the mitogen response is the ability of daughter cells of the primary responding cells to continue the proliferative response in vitro. Cells which are initially in contact with mitogen give a burst of proliferative activity with subsequent generation of daughter cells. The daughter cells continue to divide since the mitogen is still present. Pulsing of the cultures at day 3 or 4 after initiation is actually measuring the uptake of isotope by the daughters of the originally responding cells, and the number of these cells will then determine the level of a mitogen response. Experiments designed to test the adequacy of daughter cells to proliferate in response to a mitogen have shown a marked deficiency of cells from the older mouse spleen. In these experiments spleen cells from different-aged mice were placed in culture with mitogens. After 4 days the cell cultures were washed and new mitogens added, and after a further 3 days the cultures were pulsed with tritiated thymidine. As

Table 1

Cells in culture[a]		Number added X-irradiated cells	+ 1 × 10⁶ X-Irradiated spleen cells from old mice[b]	+ 1 × 10⁶ X-Irradiated spleen cells from young mice
1 × 10⁵ Spleen	BKG	580[c]	333	908
cells from old mice[d]	+ PHA	2,516	2,211	5,822
2.5 × 10⁵ Spleen	BKG	980	1,761	2,429
cells from old mice	+ PHA	6,337	6,801	14,520
5 × 10⁵ Spleen	BKG	4,868	6,974	5,329
cells from old mice	+ PHA	18,390	18,520	32,382
7.5 × 10⁵ Spleen	BKG	7,454	10,269	7,456
cells from old mice	+ PHA	30,576	34,543	51,055
1 × 10⁶ X-Irradiated	BKG	164		
cells from old mice	+ PHA	763		
1 × 10⁶ X-Irradiated	BKG	323		
cells from young mice	+ PHA	1,560		

[a] All cultures were in 0.2 mℓ medium and for a period of 3 days 3H-TdR was added for the final 16 hr of culture.

[b] X-irradiated cells received a total of 800 R.

[c] Results are expressed as the mean counts per minute of triplicate cultures in each group of PHA stimulated or background nonstimulated cultures.

[d] Old C57BL/6 mice were 20 months of age at the time of the experiment. Young C57BL/6 mice were 6 months of age.

shown in Figure 5, the degree of proliferation in the daughter cell cultures that were initiated from the spleens of young animals is equal to or slightly better than a primary response from those same spleens. However, the cells obtained from 24-month-old mice demonstrate both a low initial response and absolutely no response to a secondary stimulus. These findings can be interpreted as showing a marked deficiency of daughter cells from older animals to continue proliferation in the culture system. The reasons for this are unknown, but in most immune function assays that require proliferation, one can predict that cells from older animals will demonstrate an inadequate level of performance.

III. DISCUSSION AND FURTHER CONSIDERATIONS OF THE MITOGEN ASSAY

The considerations outlined in this paper relate directly to the parameters necessary to perform the mitogen assay and obtain results which are able to be interpreted. There are further considerations which are not of primary importance, but which are necessary in determining the interpretation of results. A primary factor in any mitogen assay is the determination of cell types in the culture. In aging research, a mitogen response that is less than normal (young) can be an abnormal functioning of a population of cells which should respond in the assay system. However, with aging, cell populations within lymphoid organs may change, and the types of cells in populations of human peripheral blood lymphocytes or mouse splenic lymphocytes may change, and may be types of cells which do not ordinarily respond to a mitogen. Therefore, there could be two entirely different interpretations of a low response: 1. the cells are there which should respond but don't; 2. the responding population is absent. The effects of pop-

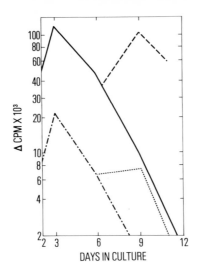

FIGURE 5.   In these experiments 5 ×
10⁵ mouse splenic lymphocytes were
cultured in 0.2 ml media. Spleen cells
were obtained from 2-month-old
C57BL/6 mice (————) and from
24-month-old mice (·—·—·—). The
initial cultures were stimulated with
PHA (———, · —) and on day 5, after
washing, the cultures were stimulated
with 5 × 10⁵ mitomycin-treated DBA/
2 spleen cells (····, — — —). After a pre-
ceeding 16-hour-pulse with 1 μCi tritiated thymidine, sets of cultures were
harvested at days 2, 3, 4, 6, 8, 9, 11,
12, and levels of radioactivity in DNA
isolates were determined. Results are
expressed as mean CPMs in five replicate-stimulated cultures less the
mean CPMs in five background non-
stimulated cultures. Cultures which
did not receive an initial PHA stimulation would not respond to the allogeneic spleen cells added on day 5.

ulation shifts can be shown in experiments utilizing animals which have been immunized or are carrying a tumor. Spleen cells from immunized or tumor-bearing mice
respond poorly in vitro to a mitogenic stimuli,[12] but there are marked changes in these
populations.[13] This is an important consideration in aging research, since many of the
older animals will have developed tumors. It also precludes the use of sick, old mice
for determining cellular responses in vitro. This consideration also applies to a study
of a human population, because a tumor or infection can change the types of cells
present in peripheral blood.

It is also possible that there are age-related changes in the presence of a suppressor
cell population or a release of suppressor factors which can cause a decrease in the
mitogen response in vitro. There is evidence that interferon, an inhibitor of proliferation, is released in larger quantities by spleen cells from older mice.[14] (See Chapter
13.) Growth regulating factors can be present in varible amounts which may be age
related. Regulation of proliferation in cultures can also be mediated by cell populations, such as suppressor cells, which may also have an age-related representation.

Incorporation of tritiated thymidine depends upon the amount of cold thymidine present in a culture. Cold thymidine will compete for incorporation into DNA synthesized by cells, and even though cold thymidine is not added by the investigator, it may be present. Cellular degradation in cultures releases cold thymidine. Competition between the isotope and cold thymidine leads to lower isotope incorporation in DNA even though cells may proliferate normally. It is also possible that a sufficiently large concentration of cold thymidine can slow or stop cellular proliferation. Elimination of cold thymidine in cultures can be accomplished by washing the cell cultures daily throughout the culture period, especially prior to the addition of isotopes. The washing will also remove any of the growth or inhibitory factors which may be present.

A final consideration is the role that the mitogen assay plays in diagnosing the level of immune function in mice or humans. Previous work comparing the mitogen response of mouse spleen cells with other assays of immune activity of the same population has shown no correlation.[15] The reasons for a noncorrelation may be that different assays rely either on a population of cells which are not mitogen responders, or a population of cells which are present in a low but sufficient concentration and have normal function. It is also possible that the necessity for cellular proliferation is different in each type of assay. However, since the T-cell mitogen response does not correlate with other T-cell assays, such as helper function or cytotoxicity, it is questionable that the mitogen assay is useful in predicting immune function of the whole animal or human. This may be especially true in evaluating human immune function when lymphoid organs are not routinely examined using the mitogen analysis. Peripheral blood lymphocyte mitogen responses may not accurately reflect the immune function potential of the individual. In the mouse, the comparison of spleen cell reactivity to a mitogen, and lymph node reactivity to the same mitogen using cells from the same mouse, shows a disturbing noncorrelation.[7] It is possible to find a low mitogen response using spleen cells, and a lymph node response to the same mitogen which is at the same level as found using cells from young mice. This may help to explain why a cellular mitogen response does not correlate with a level of other types of immune function assays.

The proliferative response of lymphocytic cells in vitro to a mitogenic stimulus can be a useful assay for the detection of a specific subtype of cell in mixtures of mononuclear cells. It is also a useful measure of proliferative ability and is easily accomplished in most laboratories. It is one of the few assays in humans which can easily demonstrate a T-cell deficit. With its inherent drawbacks, however, it may only be useful as a preliminary assay for T-cell function, and subsequent analysis of T-cell activity is necessary for an overall view of immune function. It is also useful as a probe for detecting membrane changes with age in which case proliferative function is not necessarily the end point. Experiments utilizing lectin probes for the presence of receptors on membrane or for the metabolic activity and synthesis of membrane receptors, may be quite useful for showing changes in cells during aging. (See Chapter 14.) It is also possible that the mitogen assay is giving us results which we do not fully understand at present. The inability to correlate mitogen results and other T cell functions does not necessarily mean that the results of a mitogen assay are false, inaccurate, or misleading. A better understanding of the results of mitogen assays and of cellular events within the culture system will lead to a greater usefulness of the mitogen assay in aging research.

REFERENCES

1. **Hungerford, D. A., Donnelly, A. J., Nowell, P. C., and Beck, S.,** The chromosome constitution of a human phenotype intersex, *Am. J. Hum. Genet.,* 11, 215, 1959.
2. **McIntyre, O. R. and Cole, A. F.,** Variation in the response of normal lymphocytes to PHA, *Int. Arch. Allergy Appl. Immunol.,* 35, 105, 1969.
3. **Adler, W. H., Takiguchi, T., Marsh, B., and Smith R. T.,** Cellular recognition by mouse lymphocytes in vitro I. Definition of a new technique and results of stimulation phytohemagglutinin and specific antigens, *J. Exp. Med.,* 131, 1048, 1970.
4. **Cleveland, W. W., Fogel, B. J., Brown, W. T., and Kay, H. E. M.,** Foetal thymic transplant in a case of DiGeorge's syndrome, *Lancet,* ii, 1211, 1968.
5. **Takiguchi, T., Adler, W. H., and Smith, R. T.,** Cellular recognition in vitro by mouse lymphocytes: effects of neonatal thymectomy and thymus graft restoration on alloantigen and PHA stimulation of whole and gradient-separated subpopulations spleen cells, *J. Exp. Med.,* 133, 63, 1971.
6. **Hori, Y., Perkins, E. H., and Halsall, M. K.,** Decline in phytohemagglutinin responsiveness of spleen cells from aging mice, *Proc. Soc. Exp. Biol. Med.,* 144, 48, 1973.
7. **Adler, W. H., Jones, K. H., and Nariuchi, H.,** Ageing and Immune Function, in *Recent Advances in Clinical Immunology,* Thompson, R. A. Ed., Churchill Livingstone, Edinburgh, 1977, 77.
8. **Pisciotta, A. V., Westring, D. W., DePrey, C, and Walsh, B.,** Mitogenic effect of phytogemagglutinin at different ages, *Nature (London),* 215, 193, 1967.
9. **Iscove, N. N. and Melchers, F.,** Complete replacement of serum by albumin, transferrin, and soybean lipid in cultures of lipopolysaccharide - reactive B lymphycoytes, *J. Exp. Med.,* 147, 923, 1978.
10. **Boyum, A.,** Isolation of mononuclear cells and granulocytes from human blood, *Scand. J. Clin. Lab. Invest.,* 21 (Suppl. 97), 51, 1968.
11. **Adler, W. H. and Chrest, F. J.,** The Mitogen Response Assay as a Measure of The Immune Deficiency of Aging Mice, in *Developmental Immunobiology,* Siskind, G. W., Litwin, S. D., and Weksler, M. E., Eds., Grune & Stratton, New York, 1979, 233.
12. **Adler, W. H., Takiguchi, T., and Smith, R. T.,** Phytohemagglutinin unresponsiveness in mouse spleen cells induced by methylcholanthrene sarcomas, *Cancer Res.,* 31, 864, 1971.
13. **Adler, W. H., Peavy, D., and Smith, R. T.,** The effect of PHA, PPD, allogeneic cells and sheep erythrocytes on albumin gradient-fractionated mouse spleen cell populations, *Cell. Immunol.,* 1, 78, 1970.
14. **Heine, J. W. and Adler, W. H.,** The quantitative production of interferon by mitogen stimulated mouse lymphocytes as a function of age and its effect on the lymphocytes proliferative response, *J. Immunol.,* 118, 1366, 1977.
15. **Nordin, A. A. and Adler, W. H.,** The Effect of Aging on In Vitro Cellular Interactions, in *Developmental Immunobiology,* Siskind, G. W., Litwin, S. D., and Weksler, M. E., Eds., Grune & Stratton, New York, 1979, 215.

Chapter 13

THE INFLUENCE OF INTERFERON PRODUCTION BY LYMPHOCYTES ON THE INTERPRETATION OF MITOGEN RESPONSE ASSAYS

Jochen W. Heine

TABLE OF CONTENTS

I. INTRODUCTION

To gain a better understanding of the well-documented decline in proliferative response of mouse T cells to mitogen stimulation with age of the cell donor, it has been necessary to develop more quantitative assays of lymphocyte kinetics in tissue culture.

It has been reported that the uptake of H^3-thymidine does not always indicate the degree of blast transformation. This is also a drawback, besides being a very involved technique of the autoradiographic method.

One, the virus plaque forming cell (V-PFC) assay described by Jimenez and Bloom[1] showed great potential due to its simplicity. With this assay only activated lymphoid cells are capable of replicating viruses, and thus a direct correlation exists between the number of mitogen-activated cells and the number of V-PFC. A limitation of this assay is its greater sensitivity to the influence of interferon than the radioisotope incorporation assays.

Since interferon, an antiviral agent, has been identified as both a product of immunocompetent cells and as a naturally occurring material which can inhibit or influence lymphocyte functions, particularly T-lymphocytes, the kinetics of cellular activation as assayed by both the radioisotope assay and, in particular, the V-PFC assay, have to be related to the kinetics of interferon production for each system to be studied. (Heine and Adler.[2]) This is of increasing importance when studying mitogenesis with the aging system, as the spleen cells from older mice elaborate a greater amount of interferon than do spleen cells from younger mice.[3]

II. MATERIAL — METHODS, APPLICATION, AND RESULTS

A. Chemicals

Succinyl-concanavalin A (Suc-Con A) was used for the stimulation procedure of mouse spleen cells, since the dose-response characteristics are more convenient; it is not toxic at excess concentrations, as Con A is, and has a broad response range.

Concanavalin A (Con A) was prepared from jack-bean meal as described by Agrawal and Goldstein,[5] or purchased from Pharmacia Fine Chemicals. Con A was succinylated as described by Gunther et al.[6] One hundred mg of Con A was dissolved in 25 mℓ of saturated sodium acetate at room temperature. Undissolved material was removed by low-speed centrifugation. Then the solution was transferred to a 50-mℓ flask containing 30 mg of succinic anhydride (Sigma) and stirred on ice for 1 hr. Next, it was dialyzed overnight against distilled water and lyophilized. The above was repeated by dissolving lyophilized material in 20-mℓ saturated sodium acetate, removing the precipitate by low-speed centrifugation, adding 30 mg of succinic anhydride, and stirring at room temperature for 1 ½ hr. It was dialyzed exhaustively against distilled water and lyophilized.

Phytohemagglutinin (PHA) was purchased from Difco or other sources. Both lectins were dissolved in PBS and diluted to workable concentrations upon establishing the dose-response curve and stored at −20°C.

Standard mouse interferon (G-002-904-511) and standard human leukocyte interferon (G-023-901-527) was acquired from the Research Resources Branch of National Institute of Allergy and Infectious Diseases (NIAID), NIH, Bethesda, Md. The interferon standards were reconstituted, diluted to desirable experimental titers in PBS containing 0.1% bovine serum albumin as a stabilizer, and stored in small aliquots at −70°C in capped propylene tubes (Falcon, 12 × 75 mm).

The isotopes, H^3-thymidine (^{3}H-methyl, 1.9 Ci/mmol) and H^3-uridine (5-^{3}H, 21 Ci/mmol) were purchased from Schwarzmann, Orangeburg, New York.

B. Virus

The Indiana serotype of vesicular stomatitis virus (VSV) (American Type Culture Collection) used in the assay was propagated, quantitated, and stored, as described by Heine and Galasso,[7] and Jimenez and Bloom.[1] Stock virus was produced in confluent monolayers of chicken embryo fibroblast (CE) cells which were infected at low multiplicity of infection (one plaque-forming unit, PFU, per cell) to yield preparations with negligible amount of interfering-B particles.

Mouse fibroblast L-929 cells should not be used, as they are contaminated with "C" particles, and thus the virus yield is low and of poorer quality, containing a high percentage of defective particles which can interfere with the assay. The growth medium was harvested after 20 to 24 hr, sonicated for 3 min with a Raytheon sonic oscillator operating at 9 kc or ½ min operating at 10 kc. The samples were dispensed and stored at $-70°C$ until they were used. The virus was stable at this temperature and the average yield was about or better than 10^9 PFU per mℓ. A virus yield below 1×10^8 PFU per mℓ is of low quality and should not be employed.

Chick embryo fibroblast cells were purchased from biological companies at 1×10^6 cells per mℓ in requested media and were plated at 2.5×10^5 cells per mℓ in 0.5% lactalbumin hydrolysate medium (LA) supplemented with 5% fetal calf serum in suitable tissue-culture flasks or tissue-culture dishes. The monolayers were confluent, a requirement for good virus yield and quality, upon incubation for 24 hr at 37°C and humidified 5% CO_2.

C. Preparation of Anti-Virus Antisera

For the production of antisera, virus should be propagated in cells other than those employed in the biological assays to eliminate nonspecific cross reaction. Thus partially purified VSV, propagated in CE cells was employed for the production of antiserum in rabbits. To low-speed centrifuged growth medium from 20-hr infected CE cells, polyethylene glycol (PEG) 6000 was added to yield a 6% suspension and NaCl to a final concentration of 0.5 M to precipitate the virus as described by McShary and Benzinger.[8] The suspension was stored overnight at 4°C and centrifuged at 1000 × g for 10 min. The pellet was gently resuspended (to prevent osmotic shock) in 1/100 of its original volume in LA and sonicated for 1½ min at 9 kc in the Raytheon sonicator to de-aggregate the virus. The virus preparation was washed twice with LA by centrifugation at 66,000 × g for 90 min in a type 30 rotor in a Beckman® L2-65 centrifuge. The pellets were redispensed by sonication. Virus was suspended in LA and stored in small aliquots, about 1 mℓ containing 5×10^{10} PFU mℓ at $-70°C$.

Rabbits were given intramuscular injections into the flask as described by Heine and Schnaitman[9] at weekly intervals for 3 weeks of 0.5 mℓ of Freund's adjuvant containing 10^{10} PFU of VSV. After a rest period of 2 months, each rabbit received two additional intravenous injections 1 week apart, each consisting of 2×10^{10} PFU in 0.5 mℓ LA. The rabbits were bled 7 days after the last injection. The antiserum was heat-inactivated at 56°C for 30 min prior to experimental use and for determination of the neutralization titer of VSV. The antiserum was diluted serially in medium with antiserum and incubated with a known concentration of VSV (100 PFU) for 1 hr at room temperature, and then the virus was plated on L-cell monolayers as described in Section E for determination of reduction in plaque forming units. The neutralization titer was the antiserum dilution at 50% reduction of PFU.

D. Preparation of Cell Cultures

Spleens from mice of ages ranging from 2 to 28 months (C57B1/6, CBA) were minced on fine stainless steel wire screens, washed twice in RPMI-1640 (Gibco®) by centrifugation at 1000 × g for 10 min at 12°C. For partial purification, one volume of cell pellet was suspended by vortexing in ten volumes of sterile glass distilled water and upon complete suspension diluted with an equal volume of 2 × media. The cells were then centrifuged as above and suspended in a small volume of complete RPMI-1640 which was spupplemented with 5% heat-inactivated fetal calf serum, 50 units/ mℓ of penicillin and 50 μg/mℓ of streptomycin for passage over a lucopak column. The lucopak column was prepared by extensively washing the lucopak in saline, followed by overnight soaking and repeated washing until the saline rinse was clear. The lucopak was then washed with glass distilled water. Columns were prepared by packing 12-mℓ plastic syringes with the lucopad to the 6 mℓ mark with the aid of the plunger. The syringes were then placed in their plastic holder without the plunger and autoclaved for 15 min in a pressure cooker and stored at 4°C. For use, the column was enclosed in a water jacket fabricated from a 50 mℓ plastic syringe, fitted to allow the circulation of water and was equilibrated with 40 to 50 mℓ of complete RPMI-1640 at 37°C. The spleen cells were applied in 1.5 to 2 mℓ and washed through with 30 to 40 mℓ of complete media by gravity flow. The eluent containing the cells was centrifuged, and the cells suspended in a small volume for counting and diluted for plating in tissue culture plates at the appropriate cell density.

Human lymphocyte cultures were prepared by mixing 50/50 (v/v) heparinized blood samples from donors varying in age from 19 to 90 years with 4% dextran 500 (Pharmacia) in 0.15 M NaCl and incubated for 45 min at 37°C. After the red blood cells had settled the top layer to the interface was removed and diluted and washed 3 times with RPMI-1640 by centrifugation at 1000 × g for 10 min at 12°C. The cells were then suspended in RPMI-1640 containing 10% fetal calf serum, 50 units/mℓ of penicillin, and 50 μg/mℓ of streptomycin.

E. Virus Plaque Assays

For the purpose of quantitating virus plaque-forming cells (V-PFC), 3 × 10⁶ mouse spleen cells, prepared as above, were grown in Linbro plates (24 wells per plate — 1.7 cm diam.) containing 0.5 mℓ of complete RPMI-1640 and Suc-Con A where applicable and incubated for the desired length of time at 37°C in humidified 5% CO₂. Suc-Con A was added in 50 μℓ containing the concentration in excess of optimum stimulatory activity as determined from the dose-response curve for the above system. The cells were washed twice with RPMI-1640 by centrifugation at 1000 × g for 10 min in 15 mℓ conical, capped plastic centrifuge tubes (Falcon) and suspended in 0.1 mℓ medium containing 10 to 30 PFU per cell of VSV and incubated for 2 hr with periodic agitation at above condition. The small volume of suspension facilitated ideal conditions for cell virus contact to yield unified infection of cells.

The pH of the medium should be close to 7.2 to facilitate the uptake of the virus by activated cells. A pH below 6.8 or above 7.6 retards the infection and thus interferes with the accuracy of the assay. Subsequently, the cells were washed three times with RPMI-1640 and reincubated at 0°C for 1 hr in 0.2 mℓ of diluted heat-inactivated anti-VSV serum, diluted in RPMI-1640 to a dilution capable of neutralizing the virus inoculation dose. The cells were then washed three times as above and plated at several dilutions on L-cell monolayers for plaque determination as described by Jimenez and Bloom.[1]

L-929 mouse fibroblast cells (need to be in good condition to yield complete monolayers, otherwise it becomes difficult to differentiate holes from plaques) were seeded at 2 × 10⁶ cell in 5 mℓ of complete MEM (modified) with Earle's salt containing non-essential amino acids, antibiotics (penicillin at 50 units/mℓ and streptomycin at 50 μg/ mℓ), 0.85 g/ℓ of sodium bicarbonate, 0.1% glutamine, and 10% heat-inactivated FCS in 60 mm plastic tissue-culture dishes 24 hr prior to use and were incubated at 37°C in humidified 5% CO_2. In the absence of CO_2, the media should be buffered with 1% of THM solution. The ingredients of THM are as follows: 5 mMTes(N-tris(hydroxymethyl) -methyl-2-aminoethane sulfonic acid), 7.5 mM HEPES (N-2-hydroxyethylpiperazine- N′-2-ethane sulfonic acid), 5 mM MOPS(morpholinopropane sulfonic acid) (Sigma).

Prior to plating the infected lymphocytes, the L-cell monolayers were drained, then dilutions of 0.2 ml virus-infected lymphocyte suspension were added and immediately mixed in the tissue culture dish with 1 ml of 1% nutrient agar kept at 46° (2% melted agar in water at 46°C mixed with equal volumes of 2 × complete MEM containing FCS, penicillin, and streptomycin at 46°C by one-time aspiration and rotation of the dish. Upon solidification (about 10 min) 1.5 ml of 1% nutrient agar was added as a nutrient layer. The agar should not be warmer than 46°C, as it will kill the cells. When the agar was solidified, the dishes were inverted and incubated at 37°C in humidified 5% CO_2 for two days.

If the CO_2 in the incubator had been too high, the nutrient agar would have become too acid (yellow), and this condition would have prevented plaque formation. The cells were then vitally stained with 1.5 ml of 1:10,000 neutral red in Hank's solution (Gibco®). Clear plaques of lysis were counted after about 3 to 6 hr of incubation as above. The increase in plaques formed over control was taken as the number of mitogen-activated cells.

Virus titration was accomplished by adding 0.5 ml of virus dilutions to drained L-cell monolayers and incubating for 2 hr for adsorption to occur. The dishes were then overlayed with 5 ml of 1% nutrient agar and incubated as above for two days. Then the dishes were stained with neutral red as above, and the plaques counted after 3 to 6 hr of incubation. The plaques were multiplied by the dilution factor and expressed in plaque forming units (PFU) per ml.

F. Thymidine Uptake and Interferon Production

Cells were cultured in microplates (Falcon microtest II) at 37°C in humidified 5% CO_2 atmosphere. Each well of the microplates contained $0.5 × 10^6$ mouse spleen cells in 0.2 ml of complete RPMI-1640 with or without 10 μl Suc-Con A. In the case of human cells, each well contained $1 × 10^5$ cells with 10 μl of PHA in media. The concentration of the lectins to be employed should be determined by a dose-response study with the above conditions. The dose of PHA is critical, as it has a very narrow optimum dose range which may even vary with cell from different donors, while Suc-Con A has a very broad range.

Six hr before harvesting the cells, 1 μCi^3H-thymidine was added to each culture. The cells were harvested with a Biomedical Research Institute (Rockville, Md.) cell harvester (model M-24V) onto glass fiber filters, washed with saline, precipitated with trichloroacetic acid (TCA), and dried with methanol. The TCA-precipitable material on the filters was solubilized in scintillation-counting vials with 0.1 ml of NCS (Nuclear Chicago solubilizer) before the addition of 9 ml toluene base 2,5-diphenyloxazole (PPO)-1, 4-bis-(5-phenyloxazolyl)benzene (POPOP) counting fluid for assaying by liquid scintillation spectrophotometry.

In the experiments in which the cell cultures were to be analyzed for the presence of interferon, $1 × 10^6$ mouse spleen cells or $1 × 10^5$ human lymphocytes were cultured as above without the radioactive label. At the end of the cultureperiod, the growth media were removed, centrifuged at 1000 × g for 10 min, and the supernatant was stored for stability reasons in capped propylene tubes (Falcon 12 × 75 mm) at −70°C until assay, Heine et al.[10]

G. Interferon Assays

A variety of interferon assays are described in the literature and their pro and contra are reviewed by Buckler.[11] The method employed by the author is a modified version of the microtest method described by Tan.[12]

For mouse interferon assay L-929 cells are ideal; for human leukocyte or fibroblast interferon, use early to medium passage (6-35) of WI-38, Hep-2 (CCL-23, American Type Culture Collection) or GM 258, a cell line trisomic for chromosome 21 if greater sensitivity is desired, such as detection, or following serum interferon levels.

The interferon dilutions for titration were performed directly in the wells of the microplates (Falcon microtest II). Complete MEM (100$\mu\ell$), as described in Section E, either for CO_2 or its absence was added to each well of the microplates. Then 25, 50, or 100 $\mu\ell$ of the interferon solution, depending on the desired serial dilution, was added to the first well of each row. This was followed by transferring with micropipettes or microdilutors 25, 50, or 100 μ ℓ each time to achieve 1:5, 1:3 or 1:2 dilutions. The last transfer was discarded. The above procedure can be simplified by employing any automatic microdilutor. The tubing of the dilutor was sterilized by pumping 70% ethanol through it. Due to the precariousness of the interferon assays in general, each sample should be titrated at least in duplicate, each tray should have its own interferon standard titration in duplicate, as well as exhibit several wells for virus and cell controls. After completion, the trays can be placed directly under a desk-type UV light for 4 to 6 min to assure sterility if the dilutions are done in the laboratory at large. Following the above, 100 $\mu\ell$ of 0.5 to 1 × 10⁶ cells per mℓ were added aseptically to each well with a 5 mℓ Hamilton syringe fitted with an 18-gauge needle and an automatic advancer of 100 $\mu\ell$ increments. The syringe was sterilized with alcohol, and just prior to using, rinsed with media. The plates were then incubated at 37°C for at least 18 hr, but not more than 24 hr. The accurate cell density will have to be determined for each cell line. The proper density should yield a confluent monolayer within 24 hr. If the monolayer is too heavy, one will loose part of it during the later washing procedure and introduce errors in the results. On the other hand, a too-light monolayer will reduce the sensitivity to the antiviral state induction by interferon.

Following the incubation, the growth medium was removed by a quick inverted shake of the culture plate and replaced with 100 $\mu\ell$ of complete MEM (2% FCS) containing 25 μg/mℓ of actinomycin D (Act-D) (Merck, Sharp and Dohme, Westpoint, Pa.), and incubated for 1 hr. If the media turns to acid due to the addition of the Act-D, adjust it with sterile 7.5% sodium bicarbonate.

Subsequently, this medium was replaced by 200 $\mu\ell$ medium containing 4 μg/mℓ of Act-D, 5 μCi/mℓ of ³H-uridine and 250 to 500 PFU per cell of VSV. Finally, after 7½ to 8 hr of incubation, the cultures were washed with PBS and prepared for the determination of ³H-uridine incorporation by liquid-scintillation spectrophotometry.

The media was removed as above, placed into a radioactive disposal container, and washed with PBS (25°C) by gentle immersion. This step was followed by fixing with one part acetic acid in four parts of ethanol for 5 min at room temperature. This was followed by washing once with 95% ethanol, water, and incubation in 2% perchloric acid for 15 min. The plate was then washed seven times with tap water to remove all of the perchloric acid. On the next day, 100 $\mu\ell$ of 0.2 *M hot* NaOH (94° to 96°C) was added to each well. Then, 50 $\mu\ell$ were removed with disposable glass micropipettes and transferred to scintillation vial, solubilized with 0.3 mℓ of NCS, and 10 mℓ of POPOP counting fluid was added. The interferon titer was calculated by multiplying the dilution of interferon at 50% reduction of viral RNA synthesis by the number of standard interferon units required to reduce the viral RNA synthesis by 50%.

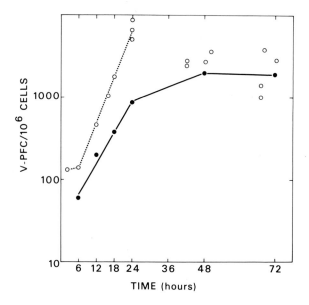

FIGURE 1. Kinetics of Suc-Con A stimulated mouse spleen cells as assayed by V-PFC. C57B1/6 (2 months males), O · · · O; CBA (2 months males), ●——● . (From *J. Immunol.*, 117, 1046, 1976. With permission.)

A faster adaptation of the above assay (32 hr vs. 72 hr) suitable for monitoring interferon elution profiles in column chromatography, quick analsis of clinical samples, or other instances where an indicative interferon titer is enough, is described by Volckaert-Vervliet and Billiau.[13]

The interferon was diluted and cells were added to the microtiter plates as described above. Upon incubation of 5½ to 6 hr, VSV at 1 to 2 PFU per cell was added in 50 µℓ to each well and incubated. When the cytopathic effect (CPE) was complete in the virus control in about 20 hr, the media were removed by inverted shaking and cells were washed as above with PBS. The plates were then dryed by placing a Kleenex® between the tray and its cover, and were again shaken in the inverted position. The cells were then vitally stained by adding a drop of crystal-violet (preparation of stain : 5 g of crystal-violet, 8.5 g of NaCl, 50 mℓ of formalin, 500 mℓ of ethanol, 1000 mℓ of distilled water, and with dissolving filter with Whatman® filter) with a pipette and allowed to stand at room temperature for 10 min. The stain was removed by extensive washing with tap water by successive submerging and inverted shaking, and finally dryed with Kleenex® as above. The plates were then read visually. The dilution at 50% CPE end point, adjusted to the 50% CPE endpoint of interferon standard for each tray, was taken as the interferon titer. For samples that prove pertinent, it is suggested to retiter them by the first method in order to obtain a more accurate titer.

H. Interpretation

The Suc-Con A mitogenic response of 2-month-old mice spleen cells employing the V-PFC assay is illustrated in Figure 1. During the first 6 to 24 hr the response is exponential with a doubling time of 3½ to 4 hr. The initial responding cells amount to 0.01% of the stimulated cell population. The observed shorter doubling time of lymphoid cells may be due to recruitment. After 24 hr of incubation, the response curve either drops off or becomes erratic and correlates with the kinetics of Suc-Con A-induced interferon production by T cells, Figure 2. The kinetics of interferon produc-

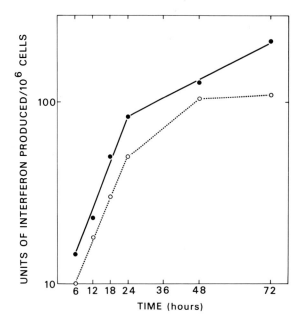

FIGURE 2. Kinetics of interferon production by mouse spleen cells stimulated by Suc-Con A. C57B1/6 (2 months males), O - - - O ; CBA (2 months males), ●——● . (From *J. Immunol.*, 117, 1047, 1976. With permission.)

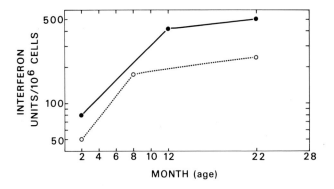

FIGURE 3.   Interferon production by mouse spleen cells incubated for 24 hours with Suc-Con A. C57B1/6, O - - - O; CBA, ●

tion during the first 24 hr of induction period is exponential. The quantitative elaboration of interferon production varies with the mouse strain used. The CBA mice are more efficient interferon producers.

The effect of interferon on the V-PFC assay was tested by adding exogenous interferon (50 units of crude homologous interferon) at the time of addition of Suc-Con A or 4 hr after induction. A 50% reduction of V-PFC was observed for both cases after 28 hr of incubation.

The kinetics of interferon production during the first 24 hr incubation period with Suc-Con A as a function of age of the cell donor is demonstrated in Figure 3. Both mouse strains (C57B1/6, CBA) elaborated a greater amount of interferon production with age and a quantitative variation was also demonstrated by the strains.

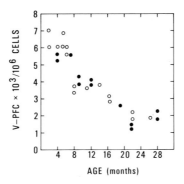

FIGURE 4. Number of viral plaque forming cells after 24 hours of Suc-Con A stimulation in spleen cell cultures from various ages of C57B1/6 (O) and CBA (•). (From *J. Immunol.*, 118, 1367, 1978. With permission.)

The decline in mitogenic-induced proliferatory response with age employing the V-PFC assay is illustrated in Figure 4. This decline in activated cells at 24 hr of incubation could reflect either an actual decrease in immuno-competent cells, or a technical artifact in the V-PFC assay due to interferon. The possibility that high multiplicity of interfering B particles present in the virus preparation may be responsible is ruled out by the quality of the VSV preparation employed (see Methods). From an experiment with cells from young mice (2 to 6 months), interferon produced during the normal course of mitogenic activation had no or minimal effect on the V-PFC assay during the first 24 hr of incubation. Thus, exogenous interferon (mouse fibroblast interferon from the National Institutes of Health, G002-904-511) was added to cultures of 2-month-old mice equivalent to concentrations found at different age levels. With the V-PFC assay, reduction was observed, but no correlation with the concentration of added exogenous interferon was found. The variability of V-PFC formation was also observed in the kinetic study between 24 to 72 hr of incubation (see Figure 1) and may be due to the differences of cellular metabolic activity required for antiviral state induction by interferon, and for the efficiency of viral infection as demonstrated by Weber and Stuart.[14] That is, resting cells are more ideal for induction of antiviral state, whereas cells actively growing are more susceptible to viral infections.

Interferon is also known to act as a cell growth inhibitor (CGI) as reported by Gresser et al.[15] The effect of exogenous interferon on the ^{3}H-thymidine assay was determined and is illustrated in Figure 5. The proliferative response to Suc-Con A stimulation, as with the V-PFC assay, declined as a function of age. Upon exposing the spleen cells of 2-month-old mice to levels of interferon equivalent to concentrations of interferon found at different ages, a similar decline was observed.

The interferon production by dextran-purified, human-blood lymphocytes stimulated by PHA indicates a similar phenomenon as with the mouse spleen cells, Figure 6. Though the increase in interferon production with age was not as pronounced. The interferon production by lymphocytes is influenced by many factors and changes observed with a homogeneous system as with inbred mice strains may be insignificant with non-homogeneous systems due to the variation in the human population.

The data suggest that the observed decline in proliferative response may be due in part to the coinciding production of interferon.

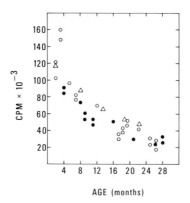

FIGURE 5. ³H-Thymidine incorporation (cpm) in 48 hour Suc-Con A stimulated mouse spleen cell cultures from various ages of C57B1/6 (○) and CBA (●) mice. In addition, the effects of age-adjusted doses of exogenous added interferon (at 4 and 24 hours of culture) were determined on Suc-Con A stimulated C57B1/6 (2 months ○) spleen cell cultures (△). (From *J. Immunol.*, 118, 1367, 1978. With permission.)

In view of the above-described observations, we believe that in order to enumerate T-lymphocyte activation, the virus plaque assay is ideal, but has to take the kinetics of interferon production into consideration. The kinetics of cellular activation should be related to the kinetics of interferon production for each system studied. From this, one can then determine the incubation time at which the number of responding cells can be accurately determined. With cells from young donors, 20- to 24-hr incubation period of the stimulation are ideal, but with cells of older donors, neither the V-PFC nor the isotype assay will give satisfactory results, except maybe at very early times. The observation that possible only a very small percentage of the cell population initially responds to mitogen stimulation makes the entertainment of attempting to isolate and study these cells unrealistic with present day methodology. Furthermore, the implication that interferon is possibly responsible for the observed aging effect on the immune system raises several questions. Why do cells from older donors elaborate more interferon? Is the possible interferon effect on the immune system also expressed in vivo? And, finally, is it possible that not only interferon, an immunogenic regulator, but an agent or process responsible for the increased interferon production elaboration is also the cause of the immune-function inhibition?

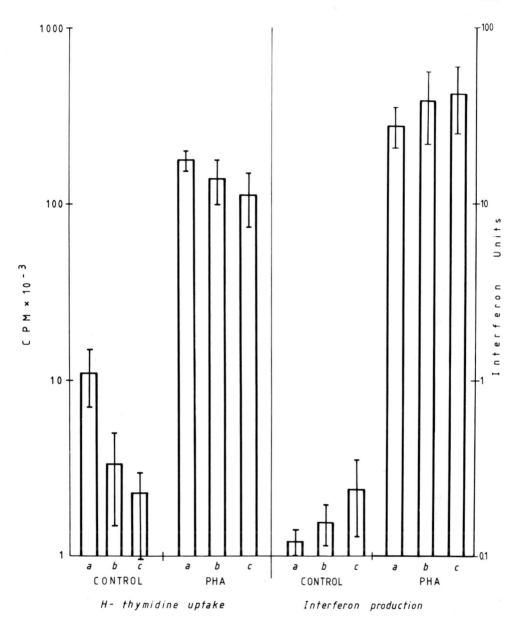

FIGURE 6. ³H-Thymidine incorporation and interferon production by 1 × 10⁵ human blood lymphocytes of donors varying in age (a = 19-35 years; b = 40-52 years; c = 75-90 years) upon PHA stimulation.

REFERENCES

1. **Jimenez, L. and Bloom, B. R.,** Virus plaque assay for antigen-sensitive cells in delayed hypersensitivity, in *In Vitro Methods in Cell-Mediated Immunity,* Bloom, B. R. and Glade, P. R., Academic Press, New York, 1971, 553.
2. **Heine, J. W. and Adler, W. H.,** The kinetics of interferon production by mouse lymphocytes and its modulating effect on the virus plaque forming cell assay as a quantitative method to determine activated lymphocytes, *J. Immunol.,* 117, 1045, 1976.
3. **Heine, J. W. and Adler, W. H.,** The quantitative production of interferon by mitogen stimulated mouse lymphocytes as a function of age and its effect on the lymphocytes proliferative response, *J. Immunol.,* 118, 1366, 1977.
4. **Adler, W. H., Takiguchi, T., Marsh, B., and Smoth, R. T.,** Cellular recognition by mouse lymphocytes in vitro. I. Definition of a new technique and results of stimulation by phytohemogglutinin and specific antigens, *J. Exp. Med.,* 131, 1049, 1970.
5. **Agrawal, B. B. L. and Goldstein, L. J.,** Physical and chemical characterization of concanavalin A, the hemagglutinin of Jack bean (*Canavalia ensiformis*), *Biochim. Biophys. Acta,* 133, 376, 1967.
6. **Gunther, G. R., Wong, J. L., Yahara, I., Cunningham, B. A., and Edelman, G. M.,** Concanavalin A derivatives with altered biological activities. *Proc. Natl. Acad. Sci. U.S.A,* 70, 1012, 1973.
7. **Heine, J. W. and Galasso, G. J.,** Effects of X-irradiated aqueous solutions on vesicular stomatitis virus, *J. Virol.,* 2, 1147, 1968.
8. **McShary, J. and Benzinger, R.,** Concentration and purification of vesicular stomatitis virus by polyethylene glycol "precipitation", *Virology,* 40, 745, 1970.
9. **Heine, J. W. and Schnaitman, C. A.,** Entry of vesicular stomatitis virus into L-cells, *J. Virol.,* 8, 786, 1971.
10. **Heine, J. W., Mikulski, A. J., Sulkowski, E., and Carter, W. A.,** Stabilization of human fibroblast interferon purified on concanavalin A-agarose, *Arch. Virol.,* 57, 185, 1978.
11. **Buckler, C. E.,** Interferon assays: General consideration, in *The Interferon System,* Texas Reports on Biology and Medicine, Vol. 35, Baron, S. and Dianzani, F., Eds., University of Texas Medical Branch, Galveston, 1977, 150.
12. **Tan, Y. H.,** Chromosome-21-dosage effect on inducibility of antiviral gene(s), *Nature (London),* 253, 280, 1975.
13. **Volckaert-Vervliet, G. and Billiau, A.,** Induction of interferon in human lymphoblastoid cells by sendai and measles viruses, *J. Gen. Virol.,* 37, 199, 1977.
14. **Weber, J. M., and Stewart, R. R.,** Cyclic AMP potentiation of interferon antiviral activity and effect of interferon on cellular cyclic AMP levels, *J. Gen. Virol.,* 28, 363, 1975.
15. **Gresser, I., Bandu, M. T., Tovey, M., Bodo, G., Paucker, K., and Stewart II, W. E.,** Interferon and cell division. VII. Inhibitory effect of highly purified interferon preparations on the multiplication of leukemia L-1210 cells, *Proc. Soc. Exp. Biol. Med.,* 142, 7, 1973.

Chapter 14

CRYOPRESERVATION OF MURINE LYMPHOCYTES

M. A. Brock

TABLE OF CONTENTS

I. INTRODUCTION

Cryobiologists and immunologists have addressed questions relating to the cryopreservation of immunocompetent cells for several years, and their experimental findings provide a firm base for the methods that will be elaborated here. Such factors as cell density and volume of the suspension, concentrations and types of cryopreservatives, rates of cooling and rewarming, as well as an array of procedures for preparation of cell suspensions, resuspenion after thawing, and demonstration of cellular function are all critical in protocols for the successful recovery of frozen-thawed lymphocytes. Despite the recent proliferation of data in this field, gaps remain in the understanding of some fundamental mechanisms of cryopreservation and of the activation of frozen-thawed lymphocytes. Where such uncertainties are known, they will also be delineated.

Some of the early studies on the cryopreservation of human and murine lymphocytes suggested the use of dimethyl sulfoxide (DMSO) as an effective cryoprotectant and established that slow cooling rates and rapid rewarming of the cell suspensions provide viable cells on which in vitro tests for function could be made (Ashwood-Smith;[1] Pegg;[2] Brody et al.[3]). These freezing procedures have been refined, and methods currently in use will be described here.

II. METHODS AND RESULTS

A. Choice of Cooling Systems

The successful cryopreservation of immunocompetent cells with a recovery of 90% or more viable and functional cells requires cooling systems that reduce freezing injury and reproduce the selected cooling slope in successive experiments. The importance of the reproducibility of cooling slopes deserves special emphasis with regard to the cryopreservation of cells from older individuals where the possibility exists that defects accompanying senescence can yield lower recoveries of one or several subpopulations of lymphocytes. Since some cooling regimens do result in the selective preservation of T- and B-cell populations, these should be avoided in the cryopreservation of cells from older animals.

The options to vary the volume of a cell suspension, cell density, and composition of the preservative medium, as might be required in cooling cells from older individuals, is an advantage achieved only with repetitious trials, if the present commercially available cooling systems are used. This is due to their basic designs that require the manual setting of predetermined periods of time for the initial rate of cooling, the rapid infusion of liquid nitrogen (LN_2) at the phase change from liquid to solid, and a second rate of cooling following the phase change. Figure 1 represents some of the types of cooling slopes described for cryopreservation systems, including that of a recently developed microprocessor-controlled system. The latter is unique because it does provide a programmable system in which only the desired cooling rate and low-limit temperature are set, regardless of the volume or composition of the cell suspension. The cooling system and the flow chart for the microprocessor-controlled rate controller have been described in detail (Baartz and Brock[4]). The principle of its operation is that the actual temperature of a reference sample of the cell suspension being cooled is continuously compared with a preselected cooling ramp of the microprocessor. A positive or negative deflection of $0.017°C$ or more activates the solenoid valves that admit LN_2 vapor into the freezing chamber. When the reference sample temperature rises $0.3°C$ above the cooling ramp, this is interpreted as the phase change from liquid to solid, and additional solenoid valves open to compensate for the heat released as ice crystallizes. The surge of LN_2 vapor drops the reference sample temperature to

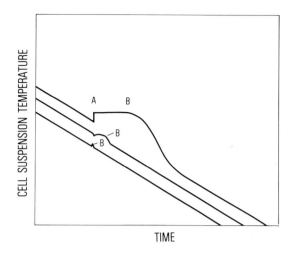

FIGURE 1. Representation of three types of cooling curves. If the temperature of the freezing chamber is uniformly lowered, the upper line depicts the temperature of the cell suspension. At the phase change from liquid to solid (A), the heat of fusion is released and the temperature of the cell suspension remains unchanged until sufficient LN_2 vapor enters the chamber to reinitiate cooling (B). The center line shows the cell suspension temperature when additional LN_2 vapor enters the chamber at the predetermined time of the phase change. The plateau is much reduced with this type of cooling which is similar to that provided by most commercial cooling systems. The lower line illustrates the cooling slopes obtained using a microprocessor-controlled cooling system. The heat of fusion (A) is automatically dissipated as additional LN_2 vapor surges into the chamber. The three lines are displaced vertically for clarity.

again equal that of the microprocessor ramp, and the initial cooling rate is restored (see Figure 1). The marked advantage offered with the use of this new cooling system is that any type of cell suspension may serve as the reference sample with repeatable and reproducible cooling slopes. The importance of rapid detection and compensation for the heat of fusion derives from the belief that a plateau in the cooling slope as shown in Figure 1 may result in cell injury. Early experiments by Rowe and Rinefret[5] and Rowe[6] in extending the time bone marrow cell suspensions remained at the elevated temperature before the selected cooling rate was restored resulted in increasing losses of viable cells. More recently, Birkeland,[7] using human lymphocytes, has compared the effectiveness of using two cooling slopes similar to the two upper curves shown in Figure 1. The thawed, cryopreserved cells exhibited markedly higher responses to mitogens and allogeneic lymphocytes in vitro when the initial cooling rate was more rapidly restored following the phase change. To avoid the possibility of cell injury and also to consistently restore the cooling rate following the phase change is of obvious importance in studies using older animals and heterogenous cell populations to minimize selective damage to certain cell types.

B. Preparation of Cell Suspensions for Cryopreservation

Single cell suspensions of murine splenic lymphocytes are prepared using most of the techniques described by Adler[8] in this volume. Only the procedures which deviate from those methods because of their special relevance to cryopreservation will be described in detail. Briefly, mice (C57BL/6) are killed by cervical dislocation, and their spleens removed to sterile RPMI-1640 media containing 10% heat-inactivated fetal calf serum (FCS) (GIBCO®, Grand Island, N.Y.). 10% FCS was routinely added to the media for the preparation of single-cell suspensions and for all the washing and dilutions required (Thorpe, et al;[9] Baartz and Brock[4]). Cellular viability before and after freezing was determined using fluorescein diacetate — ethidium bromide staining (Dankberg and Persidsky[10]). In cryoimmunology, this method is preferred to the trypan blue dye exclusion test to estimate cellular viability since high percentages of cryopreserved lymphocytes may remain unstained ("viable") yet be incapable of function (Strong;[11] Harada and Hattori[12]). The fluorescein diacetate ester is non-polar, permeates viable cells, and is hydrolyzed yielding fluorescein. This is a polar compound which is retained in cells with intact plasma membranes (Persidsky and Baillie[13]), and appears brilliant green using fluorescence microscopy.

Cell densities are adjusted to 2.5×10^6 cells per mℓ for the in vitro studies of function and to 60×10^6 cells per mℓ to prepare for cryopreservation. 50 U/mℓ penicillin and 50 μg/mℓ streptomycin (GIBCO®, Grand Island, N.Y.) are added to the media before in vitro culture and cryopreservation.

C. Procedures for Cryopreservation

The washed cell suspensions are cooled to 4°C, and cold 20% DMSO in RPMI-1640 containing 10% FCS is added slowly with gentle agitation of the cell suspension in an ice bath. Equal volumes of the suspension and cryoprotectant solutions are mixed, resulting in a final density of 30×10^6 cells per mℓ. This density is routinely used in freezing murine lymphocytes and provides sufficient cells on thawing to test for function (Strong et al;[14] Thorpe et al.[15]). Robinson and Knight,[16] however, have recovered high percentages of viable and functional Chinese hamster cells (Clone A) using densities ranging from 10^4 to 10^7 cells per mℓ with a sharp drop in survival at higher densities. Cryoprotectants other than DMSO, such as glycerol in concentrations ranging from 5 to 25% and 10% polyvinylpyrrolidone have been less effective in obtaining high recoveries of frozen cells (Strong and Sell[17]) and in preserving cellular function as judged by stimulation by mitogens and allogeneic lymphocytes in vitro (Birkeland[7]). Aliquots (1.75 mℓ) of the prepared cell suspension are pipetted into 12×32 mm Wheaton serum bottles (Wheaton Scientific, Millville, N.J.), and the bottles are sealed by crimping. The convenience of this volume for later assay of cellular function has been mentioned, however, smoother cooling slopes can be obtained with the use of smaller volumes of cell suspensions with a consequent decrease in heat released at the phase change. The use of these bottles eliminates the heat sealing of glass ampoules that requires an oxygen-gas flame and often results in undetected channels through the sealed tips. Greiff et al.[18] have described the dimensions of these channels and the movement of molecules through them, using laser dark-field and interference imaging. The sealed bottles are clipped into aluminum canes and transferred to the freezing chamber which has been precooled to 4°C. With the microprocessor-controlled rate controller, the cooling rate and the low limit of −50°C are selected. At −50°C, the samples are rapidly transferred to a LN$_2$ refrigerator at −196°C and stored in the vapor phase.

Whereas a slow cooling rate on the order of −1.0°C/min is optimal for the freezing of lymphocytes, rapid rewarming results in higher recoveries. This is accomplished by immersing the frozen samples in a 37°C water bath and agitating them until no ice crystals remain, which requires 45 sec (267°C/min warming rate) for the 1.75-mℓ samples. The seals are then removed, and the thawed cell suspensions are transferred to sterile 15-mℓ test tubes. Cold RPMI-1640 containing 10% FCS is added by drops with gentle agitation to a total volume of 15 mℓ. Slow dilution of the DMSO solution is recommended for optimal functional recovery (Strong, et al.[14]). The frozen-thawed lymphocytes are washed twice, which further dilutes the DMSO, and viability is determined with fluorescein diacetate-ethidium bromide staining. The effects of even very low concentrations of several cryoprotectants on the response of lymphocytes to mitogens in vitro have been discussed by Strong, et al.[19] They showed that DMSO at concentrations as low as 0.25% significantly altered responses to mitogens, emphasizing the importance of thorough dilution of the DMSO. The procedure given here reduced the DMSO concentrations to <0.001%.

D. Viability and Function of Unfrozen and Cryopreserved Murine Lymphocytes

The cooling velocity is a major consideration in the optimal recovery of cryopreserved cells. In a recent review, Mazur[20] has illustrated that diverse cooling rates result in maximum survival for mouse marrow stem cells, yeast, and human erythrocytes. Figure 2 illustrates some of the studies from his laboratory. The decline in the percentage of cells that survive, using a higher-than-optimal cooling rate, is thought to be due to the retention of water within the cells that would be lost by osmosis at a slower cooling rate, permitting freezing of extracellular water. Water retained in the cells freezes and may cause irreparable damage to cell membrane systems. Cellular injury at slower-than-optimal cooling rates is thought to result from the high concentrations of intra- and extracellular electrolytes produced during freezing or to cell shrinkage. The function of cryoprotectants at different concentrations in reducing cellular injury was also discussed by Mazur. Since splenic lymphocytes are a heterogeneous population, the possibility exists that T- and B-cell subpopulations may be preferentially damaged by certain cooling rates. There are three reports showing the optimal cooling velocity for cryopreservation of the subpopulations as assessed by in vitro mitogenic stimulation by phytohemagglutinin (PHA), lipopolysaccharide (LPS), and Concanavalin A (Con A), (Strong;[11] Thorpe, et al.;[9] and Farrant et al.[21]). Figure 3 is a representation of their data for murine and human lymphocytes. For both T cells activated by PHA and Con A, and B cells activated by LPS, there appear to be optimal cooling velocities which are specific for the lymphocyte subpopulation and the species. With this basic information, the survival of lymphocytes cooled over a broad range of rates using the microprocessor-controlled system may be evaluated. Furthermore, any selective injury to a subpopulation, possibly as a function of age, should be clearly distinguishable.

1. Viability of Cells Cooled at Rates Ranging From −0.25° to −10.0°C/min

The recovery of viable cells stained by fluorescein from mice 4 to 6 months old and 15 months old is shown in Figure 4. Although the older mice were just over one year of age, there were clear decreases in cellular viability in four of the ten cell suspensions.

Data of this nature are available from just a few previous studies of the cryopreservation of human lymphocytes cooled at −1°C/min. Flynn et al.[22] and Mangi and Mardiney[23] recovered 69 to 95% and 66 to 94%, respectively, of the frozen-thawed cells, with the trypan blue dye exclusion procedure as an estimate of cellular viability. Strong et al.[24] reported 75 to 100% recovery, using an autocytometer. The data in Figure 4 showing from 66 to 100% of the cryopreserved murine lymphocytes viable after cooling at −1°C/min may well represent substantially better recoveries than the previous reports on human lymphocytes due to their possible overestimation of viable cells using the procedures mentioned.

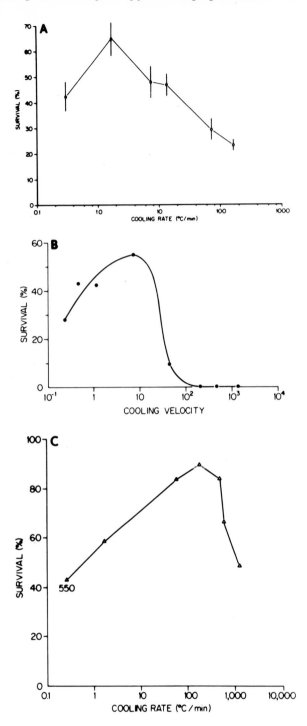

FIGURE 2.   Survival of frozen-thawed mouse marrow stem cells (A), yeast (B) and human red cells (C) as a function of the cooling rate. The cells were frozen at constant velocities to −75°C, transferred to LN₂ at −196°C, and rapidly thawed at 500 to 1000°C/min. (From Mazur, P., The role of intracellular freezing in the death of cells cooled at supraoptimal rates, *Cryobiology,* 14, 251, 1977, Academic Press, New York. With permission.)

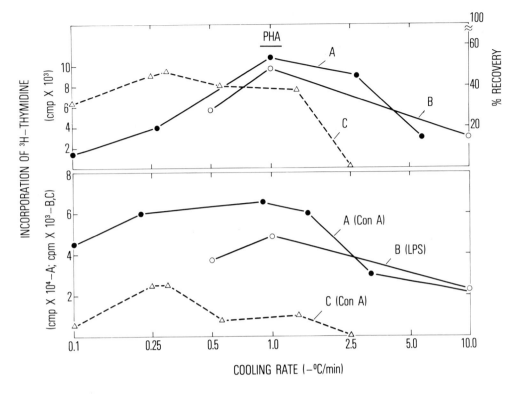

FIGURE 3. The recovery of T- and B-lymphocyte function at each of the cooling rates shown is for cells frozen in 10% DMSO; the volumes of the cell suspensions frozen, the cell concentrations, and the cooling regimens differed in each of the three studies. The curves labeled A are for mouse lymph node cells from Thorpe, et al.[9] The values for T-cell responses to PHA stimulation are expressed as the percent recovery of the unfrozen cells' response; their responses to Con A stimulation are shown as incorporation of ³H-thymidine (cpm × 10⁴). Strong[11] cooled murine splenic lymphocytes at three rates, −0.5, −1.0, and −10.0°C/min (curves B) and showed maximum incorporation of ³H-thymidine (cpm × 10³) at −1.0°C/min for T- and B-cells activated by PHA and LPS. Lymphocytes from human peripheral blood (curves C) were cooled by Farrant, et al.[21] Their data is expressed as incorporation of ³H-thymidine (cpm × 10³) by PHA- and Con A-stimulated cells. The actual values for ³H-thymidine incorporation reported in each of the three studies differed, accounting for the use of different units on the ordinates to show the curves in closer proximity.

2. Functional Recovery of Cryopreserved Cells

The key test of the effectiveness of any cryopreservation procedure is the demonstration of functional recovery of each of the frozen-thawed cell types or tissues. A variety of established tests for lymphocytic function have been used with cryopreserved cells (Strong, et al.[24]). For the studies to be reported on, murine lymphocyte freezing, the ability of the T cells to respond to PHA and Con A, and the B cells to respond to LPS in vitro, was assessed by the incorporation of ³H-thymidine to evaluate mitotic activity. These methods are discussed by Adler[8] in this volume. Both the unfrozen and cryopreserved cell suspensions are adjusted to 2.5 × 10⁶ cells per mℓ and 200 µℓ are dispensed into each well of a sterile Microtest II® tissue culture plate (Falcon Plastics, Oxnard, Calif). An Eppendorf standard fixed volume pipette fitted with disposable sterile tips is used to dispense the cells, while a Hamilton repeating dispenser and syringe unit delivers the mitogens in a total volume of 10µℓ. The mitogens are diluted with sterile RPMI-1640 to the desired concentrations, and triplicate cultures are stimulated by graded concentrations of the three mitogens. PHA-P (Difco Laboratories, Detroit, Mich.) is reconstituted in 5-mℓ sterile, distilled water and diluted to 0.1, 0.25,

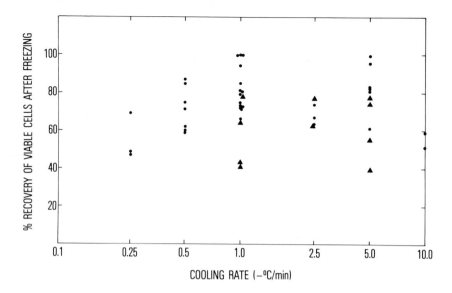

FIGURE 4.   The percentage of the original number of unfrozen cells that were viable following cryopreservation is shown for six cooling rates. The solid circles refer to 4- to 6-month-old C57BL/6 mice while the triangles represent data for 15-month-old mice.

0.50, 0.75, and 1.0% v/v; Con A (Pharmacia Inc., Piscataway, N.J.) is diluted to 0.5, 1.0, 1.5, and 2.0 μg/10 μℓ; LPS (S. Minnesota R595 supplied by Dr. Robert Wheat, Duke University) is adjusted to 2.5, 5.0 and 10.0 μg/10 μℓ. A loose-fitting Microtest II® lid covers the culture plates which are incubated at 37°C for 68 hr in a 5% CO_2 humidified air atmosphere. 0.5 μCi methyl-^{3}H-thymidine (Schwarz-Mann, Orange-burg, N.Y.), 6 Ci/mm, in 5.0 μℓ of media is added to each culture well 18 hr prior to the end of the incubation. The cultures are harvested with the Brandel Cell Harvester (Biomedical Research and Development Laboratories, Inc., Rockville, Md.) and washed with 5.0% trichloroacetic acid. The dried samples in 9 mℓ glass scintillation bottles are solubilized with Nuclear Chicago Solubilizer (Amersham Corp., Arlington Heights, Ill.), and 5 mℓ of toluene-based rpi scintillator (Research Products International Corp., Elk Grove Village, Ill.) are added. Samples are counted in a Beckman LS-250 Liquid Scintillation System. Data are expressed as counts per minute (cpm) for triplicate samples of the stimulated cells and for the nine non-stimulated cultures routinely used.

Some special precautions not usually emphasized in cryoimmunological studies should be mentioned. The first concerns the FCS which is added to the culture media of unfrozen and cryopreserved cells. Strong[11] has shown that different lots of FCS from the same supplier support the stimulation of murine lymphocytes by PHA and pokeweed mitogen to different degrees. In preliminary experiments to determine the degree of support by each lot of FCS used in the present studies, a difference related to the age of the mice was also observed (Figure 5A). Therefore, FCS of one lot was frozen in aliquots to be thawed and added to the culture media on the day either the control non-frozen or the cryopreserved cells were to be used. The use of media containing FCS stored above freezing temperatures resulted in a depressed proliferative capacity of cells cultured in it.

Another area for concern became apparent in analyzing the recoveries of cryopreserved lymphocytes. All in vitro tests for function were made with graded concentrations of the three mitogens. Figure 5B illustrates the responses to PHA observed in

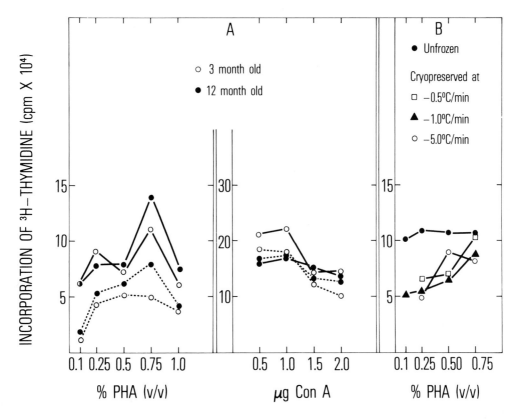

FIGURE 5. (A) Murine splenic lymphocyte responses to PHA and Con A. The solid and dashed lines are for cell suspensions in media containing 10% FCS from Flow Laboratories (McLean, Va.) and GIBCO®, respectively. Media containing FCS from Flow Laboratories supported proliferation in response to stimulation by PHA better than that from GIBCO®, however FCS from both sources was equally effective in supporting the responses to Con A by lymphocytes from a 12-month-old mouse. (B) The responses to graded concentrations of PHA by unfrozen and cryopreserved lymphocytes from 5-month-old C57BL/6 mice are shown. The concentration of PHA required for maximum incorporation of ^{3}H-thymidine differed depending on the treatment of the cells.

control unfrozen cells and in those cryopreserved at three different cooling rates. It is apparent that any one concentration of mitogen would not evoke maximum incorporation of ^{3}H-thymidine in the control and experimental groups. Changes in the dose-response curves after cryopreservation were observed frequently in the responses to PHA and Con A stimulation. It seems evident that the use of graded concentrations of mitogens is required for the assessment of functional recovery, yet this aspect of the experimental protocol is largely ignored in cryoimmunological studies. Whether these changes in responsiveness are due to alterations in the plasma membrane or cellular organelles is unresolved.

The functional recovery of murine lymphocytes from young animals using the microprocessor-controlled freezing system has been reported for cells cooled at −1°C/min (Baartz and Brock[4]) and for cells cooled at a range of rates (Brock and Baartz[25]). The incorporation of ^{3}H-thymidine by stimulated lymphocytes cryopreserved using cooling rates ranging from −0.25 to −10.0°C/min is shown in Figure 6. In contrast to the earlier studies of murine lymphocytes shown in Figure 3, high levels of ^{3}H-thymidine were incorporated by stimulated cells cooled at rates slower than −1°C/min. The levels of incorporation attained by stimulated lymphocytes from older animals (15

Table 1
THE EFFECT OF DIFFERENT COOLING RATES ON THE PROLIFERATIVE CAPACITY OF LYMPHOCYTES FROM 15-MONTH-OLD MICE STIMULATED BY PHA, LPS, AND CON A

Cooling rate (−°C/min)	Incorporation of ³H-thymidine (% of unfrozen cells)[a]		
	PHA	LPS	CON A
−1.0	19.5	74.0	7.4
	35.2	72.7	9.4
	5.0	99.9	8.2
	3.0	29.9	4.9
−2.5	7.2	133.4	8.2
	3.9	37.7	4.5
−5.0	87.3	70.6	52.9
	65.4	56.6	41.4
	6.3	96.7	5.7
	3.2	35.2	2.4

[a] $\dfrac{\text{cpm frozen-thawed cells} - \text{cpm nonstimulated cells}}{\text{cpm unfrozen cells} - \text{cpm nonstimulated controls}} \times 100$

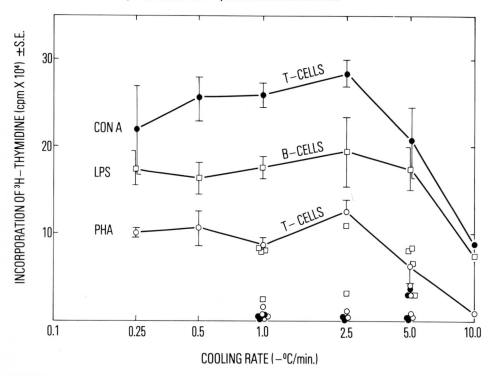

FIGURE 6.　The incorporation of ³H-thymidine by 0.5 × 10⁶ C57BL/6 spleen cells in response to stimulation by PHA, LPS, and Con A. The standard error is shown for the means of all cryopreserved samples from 3- to 6-month-old mice at each rate. The number of samples frozen-thawed at the rates −0.25, −0.5, −1.0, −2.5, −5.0, and −10.0°C/min were 3, 4, 9, 3, 4, and 1, respectively. The solid lines connect the means for 3- to 6-month-old mice; the solitary symbols represent data for 15-month-old mice.

months old) are lower for unfrozen cells as has been reported previously (Adler;[8] Adler and Chrest[26]) and, interestingly, the proliferative capacity of cryopreserved T cells, but not B cells, appears to be depressed at a cooling rate of $-1°C/min$, which is not expected to be a suboptimal rate. When these data for cryopreserved cells are compared with the incorporation of ^{3}H-thymidine by their unfrozen controls, lymphocytes from the younger mice stimulated by all three mitogens reached 70 to 100% of control levels at cooling rates ranging from -0.25 to $-5.0°C/min$. Data for the 15-month-old mice are shown in Table 1. The selective injury to the T-cell subpopulations of lymphocytes from the older mice is clear. This is interesting because the viability of the frozen-thawed cells and the percentage of the unfrozen cells recovered were similar at the different cooling rates, but obviously the cells from the older mice were damaged. The major sites of freezing damage are considered to be plasma membranes, organelle surface membranes, and/or cellular biomembrane systems (Mazur[20]). Although the retention of fluorescein by the lymphocytes cryopreserved at the different cooling rates indicates that plasma membranes were intact, injury to the recognition mechanism could occur. This may provide a tool for detecting aging changes in mammalian cellular structure and function. Presently, the sites of injury are unresolved.

III. DISCUSSION

Detection of selective freezing injury to either T- or B-lymphocyte subpopulations in cell suspensions from older animals requires reproducible cooling regimens and stringent testing of the viability and function of the cryopreserved cells. The procedures given above stress the specific methods often unemphasized in cryoimmunology which provide comparative information. The microprocessor-controlled freezing system has advantages in its operation and use for the cryopreservation of murine lymphocytes as well as other cell types, and it is being developed commercially by Polaron Instruments Inc. The lack of selective injury to one or more subpopulations of lymphocytes in young mice with this cooling system made its use imperative for detecting the changes following cryopreservation that were observed in lymphocytes from older mice. The fact that T lymphocytes from the 15-month-old animals were damaged even under what are considered to be optimal cooling conditions initiates investigations for methods of cryopreservation of cell types from older animals, both for immediate experimental purposes and for later use. Areas that can be probed include additional analysis of the cooling and rewarming velocities and of cryoprotectants other than DMSO.

Some cautions in the in vitro assessment of cellular viability and function should be stressed again. The use of the fluorescein diacetate — ethidium bromide assay for cellular viability has proved to be significant in order to avoid overestimation of the percentage of viable cells in cryopreserved cell suspensions and in the dependent calculations of cell densities for in vitro tests of cellular function. Determinations on thawed cell suspensions cooled at rates ranging from $-0.5°$ to $-10.0°C/min$ resulted in a 10 to 20% overestimation of cellular viability using the trypan blue dye exclusion test as compared with fluorescein diacetate — ethidium bromide. Subsequent calculations of the recovery of viable cells in the suspensions frozen were excessively high if based on the dye-exclusion test data. It is also clear that reliable assessment of cellular responses to mitogens in vitro requires the use of graded concentrations of the mitogens, particularly PHA and Con A, in addition to the use of the same lot of FCS for unfrozen and frozen-thawed cells from one suspension. Some of the low recoveries of function reported by others for PHA-stimulated cryopreserved lymphocytes could be due to the use of only one, nonoptimal concentration of the mitogen. The importance of these procedures for discerning differences in in vitro cellular viability and function was evident when cryopreserved lymphocytes from young and older mice were compared. Although the plasma membranes of cells from both groups retained intracellular fluorescein, an indication that the membranes were intact, the function of T cells from the older animals was selectively impaired after cooling at certain rates. This suggests that there are discrete changes in cellular structure and/or function with age which were revealed after cryopreservation and prevented the restoration of cellular integrity.

REFERENCES

1. **Ashwood-Smith, M. J.,** Low temperature preservation of mouse lymphocytes with dimethyl sulfoxide, *Blood,* 23, 494, 1964.
2. **Pegg, P. J.,** The preservation of leucocytes for cytogenetic and cytochemical studies, *Br. J. Haematol.,* 11, 586, 1965.
3. **Brody, J. A., Harlem, M. M., Plank, C. R., and White, L. R.,** Freezing human peripheral lymphocytes and a technique for culture in monolayers, *Proc. Soc. Exp. Biol. Med.,* 129, 968, 1968.
4. **Baartz, G. and Brock, M. A.,** A microprocessor-controlled rate controller for use in cryopreservation, *Cryobiology,* 16, 497, 1979.
5. **Rowe, A. W. and Rinfret, A. P.,** Controlled rate freezing of bone marrow, *Blood,* 20, 636, 1962.
6. **Rowe, A. W.,** Biochemical aspects of cryoprotective agent in freezing and thawing, *Cryobiology,* 3, 12, 1966.
7. **Birkeland, S. A.,** The influence of different freezing procedures and different cryoprotective agents on the immunological capacity of frozen-stored lymphocytes, *Cryobiology,* 13, 442, 1976.
8. **Adler, W. H.,** The use of the mitogen response assay in studies of immunology and aging, in *Methods in Immunology and Aging Research,* Adler, W. H. and Nordin, A. A., Eds., CRC Press, Inc., Boca Raton, Fla, 1980.
9. **Thorpe, P. E., Knight, S. C., and Farrant, J.,** Optimal conditions for the preservation of mouse lymph node cells in liquid nitrogen using cooling rate techniques, *Cryobiology,* 13, 126, 1976.
10. **Dankberg, F. and Persidsky, M. D.,** A test of granulocyte membrane integrity and phagocytic function, *Cryobiology,* 13, 430, 1976.
11. **Strong, D. M.,** Differential Cryobiological Effects on Murine T and B Lymphocytes, Ph.D. thesis, Medical College of Wisconsin, Milwaukee, Wis., 1973.
12. **Harada, M. and Hattori, K.,** Does the dye exclusion test indicate true viability?, *Cryobiology,* 15, 681, 1978.
13. **Persidsky, M. D. and Baillie, G. S.,** Fluorometric test of cell membrane integrity, *Cryobiology,* 14, 322, 1977.
14. **Strong, D. M., Ahmend, A., Sell, K. W., and Greiff, D.,** Differential susceptibility of murine T and B lymphocytes to freeze-thaw and hypotonic shock, *Cryobiology,* 11, 127, 1974.
15. **Thorpe, P. E. and Knight, S. C.,** Microplate cultures of mouse lymph node cells. I. Quantitation of responses to allogeneic lymphocytes, endotoxin and phytomitogens, *J. Immunol. Methods,* 5, 387, 1974.
16. **Robinson, D. M. and Knight, C.,** Population - density - dependent survival from freezing in mammalian cells, *Cryobiology,* 10, 528, 1973.
17. **Strong, D. M., and Sell, K. W.,** Functional properties of cryopreserved lymphocytes, in *Cryoimmunologie,* Simatos, D., Strong, D. M., and Turc, J-M., Eds., INSERM, Paris, 1977, 81.
18. **Greiff, D., Melton, H., and Rowe, T. W. G.,** On the sealing of gas-filled glass ampoules, *Cryobiology,* 12, 1, 1975.
19. **Strong, D. M., Ahmend, A. A., Sell, K. W., and Greiff, D.,** In vitro effects of cryoprotective agents on the response of murine T and B lymphoid subpopulations to mitogenic agents, *Cryobiology,* 9, 450, 1972.

20. **Mazur, P.,** Mechanism of injury and protection in cells and tissues at low temperatures in *Cryoimmunologie,* Simatos, D., Strong, D. M., and Turc, J. M., Eds., INSERM, Paris, 1977, 37.

21. **Farrant, J., Knight, S. C., and Morris, G. J.,** Use of different cooling rates during freezing to separate populations of human peripheral blood lymphocytes, *Cryobiology,* 9, 516, 1972.

22. **Flynn, R., Troup, G. M., and Walford, R. L.,** Cytotoxicity test with frozen lymphocytes, *Int. Arch. Allergy Appl. Immunol.,* 29, 478, 1966.

23. **Mangi, R. J. and Mardiney, M. R., Jr.,** The in vitro transformation of frozen-stored lymphocytes in the mixed lymphocyte reaction and in culture with phytohemagglutinin and specific antigens, *J. Exp. Med.,* 132, 401, 1970.

24. **Strong, D. M., Woody, J. N., Factor, M. A., Ahmend, A., and Sell, K. W.,** Immunological responsiveness of frozen-thawed human lymphocytes, *Clin. Exp. Immunol.,* 21, 442, 1975.

25. **Brock, M. A. and Baartz, G.,** Cryoprotection of Murine lymphocyte subpopulations using a microprocessor-controlled cooling system, *Cryobiology,* 17, 439, 1980.

26. **Adler, W. H., and Chrest, F. J.,** The mitogen response assay as a measure of the immune deficiency of aging mice, in *Developmental Immunobiology,* Siskind, G. W., Litwin, S. D., and Weksler, M. E., Eds., Grune & Stratton, Inc. New York, 1979, 233.

INDEX